Health Informatics
(formerly Computers in Health Care)

Kathryn J. Hannah   Marion J. Ball
Series Editors

Health Informatics Series
(formerly Computers in Health Care)

Series Editors
Kathryn J. Hannah   Marion J. Ball

(continued after index)

Krzysztof Zieliński   Mariusz Duplaga
David Ingram
Editors

Information Technology Solutions for Healthcare

With 98 Figures
(3 in Color)

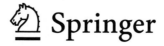 Springer

Professor Krzysztof Zieliński
AGH University of Science & Technology
Kraków
Poland

Professor Mariusz Duplaga
Jagiellonian University Medical College
Kraków
Poland

Professor David Ingram
Centre for Health Informatics and
    Multi-professional Education
University College London
London, United Kingdom

Series Editors:

Kathryn J. Hannah, PhD, RN
Adjunct Professor
Department of Community Health Science
Faculty of Medicine
The University of Calgary
Calgary, Alberta T2N 4N1
Canada

Marion J. Ball, EdD
Vice President
Clinical Solutions
2 Hamill Road
Quadrangle 359 West
Healthlink, Inc.
Baltimore, MD 21210
and
Adjunct Professor
The Johns Hopkins Universi
School of Nursing
Baltimore, MD 21205
USA

British Library Cataloguing in Publication Data
Information technology solutions for healthcare. - (Health informatics)
    1. Medical informatics
    I. Zieliński, Krzysztof   II. Duplaga, Mariusz   III. Ingram, David
    362.1′0285
ISBN-10: 1852339780

Library of Congress Control Number: 2005927242

ISBN-10: 1-85233-978-0   e-ISBN 1-84628-141-5   Printed on acid-free paper.
ISBN-13: 978-1-85233-978-4

© Springer-Verlag London Limited 2006

Printed in the United States of America   (TB/MVY)

9 8 7 6 5 4 3 2 1

Springer Science+Business Media
springeronline.com

Series Preface

This series is directed to healthcare professionals who are leading the transformation of health care by using information and knowledge to advance the quality of patient care. Launched in 1988 as Computers in Health Care, the series offers a broad range of titles: some are addressed to specific professions such as nursing, medicine, and health administration; others to special areas of practice such as trauma and radiology. Still other books in the series focus on interdisciplinary issues, such as the computer-based patient record, electronic health records, and networked healthcare systems.

Renamed Health Informatics in 1998 to reflect the rapid evolution in the discipline now known as health informatics, the series continues to add titles that contribute to the evolution of the field. In the series, eminent experts, serving as editors or authors, offer their accounts of innovation in health informatics. Increasingly, these accounts go beyond hardware and software to address the role of information in influencing the transformation of healthcare delivery systems around the world. The series also increasingly focuses on "peopleware" and the organizational, behavioral, and societal changes that accompany the diffusion of information technology in health services environments.

These changes will shape health services in the new millennium. By making full and creative use of the technology to tame data and to transform information, health informatics will foster the development of the knowledge age in health care. As coeditors, we pledge to support our professional colleagues and the series readers as they share the advances in the emerging and exciting field of health informatics.

Kathryn J. Hannah
Marion J. Ball

598 78547

Preface

The 1998 UK Foresight Report described the field of Health Informatics thus: "Health Informatics examines the organisational, professional and technical issues involved in the use of information systems to support patient-centred healthcare delivery. It includes activities like clinical decision making, efficient information management, knowledge acquisition and dissemination, and informed patient participation."

Health informatics is evolving quickly, driven by:

- rapid pace of innovation in information and communications technologies and their increasingly pervasive deployment in biomedicine and healthcare,
- exponential growth of knowledge in the biomedical and clinical sciences, and associated need to structure and organise this knowledge as an accessible, up-to-date and coherent electronic resource,
- rapid change in social, professional, legal and organisational contexts of healthcare, associated with greater focus on cost-effectiveness, safety and governance of treatments and services.

Though by no means yet a mature discipline, innovation in the field, over several decades, has proven most successful where pursued locally, under the leadership of successful healthcare professionals, engineers and scientists. As with much investment in IT, the specification and effective delivery of large-scale national projects has been hazardous, reflecting lack of knowledge about generic clinical service requirements and clinical, technical and management discipline needed to support innovation at this level.

To meet national and international healthcare needs, an information infrastructure must join up clinical process and meaning across the many services, professions, organisations and locations of healthcare that provide services and support for individual patients and the communities in which they live. To do this reliably and confidentially, in timely fashion, is the nature of the complex, 2020 challenge we now face. The scale and precision of operational performance of systems that is needed, the necessary clinical and technical standardisation of data, systems and services and the educational and organisational development required to manage the implied change and enable effective deployment and use of the new infrastructure, by patients and professionals alike, are key aspects. Innovation, driven by diversity and local requirement, from the bottom up, must now grow upwards and find accommodation with standardisation and nationally coordinated procurement and implementation of new systems and services, driven from the top down.

Health informatics has now reached a crucial stage of collision between these, hitherto rather damagingly disconnected, bottom-up and top-down evolutionary strategies. The requirement for a comprehensive, coherent and patient focused health information infrastructure has risen to the highest level in the scale of priorities of health services internationally. Investment on a national scale is now forthcoming in some countries and from it can come benefits from:

- Evidence-based underpinning of health information standards and services and their evolution, over time,
- New professionalism in the management of information, across the whole healthcare enterprise,
- New industrial capacity for relevant supporting products and services,
- Enhanced international collaboration on global health issues.

Research is vital in health informatics because we must learn, practically and by careful experiment, about the necessary underpinning discipline of health informatics. There are no available and proven blueprints of design for such a comprehensive infrastructure and, moreover, the target is shifting all the time.

Science moves on:

- E.g. advances in genomics are leading to potentially huge new personal health data collections, correlating genotype and phenotype of disease with treatment and outcome.

Healthcare services move on:

- E.g. there are increasing concerns for improved patient safety, for achievement of best possible clinical outcomes and for security and confidentiality of personal health data.

Society and the law move on:

- E.g. the cost–effectiveness of chronic illness services for ageing populations, the need to respond globally to new epidemics of infectious diseases, the requirement to show due diligence within a markedly sharper legal framework for management of personal health data.

Introduction

The main concept behind this book is to present the transformation of healthcare services in the Information Society age. These changes are catalysed by conducting professional and social activities with the use of the Internet and mobile tools. The synergy of computer technologies and medical services opens up new, fascinating possibilities in the areas of continuing care, chronic disease treatment, home monitoring of elderly people, etc. The understanding of the nature of this IT-accelerated healthcare transformation is a key factor in improving medical standards and reducing costs. The book addresses this issue as a priority of the Information Society and presents a complete survey of many promising e-health technologies, implemented as real-life applications. Our focus is on providing an integrated overview of the medical, social and technical aspects of e-health. Applying information technologies to healthcare promises fundamental changes in existing models of care delivery and system performance. Hence, an in-depth presentation of how healthcare services are enhanced by the Internet and mobile tools is one of the essential objectives of the book. This unique analysis of the evolution of healthcare services is illustrated by numerous examples; the book also contains a description of available telecare solutions.

The scope of our work is both complex and innovative. The editors have decided to invite leading experts in the field to author individual chapters, related to the deployment of IT tools for solving important problems in 21st century healthcare systems. This approach guarantees high scientific and professional value of the book.

The idea of publishing a book on the use of information technology solutions for improving healthcare delivery systems originates from the PRO-ACCESS initiative (ImPROving ACCESS of Associated States to Advanced Concepts in Medical Telematics, IST-2001-38626) focused on providing better access for new EU Associated States (now full EU members) to modern e-health technologies developed at leading European centres.

Chapter 1, *Evolution of IT-Enhanced Healthcare: From Telemedicine to e-Health*, introduces the concept of telemedicine, including definitions and requirements of telemedical systems. The evolution of contemporary telemedical systems and challenges faced by future technologies are also shown. Additionally, this chapter reviews speciality-specific applications, including formal and legal aspects of telemedicine as well as its acceptance among users. An important item is the cost/benefit analysis of telemedical services.

Chapter 2, *Access Technologies in Telecare*, overviews access telecommunication technologies. Basic requirements for such communications are considered, both in the hospital-to-patient scenario and in the hospital-to-hospital scenario. The available and emerging solutions are also briefly presented.

Chapter 3, *Internet Technologies in Medical Systems*, presents the requirements and architectures of Internet-based medical systems, with focus on Internet telemedical services, Web services and portal technologies. The next-generation point-of-care information systems are also described and the shift in the methodology associated with medical systems to suit new software architectures is analyzed. As a case study, the TELEDICOM system for collaborative teleradiology is presented.

Chapter 4, *Security and Safety of Telemedical Systems*, describes the requirements related to this important area, analyzing them in the context of legal acts affecting the security of e-medical systems. Subsequently, security system architecture modelling and techniques for securing e-medical systems are described.

Chapter 5, *Wireless Systems in e-Health*, focuses on modern wireless technologies. Security aspects and wireless interference issues are discussed. Wireless hospital and telecare applications are also described and the requirements for mobile access from PDA devices to medical databases are considered in more detail. As a case study, a wireless emergency system is presented.

Chapter 6, *Relevance of Terminological Standards and Services in Telemedicine*, describes medical terminology standardization on several levels of granularity and overviews existing classifications and nomenclatures. As a case study, this chapter presents the TOSCA Project dedicated to establishing a common terminology.

Chapter 7, *Electronic Health Records*, describes the progress in constructing a common set of data structures contained in medical records and reports on the main standardisation efforts in this area. The Electronic Patient Record has fundamental significance for the implementation of medical information systems and telemedical applications.

Chapter 8, *Decision Support Systems in Medicine*, covers knowledge-based and expert systems which support physicians in making medical decisions by providing interactive tools. A classification of such systems is presented and their internal structures and architectures are evaluated. Several classes of expert systems are described and compared.

Chapter 9, *Health Telematics Networks*, briefly describes the requirements and architecture of telematics networks and the organisational models for such networks. It also overviews e-health network services available over the Internet.

Chapter 10, *IT Applications for the Remote Testing of Hearing*, presents innovative telemedical systems for sensory self-diagnostics over the Internet. The preconditions and structures of successful nationwide programs based on these systems are also described.

Chapter 11, *Model of Chronic Care Enabled with Information Technology*, defines the scope of the problem, describing Web-based and telemonitoring solutions as the most commonly used technologies in the area. Subsequently, issues relating to patient empowerment and formal aspects of electronic patient-physician communications are described. The chapter is summarized by an overview of benefits and real-life applications.

Chapter 12, *Computer-Aided Interventions*, presents image-guided surgery as an evolving technology used to carry out minimally-invasive procedures. Such procedures enable access to difficult-to-reach organs and minimise trauma to the patient. This area combines high-speed computer systems with specialised software and tracking technology.

Chapter 13, *Biosignal Monitoring and Recording*, concerns monitoring and recording biosignal data as an extension of medical investigations which takes into consideration their changes over time. This information is used to develop a diagnosis or if it is not sufficient to request more investigations. By this approach a better understanding of physiological control systems can be achieved.

Chapter 14, *Enhancing Medical Education through Telelearning*, specifies telelearning standards and requirements for medical telelearning platforms. The chapter contains an overview of existing telelearning platforms and multimedia material. The process of preparing educational materials for medical e-learning is described, as are the technical aspects of handling multimedia in e-learning medical systems. As a case study, the Medical Digital Video Library and the Virtual Video File System are presented.

Acknowledgments

All books are collaborative efforts, and this one is no exception. Numerous people have contributed ideas, comments and inspiration, helping turn our concept into reality.

Many chapters of this book have been inspired by discussions during the three "E-health in Common Europe" conferences organized as part of the PRO-ACCESS IST Project in June 2003, March 2004 and December 2004 respectively. The chapters are not selected papers from these conferences, nor do they duplicate the contents of invited lectures - they are intentionally written by leading experts, using materials which detail the most relevant emerging problems in modern telemedicine.

Contents

1 Evolution of IT-Enhanced Healthcare: From Telemedicine to e-Health

Mariusz Duplaga², Krzysztof Zieliński¹

¹   Department of Computer Science, AGH University of Science and Technology, Krakow, Poland
²   Jagiellonian University Medical College, Krakow, Poland

The use of information and telecommunication technologies in healthcare results from the endeavour for improvement of the quality and availability of services as well as their cost-effectiveness. Availability of consecutive technologies enabling communication between distant parties had an impact on the development of the new domain called telemedicine. Even now the most popular form of telemedical contact between patient and physician as well as between health professionals is the phone call. It seems to be so natural that hardly anybody realizes that telephone communication may be perceived as telemedicine.

First examples of telemedical solutions were clearly linked to technical innovations and such inventions as the telephone or telegraph were usually quickly picked up by healthcare. However, telemedicine as a field of knowledge started to develop from the late 1940s. In 1948, the transmission of radiological images was carried out through a telephone line between West Chester and Philadelphia in Pensylvania in the USA. In 1959, closed-circuit television systems were applied for transmission of a neurological examination for educational purposes in another location. Three years later, a microwave connection was implemented between Nebraska Psychiatric Institute and Norfolk State Hospital. This connection was used for teleconsultations for about 6 years. In the late 1960s a telemedical link was established between Massachusetts General Hospital and surgery performed in Boston's Logan International Airport. It enabled transmission of the video and interaction between both sides of the connections. The scope of teleconsultations covered dermatology, radiology, cardiology and psychiatry.

Telemedical services were financed from federal funds in 15 centres in the USA from the 1970s to the early 1980s. The results obtained in some of these large projects seemed to support the feasibility of telemedical services. The use of satellite connections for care delivery in Canada or Alaska could be an example of telemedicine usefulness. The project relying on the use of satellite links for delivery of medical services to Papago Indians was conducted by the National Aeronautics and Space Administration for 20 years. It yielded important indications about the possible use of various technologies in telemedicine. Most of these initial telemedical projects conducted in the USA were based on the use of standard analog television and required complex, relatively expensive infrastructure. Furthermore, these were demonstrative projects and comparisons with standard care usually were not conducted. Long-term maintenance of test telemedical systems was not assured and most of the projects did not survive after the period of financement from external funds.

In the late 1980s and early 1990s the number of references in the literature related to telemedicine showed a decreasing trend. Simultaneously, the progress in digital technology was so great that with time new technologies feasible for telemedicine became less expensive and commonly available. Finally, the market was filled with teleconferencing systems based on computer equipment. The costs of appropriate bandwidth for transmission of data also decreased. Technological progress had an impact on the definition of the objectives realized in telemedical projects. The researchers focused on such aspects which could influence significantly further development of telemedicine as lack of appropriate standards and regulations of the reliability issues, security and confidentiality and failing financing models. Considerable attention was directed to the telemedical application bringing better care to rural and remote areas. Furthermore, the scenarios for supplying specialistic competencies to primary care were explored. In the 1990s the objective of information systems development for healthcare became one of the priorities of the research and development framework programs of the European Union. This strategy had considerable impact on the search for appropriate solutions and applications in telemedicine in Europe.

Since the mid-1990s, the growth of the Internet community has accelerated tremendously. Internet expansion has also brought a new vision of telemedical services; the concept of e-health arises in relation to the complex environment of electronic transactions in healthcare. Modern information technologies appearing in this time, e.g. wireless and mobile systems, are quickly adapted by research teams targeting medicine as user domain. More and more emphasis is placed on the costs of implemented solutions as well as on the quality of care delivered with telematic technologies. Enhanced availability of medical services also becomes a key issue.

Definitions of telemedicine were gradually developed and modified over the years. The first formal definition of telemedicine was proposed by Bird in 1971[3]. The aspect of medical practice carried out without traditional contact between physician and patient but with the use of interactive audiovisual transmission was underlined by him. Willemain and Mark pointed out that every system used by physician and patient who are in different locations is contained in telemedicine[30]. A more complex definition was proposed by Bashshur. He postulated that telemedical systems should fulfill several criteria including geographical distance between centres participating in transmission of medical information, the use of teleinformatic technology as a substitute for direct contact, employment of dedicated personnel for system maintenance and application of clinical guidelines regulating diagnostics and treatment of patients[2].

In the range of the program "Advanced Informatics in Medicine" financed by the European Union the definition was formed which states that telemedicine relies on diagnostics, monitoring and treatment of a patient with the use of systems which allow for access to expert advice and patient data regardless of where the patient and information about him or her are located. Furthermore, in a publication issued by the Institute of Medicine in the USA, telemedicine was defined as the use of information in electronic form and communication technologies for provision of medical care when the participants of interaction are located in different places[8]. And finally, in the WHO report titled "A Health Telematics Policy in Support of WHO's Health-For-All Strategy For Global Health Development" prepared in 1997, telemedicine was described as the form of healthcare provided by all health professionals using information and communication for the exchange of essential data on diagnostics, treatment and prevention of diseases, on scientific research and for assuring the continuity of medical education, in situations when distance is the critical factor[31].

The wide scope of implementations of modern teleinformatic technologies in various areas of healthcare results in difficulties with a comprehensive, descriptive definition of telemedicine. Interaction within the telemedicine domain may be carried out between various participants of the healthcare arena. Specifically, these contacts can be accomplished between health professionals, between patients and health professionals, between patients assisted by health professionals and other health professionals, between health professionals and organizations responsible for health maintanence, between providers and payers and many others. It is difficult to predict how long the term "telemedicine" will remain in our vocabulary as we face nowadays trends for technology convergence. In the future, separation of telemedicine from other areas of electronic activities will probably be impossible. Some experts also predict the disappearance of the concept of telemedicine because they stipulate that at some moment most healthcare services will be based on the use of information and communication technologies.

There is no doubt that telemedicine is characterized by a multidisciplinary approach. Most existing definitions place stress on communication as well as on exchange of medical information with benefit for health or education status of patients and/or providers. The spectrum of terms with similar meaning is quite wide nowadays. Telehealth and e-health seem to be the broadest ones. Telehealth is a more generic term applied in the context of the use of information and communication technology (ICT) to deliver health services, expertise and information over a distance[28]. It seems that currently, among all terms related to the use of information and communication technologies in the context of health maintenance, the concept of e-health has become the most universal one. Specifically, it is broader than telemedicine and can be described as an emerging field in the intersection of medical informatics, public health and business, that enables health services and information to be delivered or enhanced through the Internet and related technologies[7].

Regardless of the definition of telemedicine we choose, its three main dimensions remain health service, telecommunications and computer technology. The wide scope of telemedicine adds to difficulties faced during the processes of development, implementation and deployment of telemedical solutions. Potential benefits from telemedicine are frequently underlined as the rationale for further development of this domain. They can be summarized as [19]:

- Improved access: telemedicine can provide and improve access to healthcare in underserved or neglected areas.
- Reduced cost: potential savings depend on the participant in the telemedical interaction. They include smaller transportation costs for patients seeking speciality care or healthcare providers referring their patients for consultation to another medical centre. Expenditures for speciality care facilities in peripheral locations may also result from the opportunity of obtaining expert medical advice with telemedicine link.
- Reduced isolation: telemedicine may be perceived as a medium for maintaining contacts with peers and medical experts during patients' consultations and educational sessions. It has been reported that color, full-motion video is critical to health professionals in simulating face-to-face communication between colleagues in consultations and between patients and physicians[4]. Furthermore, it supports existing provider-

patient relationships and simultaneously facilitates access to speciality care.

- Improved quality of care: access to expert advice with real-time interaction when needed, seems to be important in achieving the better quality of care through telemedicine. Continuous care quality improvement results from education through telemedical contacts between health professionals in remote locations and specialists employed in medical referential centres.

- Enhanced continuity of medical education: teleconsultations and interactions with other health professionals bring important benefits for competency building. Telemedical links may also be used for telelearning activities addressed to health professionals practicing in distant medical centres diminishing their feeling of professional isolation.

- Effective utilisation of medical resources: appropriate use of telemedicine may result in better integration of healthcare on various referential levels and support continuity of care.

Despite considerable progress in communication technology, the transmission of medical data is still a challenge due to security requirements, required quality of service (QoS) and vast volumes of medical data. Furthermore, transmission of medical data over telecommunication links is subject to special legal regulations in many countries. The interaction in telemedicine conducted with the objective of obtaining diagnosis or getting expert advice is an inherently complex process. It may be achieved in various scenarios: from off-line communication via e-mail or ftp, through Web coordinated medical data exchange to on-line interactive multiparty video-conferencing.

The educational aspect of telemedicine is also a challenge in terms of computer-based training. It may require access to multimedia document repositories, high-resolution digital images, 3D reconstructions of the human body, and real-time or off-line video transmission of medical procedures. Appearance of ambient computing and easy access in our everyday life to mobile wireless communication technology open a new promising application field in telemedicine, particularly in the area of remote patient monitoring and care delivered to patients with chronic medical conditions.

1   Conditions for Telemedicine Development

Telemedicine systems should fulfill a unique set of requirements which in many respects distinguishes them from a standard teleconferencing system[16]. In the case of consultation for obstetrical ultrasound in potentially high-risk pregnancy, the ultrasound study consisting of images, color flow, and Doppler spectral and auditory information of good quality needs to be transmitted in real time. For dermatology applications, a high-resolution camera with either a low frame rate or still image capture capability rather than standard video at 30 frames/sec might be required. Many image processing and graphics functions are often necessary when analyzing medical images with intent of establishing a primary diagnosis or a plan of treatment. They range from window and level adjustment, magnification and minification, digital magnifying glass, image mensuration, adaptive histogram equalization, unsharp masking, and convolution to 3-dimensional visualization, texture measurements, volume measurements, spatial registration, lung nodule screening, microcalcification detection and stereotactic surgical planning. Modern digital radiology requires DICOM standard for image processing[20]. It is commonly used by medical equipment vendors and enables sophisticated processing and analysis of digital medical data provided during telemedical consultation.

Telemedicine is used for transmission of necessary information about patients via telecommunication channels and thus diminishes the need for patient and health professional transportation. However, if communicating medical facilities are moderately distant, the quality of the system should assure better functionality in comparison to traditional forms of cooperation employed by these facilities. Telemedical systems should offer fast and reliable services, intuitive functionalities and reliability of transferred data, e.g. high image quality, to be a competitive option for health professionals.

The requirements for modern telemedical systems could be grouped according to three categories: telemedical workstation, communication network and human perception of media.

- Telemedicine workstation: telemedical systems require programmable video, audio, image handling and compression to support applications ranging from typical video teleconferencing to those providing "diagnostic-quality" video, audio and medical images in interactive way. Telemedical systems should usually provide use of the following standards and formats: MPEG (for a high-quality audio/video compression), JPEG (for still image compression), H.320 (for videoconferencing over ISDN), and H.324 (for videoconferencing over POTS). In addition, the acquisition, compression and processing, and the communication interface need to be tightly integrated to assure necessary system efficiency. Support for data acquisition from peripheral medical devices, e.g. electronic stethoscope as well as images from medical imaging equipment and high-resolution cameras is also critical. Appropriate high-resolution displays are necessary in some applications.
- Communication network: telemedical systems should adapt to a wide variety of bandwidths (e.g., from 28 kbps to over 155 Mbps), depending

on the clinical application, the available telecommunication channels (ISDN lines, land-based fiber optic cable, satellite link) and the desired interaction level in order to achieve optimum utilization of available transmission medium while providing the best quality video and audio. For example, basic teleconsultation applications can usually be accomplished at low bitrates with available compression and processing hardware. However, real-time consultation based on the transmission of high-quality video or DICOM images requires higher bitrates and specialized hardware. Of course, with more challenging subjects of teleconsultations, higher bandwidths will be required to provide adequate quality of service.

- Human perception of media: the latency of communication should be minimized in order to support an effective interaction within the telemedical system. It has been reported that lead/lag between the audio and video playback should be less than 80 msec to be perceived as synchronized by human observers[21]. In case of full duplex communication, both audio and video should arrive no later than 80 msec, which is not easy to achieve. Although the criteria vary depending on the situation, transmission of a very large image should usually be done in less than 10 seconds if user distraction is to be avoided. These requirements call for network connections that feature guaranteed bandwidth and maximum delays at a given bitrate such as ATM[12].

2   Types of Applications

Critical factor in the evaluation of telemedical systems is the time span required for obtaining a response from the expert on the other side of the telemedical connection. Furthermore, this criterion determines two basic types of applications in telemedicine (Figure 1-1): store-and-forward and real-time systems.

Store-and-Forward Telemedicine. This is commonly used for transferring digital images from one location to another. Images are captured with digital cameras or still video and sent to another location. They have attached a text summary of the case and are sent by email or WWW. This type of application is usually not feasible for emergency interventions, as a specialist reviews cases when convenient. There is no limit to the geographical distance between origin and destination of the image.

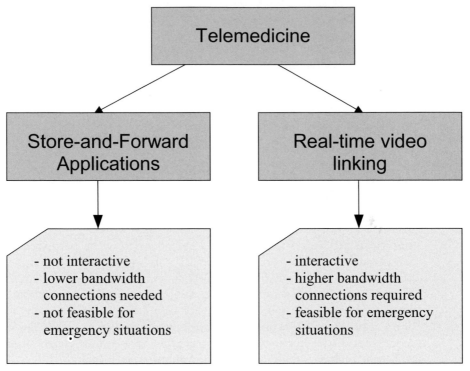

Figure 1-1 Two basic types of systems used in telemedicine.

Real-Time Video Linking. This approach is used when a "face-to-face" contact and interaction are necessary. The scenario may encompass a session between a patient and assisting health professional in one location and a specialist in another location or a session between health professionals on both sides. In some specific applications, a patient may be the sole participant in the teleconferencing session, e.g. in homecare applications. Specialized video conferencing equipment at both locations allows for real-time consultation. High-bandwidth communication channels are necessary, although this type of telemedicine is now within the reach of the desktop computers connected to the Internet.

Store-and-forward telemedicine has become increasingly more popular as it is well-suited to Web technology. It is particularly suitable for teleradiology. Teleradiology is the electronic transmission of radiological images e.g. CT or MRI scans, X-rays, from a remote site where the image is captured to a central site for the purpose of their interpretation or consultation. Teleradiology requires rapid interpretation and report turnaround of the images sent for consultations. From a technical point of view, medical data can be uploaded on a Web server and then accessed via Web browser at a convenient time. In the same way, the diagnosis could be attached to the medical data exposed by the Web server. This model may be further elaborated by storage of the patient's record in the database. Such approach assures scalability of the solution. Access to medical data via WWW has many advantages. Data are available on virtually any computer terminal with thin client technology. This solution could be adjusted with security mechanisms which support authentication and authorization. Notification function is a valuable extension of this non-interactive telemedical solution. It enables distribution of the messages in the form of SMS or e-mail to the physician or other health professional that the package of medical data for teleconsultation has been setup or the teleconsultation has been performed by the expert.

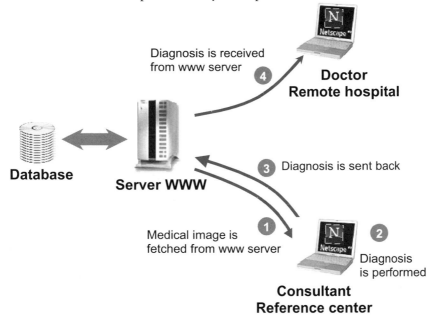

Figure 1-2 Web-centric teleradiology.

The basic steps performed in this model are as follows:

1. A selected radiology image is fetched from a database by dedicated software installed over Web server and sent to the evaluator's Web browser.
2. Consultant evaluates the image.
3. Image description and suggested diagnosis is posted back to Web server and stored in the database.
4. Then the description/diagnosis may be read by the referring physician when needed.

Store-and-forward approach may be implemented between the medical institutions over relatively narrow bandwidth links. The upload of data can be carried out at night in order to make it available for teleconsultation taking place in the morning.

Real-time video linking paradigm presents only a basic model which could be easily expanded. Medical data, e.g. DICOM images or as JPEG files, can be sent over in parallel to real-time video and audio transmission. Such scenario requires high-speed computer network communication and powerful medical station to perform on-demand necessary graphical data transformation. The basic point-to-point scenario may be further expanded to group or multi-point model shown in Figure 1-3.

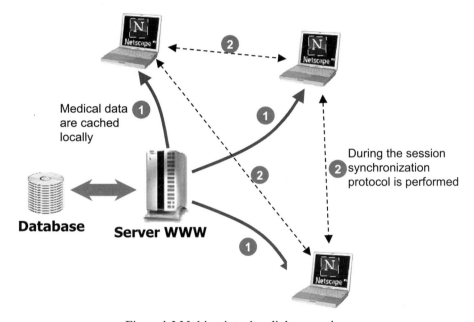

Figure 1-3 Multi-point teleradiology session.

It is necessary to point out that this model could also be applied when no high-speed computer networks are available. The medical data could be distributed before the teleconsultaion session is started and cached on local servers. Such approach reduces the delay of getting the data during the session. Interactive processing of large files, e.g. in DICOM format, is particularly important for the impact of the teleconferencing session. The solution proposed by Zielinski et al. relies on synchronization protocol used for distribution of local transformations on medical data to other session participants[32]. This protocol does not require broadband connections. It enables sharing of the medical documents between all the session participants as depicted in Figure

1-4. The markings introduced on the image by participants of the teleconferencing session can have different colours. The interactive teleconsultation session should be preceded by scheduling process which may include session announcement, invitation of medical experts and data distribution. The session may be performed on contractual planned basis or ad hoc in emergency situations.

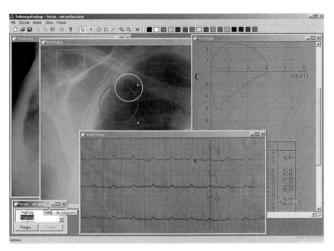

Figure 1-4 Example of "whiteboard" application for sharing medical documents during teleconferencing sessions.

3 E-health as Ubiquitous Environment for Transactions

The term "e-health" emerged in the 1990s, by analogy to e-business, in relation to medical services offered through the Internet. It designates the continuum of various types of electronic transactions related to the healthcare carried out through the use of Internet technologies. Nowadays, a general understanding of e-health covers areas which rely not only on the use of the Internet, but also on other telematic technologies. The pressure on the use of alternatives technologies is particularly high in regions where Internet penetration is low. The use of mobile telephony is one of the promising trends in healthcare-related communication. E-health covers both provision of contents and services targeting health professionals, patients and citizens. This environment of transactions in healthcare has become more and more complex. Additionally, the e-health area is far more attractive for investors than traditional telemedicine. It is underlined that development of e-health services is usually propelled by the desire to achieve financial profits. In general understanding, the e-health area is much broader than telemedicine. In some way, it results from application of rules governing e-business to the sphere of telemedical application.

Such wide concept of e-health was promoted by Mitchell[18]. He defines e-health as electronic transmission, storage and access to data available in digital form for clinical, educational and administrative purposes, both locally and from a distance. In a 2001 report published by the e-Health Institute titled "eHealth after the Bubble Period", e-health was defined as the use of modern information and communication technologies, specifically the Internet, for maintaining health and improvement of healthcare[5].

The brief definition of e-health proposed by Lee et al. is based on five key elements: the provision of the contents, assuring the connectivity, inclusion of economic mechanisms (commerce), creation of community and support for clinical care. The cluster of services based on the provision of the contents encompasses presentation of the information, assistance at information search, decision support and telelearning. The aspect of connectivity is particularly important in medical information systems, medical services and systems integration, electronic transactions and clinical trials. Social interactions in the context of e-health comprise personal contacts, information exchange, emotional support and development of communities. Essential in the e-health environment, according to some authors, is the capability of income generation and self-financing of the enterprise. The rationale for e-health development results not only from a desire to achieve returns from investments but also from general phenomena such as increasing prevalence of chronic disease, aging of the population, and growing costs of healthcare. E-health environment also favours the empowerment of citizens as to perception of their health status, coordination of medical care (continuity of care, shared care) and enabling access to electronic patient record[25]. The motive of making clinical decisions by interdisciplinary teams is also frequently underlined. Growth of the e-health area remains in synergy with modern strategies of prevention, diagnosis and treatment of diseases.

E-health industry is focused on delivery of tools, solutions and services linked to specific aspects of healthcare and e-business. The areas of the most intensive e-health industry development include administrative systems, clinical information systems, telemedical systems and purchases of products associated with medical care. The scope of possible e-health application is vast, however, the portals for citizens, patients and health professionals still remain the commonest companies active in this area. E-health companies derive income from their activities through sponsors, paid advertisements, payment for services, the offers of subscription systems and payment per transaction.

The market for electronic transactions in healthcare results from interaction between its active actors like organizations maintaining the health status of the community, providers of medical services and consumers (patients, citizens) as well as providers of e-health applications, public health institutions, health policy makers and employers.

Two main models of e-health companies exist: services for business partners (business-to-business) and for consumers (business-to-consumer). Most organizations active in the area of public health show a passive approach in modification of workflow processes through implementation of computer technologies. Such situation is related to costs of the undertakings, but also to shortage of appropriate tools for the public health field. The status of information technology adaptation in medical institutions is highly inhomogeneous and dependent on general economic circumstances and status of healthcare facilities in a specific country. Furthermore, information systems are quite slowly accepted by clinicians, even if they show meaningful interest in Internet and related technologies. Not many of them see opportunities resulting from Internet use for improvement of medical practice, even in those countries with high Internet penetration.

The potential benefits from the use of Internet applications in each practice could be savings, acceleration of service delivery and improved quality of healthcare. However, these benefits, intuitively expected, are quite difficult to evidence. Many barriers to e-health growth could be removed by organizational changes, appropriate economic strategies and open attitude to emerging technologies. Some authors underline the following obstacles in e-health development: the threats to confidentiality of medical data, inefficient integration of different technologies, the need for development of technical and clinical standards and reimbursement for services offered electronically.

Growth of the e-health environment is promoted by the pressure on improvement of efficiency both in healthcare activities and on the economic side of healthcare services. Patients and citizens are also vitally interested in better access to reliable health-related information. Questionnaire studies conducted in the USA indicate that at least 50% of all adults accessing the Internet searched for information related to health and medicine. This pressure for access to health-related content on the Internet is linked to a wider phenomenon of influencing the modes of healthcare delivery by patients and their families. Since 2001, when the great collapse in the Internet economy occurred, the importance of a valid financing model for such activities has been well appreciated[5][14]. Currently, e-health companies remaining in the market reveal robust mechanisms for income generation. Furthermore, the awareness of the frequency of medical errors increases questions about mechanisms for improvement of care quality. In this context, the use of e-health applications is perceived as a possible remedy.

Development of the e-health area influences considerably the context of health services delivery and changes established forms of communications. One of the essential aspects of e-health environment expansion is remodeling of the relationship between health professionals and patients. Other areas undergoing quick changes include the focus on patient empowerment in the therapeutical process, the emphasis on prevention and shaping appropriate health-maintaining behaviours in society and building of supportive relations outside institutional healthcare systems, frequently in patients' homes.

4 The Impact on Relations in Healthcare

A common example of the new quality in relations between patient and physician is that of a patient suffering from specific symptoms or diseases presenting at a physician's office with many print-outs from Websites offering health-related content. For many health professionals this situation is "awkward" as he or she is immediately confronted with the information load absorbed by the patient over the course of days or even weeks. A health consumer who is aware of his or her health status and medical problem is the ideal option for the most successful care strategies developed nowadays. On the other hand, physicians should be aware that in the contacts with their patients they should play the role of partner and navigator in this information overload. The important advantages of the e-health environment supporting the self-managed role of the health consumer encompass easy access, empowerment of the patient/consumer, availability of feedback channels as well as considerable elasticity. The importance of the feedback channels was underlined by some authors[1].

A growing number of people believe the Internet is the most feasible source of health-related information; they appreciate its better access and volume of resources. However, some negligence exists in relation to the reliability issues linked to the health-related information available on the Internet. E-health may reshape modern public health strategies as information technology offers new more effective approaches to prevention. This feature goes along with trends for emphasis of consumer-driven healthcare and enables the implementation of patient-centred care models.

The perception of potential advantages of e-health solutions is diversified across the healthcare scene. Health professionals tend to put more attention on the risks resulting from access to unreliable health-related information by patients. However, around-the-clock access to specific information, especially if the website offers personification mechanisms, is highly appreciated by the patients and their families. This results from the fact that healthcare systems face substantial problems when confronted with the growing challenge of offering high-quality care in a cost-effective mode to modern societies, especially taking into account such phenomena like increased life span and percentage of people with chronic diseases in the population. The limited time that can be devoted by the physician to individual patients makes Internet health-related resources even more attractive.

The use of Internet-based health-related resources and tools yields new kinds of social relations (e.g. patient support groups) and on the other hand, enables anonymity for those who suffer from embarrassing medical conditions. Furthermore, the patient may be decidedly more active in the e-health environment than in traditional healthcare settings. This results in a shift from his or her passive role in relation to the physician to one of partnership.

Nowadays, self-management has become a well-evidenced target of national and international strategies for management of specific medical conditions (e.g. Global Initiative for Asthma GINA[9], Global Initiative for Chronic Obstructive Lung Diseases GOLD[10]). This has resulted in the eruption of e-health solutions in the area of chronic care, which offer the provision of information adjusted to patient needs, feedback communication with health professionals at monitoring centres, prompt response from health providers in case of unfavourable trends in patients' health status and opportunity to participate in support groups with other patients and their families. Even if some risk may be related to access to unreliable health-related contents on the Internet, the role of e-health solutions in patient education cannot be overestimated.

5   Evaluation of the Benefits

A systematic review of evidence for benefits resulting from telemedicine was published in the Journal of Telemedicine and Telecare in 2002. It was prepared by the Finnish Office of Health Care Technology Assessment and Alberta Heritage Foundation for Medical Research. The review was based on the literature published in the years 1966 – 1998[11][23]. It included papers in which telemedical application had been compared with standard procedures not encompassing the use of telemedicine and in which administrative changes, the impact on morbidity indicators and phfarmacoeconomic analysis were described. As the follow-up of this first systematic review, the literature from 1998 to 2000 was evaluated. From the literature search, 177 papers were selected for further evaluation. Of these, 64 fulfilled the criteria for inclusion in the review. Two additional papers related to the projects conducted by Alberta

Heritage Foundation for Medical Research were covered by review. The studies selected for review were grouped according to speciality (burns treatment, cardiology, dermatology, emergency medicine, home care and telemonitoring, teleconsultations, psychiatry, neurology, ophthalmology, pathology and radiology). Half of the studies were carried out in the USA, others in such countries as the United Kingdom, Canada, Finland, Norway, France and Australia. Singular studies came from Austria, Germany, Greece, Hong Kong, Italy and New Zealand. This systematic review showed that telemedical systems have an advantage over the traditional medicine approach. In part of the studies, benefits from telemedical applications were evidenced, but also disadvantages were found or no clear response was reported. In only five studies was the strategy based on standard care more beneficial than that based on telemedical systems. The results obtained in specific countries were considerably dependent on the local conditions. In some studies, savings and clinical benefits resulted from evasion of unnecessary transportation and resulting delays. In one study focused on burn wound treatment, the telemedical system yielded savings linked to smaller transportation costs, but simultaneously, the costs at the centre involved in burn treatment increased. Furthermore, the use of telemedical applications was linked with clinical limitations. In most studies in the field of telecardiology, limited evidence of clinical and economic benefits was gained. The cumulative analysis of teledermatology application use yielded particularly interesting results. Telemedical applications incurred additional costs on the healthcare provider, but savings to the patient. In emergency units, telemedicine use produced similar results in terms of the quality of patient care, but it accelerated the process of decision taking.

Promising results were also obtained in studies which evaluated the use of e-health applications in home care and telemonitoring of patients' status. They seem to confirm that telemedical systems may bring savings and improvement of the quality of care in chronic medical conditions. The improvement of treatment results was noted in patients with diabetes, chronic heart failure and arterial hypertension.

Considerable number of published studies focused on medical teleconsultations. The efficiency and opportunity for savings resulting from electronic referrals to hospitals as well as better availability of information for surgical consultations were confirmed[13]. Savings were also reported in studies on the use of telemedical systems in prisons.

However, the results of studies concerning benefits from the use of e-health applications conducted to date, are generally ambiguous. Particularly, the methodology of studies on telemedicine focusing on the cost-effectiveness of implemented solutions was questioned[29]. There is seen a desire in the research community to obtain solid scientific evidence of benefits from the use of e-health applications, both in terms of better quality of care as well as cost limitation. By analogy to evidence-based medicine doctrine, the search for hard evidence of benefits from e-health system implementations is called evidence-based telemedicine.

The promise of the improvement of healthcare service quality through e-health development gained a new meaning due to reports on the frequency of complications occurring in the results of medical errors. This issue was addressed by consecutive reports of the Institute of Medicine, which clearly indicated the use of modern IT strategies as a possible way of decreasing the occurrence of medical errors[15].

The evaluaton of telemedicine and e-health applications is associated with considerable difficulties. Potential benefits are perceived by actors of the healthcare scene (patients, health professionals, payors, technology providers, society, health authorities) in different ways. Furthermore, the improvement in care delivered to patients may add additional expenditures onto the healthcare providers. Some benefits are hardly measurable, even if they have profound social impact.

6 Legal and Ethical Barriers

According to many national regulations the relationship between health professionals and patients should rely on direct, face-to-face contacts. This requirement has potentially limiting effect on the growth of e-health and telemedicine applications with focused clinical context. Such situation stems from traditional concepts of medical care delivery and is not necessarily in line with progress occurring in information and communication technologies. Furthermore, the challenges facing modern healthcare systems clearly call for a new approach to care delivery and the use of information technology offers potential mechanisms for improving their effectiveness.

Nonetheless, the liability issues are a source of considerable fears expressed by health professionals when confronted with modern telemedical solutions potentially enhancing medical practice[24]. There is also wide discrepancy between overall support for information society development and specific regulations related to health professionals' codes of behaviour in many countries[26]. A systematic approach to evidence studies showing the safety and adequacy of technical solutions would be of great help in overcoming formal barriers to e-health growth.

The security and confidentiality of patient data are important aspects of implementation of e-health systems. Adhering to standard policies available within a technological framework should be parallel to appropriate organizational security maintaining measures introduced in healthcare institutions. The protection of medical information was targeted by the Health Insurance Portability and Accountability Act (HIPPA) accepted in the USA in 1996[27]. This law creates the framework for achieving the standards related to security of medical records, integrity and authentication. Generally, they are focused on electronic transmission of electronic data by the main players in the healthcare domain. The use of personal information on European grounds was addressed in the European Directive on Data Protection which was accepted in 1995 (established as law three years later). The Directive also covers the issues related to information processing, specifically the processing carried out in computer systems[6].

The issue of delivery of healthcare services within the e-health environment and specifically telemedical activities was not addressed adequately in all countries facing the growth of this field. Specific regulations and licensure practices can be a subject of considerable differences even within one country adding to the considerable mismatch of legislation. For example, the licensure practices in states of the USA may differ meaningfully, and it must usually be carefully planned if telemedicine services are to be offered across interstate borders. Countries with advanced knowledge-based economies and with rapidly spreading information society have undertaken considerable efforts to implement laws regulating e-health and telemedicine activities.

Existing situation of many local approaches to legal regulation of the issues of security and confidentiality, reimbursement and reliability was addressed within G8 project ENABLE established in order to identify and overcome obstacles on the way to healthcare services in information society crossing borders[22].

7 Reimbursement Policies

The issue of reimbursement for services offered through telemedical systems is still open. Generally, health maintaining organizations do not seem to be enthusiastic about payment for care delivered through telemedicine, even if potential benefits and savings may be impressive[17]. Such situation is undoubtedly associated with existing fears regarding potential difficulties in assuring clear service definition, quality assurance, convincing service documentation and finally, liability of service provider. The risks related to the use of telemedical systems which could hamper the quality of the service are related to technology-dependent factors (e.g. inappropriate technology, inadequate communication bandwidth or image quality) or human factors (e.g.

insufficient training, lack of acceptance, inappropriate organizational framework, shortage of competences, fear of responsibility). However, the approach to reimbursement for telemedicine-type activities underwent substantial changes in recent years, at least in some countries.

Typical applications developed in the e-health environment depend inherently on effective financing models, so the maintenance of the services results usually from the interest of potential customers (individuals or organizations). Some services may be covered also by health maintaining organizations, especially if existing evidence supports the cost-effectiveness and care quality improvement of the specific solution. Internet-based system supporting patients with long-term medical conditions is a good example of the service which can be offered on the basis of subscription by individual consumers (patients) or services offered to a population by third-party organizations, in some situations even by local health authorities. Specific arrangement depends on the healthcare system model implemented in a country.

8 Summary

Telemedicine concept originated from attempts to deliver healthcare services to patients located some distance from providers. Consecutive inventions brought by technological progress like the telephone and telegraph were early adapted in the healthcare domain. First examples of such applications come from the 1920s. In subsequent decades, more advanced systems were developed and first definitions of telemedicine were shaped in the 1970s. For a long time, telemedicine was available to a few centers able to establish expensive infrastructure. As a result of the digital revolution and explosion of the Internet which occurred in the 1990s, the cost of equipment and connections feasible for telemedicine decreased considerably. Furthermore, the concept of e-health as a diversified environment for various types of electronic transactions in healthcare was formed. Nowadays, the e-health domain is an important element of the information society. However, there are still many problems related to legal and ethical aspects of healthcare services based on electronic transmission. The use of telemedicine and e-health applications is a source of fears associated with potential risks, malpractice and liability. On the other hand, potential and evidenced benefits from specific solutions, e.g. in chronic care or in second opinion provision, start to prevail over skepticism.

9 Bibliography

[1] Anderson J.G., Rainey M.R., Eysenbach G.: The Impact of CyberHealthcare on the Physician-Patient Relationship. Journal of Medical Systems 2003; 27(1): 67 84

[2] Bashshur R.L.: Telemedicine and medical care. In: Telemedicine: Exploration in the Use of Telecommunications in Healthcare. Eds.: R.L.Bashshur, P.A.Armstrong, Z.L.Youssef, Springfield, IL, 1975

[3] Bird K.T.: Teleconsultation: a new health information exchange system. Third Annual Rep. Veterans Admin., Washington, DC, 1971

[4] Boor J.L., Schaad D.C., Evans F.W.: Communications Satellites in Health Education and Healthcare Delivery: Operation Considerations. J Educ Tech Syst 1981; 9(4): 371-377

[5] Eng T.R., Harris L.: eHealth after the "Bubble" Period: Focusing on the Value of Proposition. Seattle, Washington: eHealth Institute, April 2002

[6] European Directive on Data Protection. Directive 95/46/EC on the Protection of Individuals with Regard to the Processing of Personal Data and on the Free Movement of Such Data http://www.cdt.org/privacy/eudirective/EU_Directive_.html

[7] Eysenbach G.: What is e-health? J Med Internet Res 2001; 3(2): e20

[8] Field M.J.: Telemedicine. A Guide to AssessingTelecommunications in Health Care. Institute of Medicine, National Academy Press, Washington, 1996

[9] Global Initiative for Asthma Website: http://www.ginasthma.com/

[10] Global Initiative for Chronic Obstructive Lung Diseases GOLD Website: http://www.goldcopd.com/

[11] Hailey D., Roine R., Ohinmaa A.: Systematic review of evidence for the benefits of telemedicine. J Telemed Telecare 2002; S(Supp.1): S1:1-7

[12] Handel R., Huber M. N., Schroder S.: ATM Networks: Concepts: Protocols, Applications. Addison-Wesley, Reading, MA, 1993

[13] Hersh W.R., Helfand M., Wallace J., Kraemer D., Patterson P., Shapiro S., Greenlick M.: Clinical outcomes resulting from telemedicine interventions: a systematic review. BMC Med. Informatics Decision Making 2001;I:5

[14] Itagaki M.W., Berlin R.B., Schatz B.R.: The Rise and Fall of E-Health: Lessons From the First Generation of Internet Healthcare. Medscape TechMed 2002; 2(1): http://www.medscape.com/ viewarticle/431144

[15] Kilbridge P.: Crossing the Chasm with Information Technology. Bridging the Quality Gap in Health Care. First Consulting Group; July 2002

[16] Kim D., Cabral J.E., Kim Y.: Networking Requirements and the Role of Multimedia Systems in Telemedicine. http://icsl.ee.washington.edu/projects/gsp9/spie1095/

[17] Lapolla M., Millis B.: Is telemedicine reimbursement a real barrier or a convenient straw man? Telemedicine Today 1997; 5(6): 5

[18] Mitchell J.: From Telehealth to E-Health: The Unstoppable Rise of E-Health.

http://www.noie.gov.au/projects/ecommerce/ehealth/rise_of_ehealth
/body_unstoppable_rise.htm

[19]Moore M.: "Elements of success in telemedicine projects," Report of a research grant from AT&T, Graduate School of Library and Information Science, University of Texas at Austin, 1993

[20]National Electrical Manufacturers Association (NEMA): Digital Imaging and Communication in Medicine
2004http://medical.nema.org/dicom/2004.html

[21]Parsons D.M., Cabral J.E., Kim Y. Jr., Lipski G.L., Frank M.S.: MediaStation 5000: A Multimedia Workstation for Telemedicine. Medical Imaging, 1995; 2431: 382-387

[22]Rogers R., Reardon J. (eds): Barriers to a Global Information Society for Health: Recommendations for International Action. Report for the project G8-ENABLE. EC Information Society Project Office, Brussels, December 1998

[23]Roine R., Ohinmaa A., Hailey D.: Assessing telemedicine: a systematic review of literature. Can Med Assoc J 2001;165(6):765-771

[24]Stanberry B.: Legal ethical and risk issues in telemedicine. Computer Methods and Programs in Biomedicine 2001; 64: 225-233

[25]Talley R.C.: Impediments to the promises of e-health. Am J Health Syst Pharm 2001; 58(24):2379

[26]Terry N.P.: Improving the legal and regulatory climate for telemedicine and e-health. International Congress Series 2003; 1256: 279-284

[27]The Health Insurance Portability and Accountability Act of 1996 (HIPAA) http://www.cms.hhs.gov/hipaa/

[28]University of Calgary 2002. What is telehealth?
http://www.fp.ucalgary.ca/telehealth/ What_Is_Telehealth.htm (25 September 2003)

[29]Whitten P., Mair F., Haycox A., et al.: Systematic review of cost effectiveness studies of telemedicine interventions. BMJ 2002; 324: 1434-1437

[30]Willemain T.R., Mark R.G.: Models of healthcare systems. Biomed Sci Instrum 1971; 8: 9-17

[31]World Health Organization: A Health Telematics Policy in Support of WHO's Health-For-All Strategy For Global Health Development. Report of the WHO Group Consultation on Health Telematics, December 11-16, Geneva, 1997
http://whqlibdoc.who.int/hq/1998/WHO_DGO_98.1.pdf

[32]Zielinski K., Cala J., Czekierda L., Zielinski S.: Collaborative Teleradiology. In: Bubak M., Dick van Albada, Sloot P.M.A., Dongarra J.J. (eds.) ICCS 2004; LNCS 3039, 2004: 1172-1179

2 Access Technologies in Telecare

Marek Natkaniec[1], Zdzisław Papir[1], Rafał Watza[1]

[1] Department of Telecommunications, AGH University of Science and Technology, Krakow, Poland

Medical services and applications (like telecare) require diversified ways of access to stored resources. These could be medical databases or on-line hosts with e.g. cameras and microphones or other wired or wireless devices that help recover and monitor patient health. In this chapter we try to aggregate and recap a wide range of access techniques that are used in telemedicine both by doctors and by patients. Basically the access is performed using wired or wireless networks, but many techniques might be applied.

1 Overview of Access Techniques

The main requirements for medical institutions when sharing information are dissemination and teleconsultations between different users (doctors or patients). If any electronic database exists, an efficient way used for e-learning or telemedical activities is having a stable and fast access to its resources.

The diversified access options are possible by medical partners ranging from broadband networks (leased DSL lines, T1/E1) through medium throughput media like ISDN to narrowband and switched lines (modem, GSM). It has been found that the intensity of streams incoming and outgoing from any medical resources may vary from 10 Mb/s to several tens of kb/s, so even users accessing a medical database through narrowband connections may gain access. Moreover, the global trend is to get access via wireless networks to maintain maximum mobility of the user. A typical network structure is shown in Figure 2-1.

In the case of an institution with several branches, with a high-speed Intranet network (like LAN), one can achieve access using computer networks (IP networks). This technique is often used, because there are many such networks and there are many IP-like devices. For that reason, this method is also relatively inexpensive, so almost any hospital or medical party can decide to connect to the Internet. Security and integrity in IP-like networks can be achieved by installing firewalls, special separating devices or implementing specialized software enabling ciphering and tunnelling.

In evolving countries not many hospitals or clinics can afford having a permanent connection to the Internet or Intranet. However, a basic dial-up connection does not achieve data transmission of satisfying quality. That is why using ISDN networks seem to be a compromise solution: good data transmission rates, almost permanent connection and relatively low prices. There are many different techniques used to access medical resources, such as [1]:

- telephone networks (PSTN),
- ISDN network,
- private (corporate) network LAN/WAN,
- leased-line (channel 2 Mb/s),
- xDSL lines,
- cellular networks (GSM, UMTS),
- Bluetooth, UMTS, LMDS,
- satellite links.

Some of the criteria for deciding whether the access technique is important or not, is applied or not in a specified network, are related to the cost, availability and penetration of the service (for example the penetration of ISDN nodes). If the capital or operational expenditures of some access technique are too high for the institution, they will not be able to afford it and use that service. For that reason, some of the above-mentioned techniques are not currently applied. In the following paragraphs the most popular techniques are described.

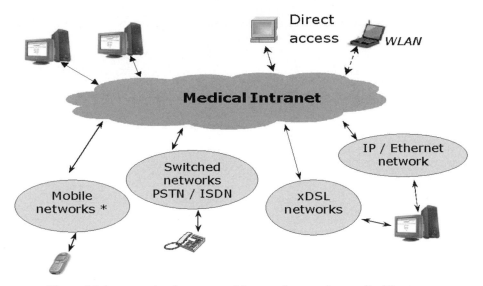

Figure 2-1 An example of current multi-network accessing medical Intranet.

*Mobile networks: GSM, UMTS, Bluetooth

1.1 PSTN Network

The traditional method of accessing any medical library or other resource is connection across a PSTN network using dial-up technique supported by a modem. This method seems to be inexpensive, but of rather poor quality and low transmission throughput. Maximum transfer rate is set to 56 kb/s but in practice achieved speed drops below 40 kb/s. Due to this main disadvantage, only less important data transmission might be transmitted via a dial-up connection. Moreover, using a PSTN dial-up connection each user has to meet low priority and security of transmitting data. For that reason, such a solution might be applied as a supplementary access method. Finally, administrative connection should not be allowed through that medium, since fault and fraud possibility can minimize the importance of system security.

Penetration of PSTN networks is usually very high, the highest among all telecommunication networks. A very important issue for end users is the high availability of point of presence to PSTN networks, especially at home. Regardless of network evolution, switched telecommunication networks are still the main medium to provide user connectivity. Not only data transmission through PSTN can occur in telecare. Sometimes voice connection may also be regarded as access to medical resources, like automatic information or registration at health centre.

1.2   ISDN Network

Another way of connecting to medical libraries via a telecommunication network is an ISDN network. A typical connection configuration is shown in Figure 2-2. This alternative connection may be used due to satisfying data throughput as well as available penetration on the market. This connection is especially significant for new or emerging parties. A single Basic Rate Access (BRA) line establishes connection speed at 128 kb/s which seems to be an advantage over PSTN networks. By combining two ISDN lines, users achieve up to 256 kb/s which is enough for browsing online webpages, downloading files (audio or video) from databases, performing teleconsultation before an operation or sending important patient's files. Increasing quality of service (higher throughput, smaller delays, higher security) is provided at higher prices for installation and connections between involved parties. In many ways this solution is the best compromise method of accessing a specialized library. In some aspects this connection technique was a kind of compromise and additional scenarios should be analyzed. Accessing medical content through an ISDN network allows more security, because each node (like a medical database) can arrange a closed list of ISDN numbers that are allowed to dial-in to the database. Moreover, each user is identified by login and password, so no-one unauthorized or from an unauthorized number can access confidential data.

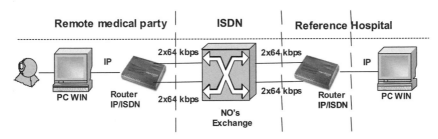

Figure 2-2 An architecture of network using ISDN technique [6].

Connections are established from time to time and for a specified period of time when access to a digital video library is required. In this case it is also possible to obtain time-to-call in less than 1 second. This method is much cheaper than leasing digital lines from a telecommunication operator and could be an important point for hospitals and other medical parties.

Two types of access connection have been defined:
- Basic Rate Access (BRA) – channel 2B+D, throughput of 144 kb/s (for personal users and home care),
- Primary Rate Access (PRA) – channel 30B+D, throughput of 2 Mb/s (for hospitals or academic centres).

Considering access to a digital video library, for example, we have to realize that a BRA interface provides low throughput and that a PRA interface may be too expensive. The optimal solution can unify at least two basic channels when multimedia streams are transmitted through an ISDN router connected to the lines and a PC (used as a digital video library terminal).

1.3 Intranet and Outer TCP/IP Networks

Some medical institutions can achieve access using a computer network (IP network). This technique is very often used and the penetration of IP-like devices is high [18]. Just for that reason, this method is inexpensive so each medical party can decide to connect to the Internet. When deciding to use IP (LAN) networks for transferring medical content, one has to perform special activities in terms of data security and integrity. This can be achieved by installing firewalls, special separating devices or implementing specialized software enabling ciphering and tunnelling.

An important aspect of LAN/WAN networks is security of data. For the standard, insecure Internet network, transmission of medical, confidential material is highly risky. Many users want to scan the network, so when using public networks, some secure protocols (like SSL) must be applied in order to isolate medical traffic. One of the best solutions is to separate (dedicated) links and devices like a router from the ISP to the medical institution to establish permanent, highly secure connections.

Not only single LAN networks can play a role in telecare. Sometimes a hospital runs LAN/WAN networks for a distributed geographical region. If many doctors or many personal computers are to be connected to the medical databases, the problem of data integrity may occur. A better effect would be achieved by designating a room or two where doctors could access medical databases. Such a place should be located as close as possible to the location of the server, in other cases significant delays will influence the total impression of the quality of the teleconsultation [15]. On the other side, a single place of work and data storage will keep all information sent by patients safe and coherent.

1.4 Fibreoptic Networks

Access to the medical library is also possible with fibre optic wires and optical interfaces. This solution usually deals with very high speed connections, permanent links to the outer limit (e.g. medical library) and low delays [12]. Unfortunately, few medical parties can afford installing permanent optical wires, and some of them share the total throughput by using it not only for connections to medical servers but also for everyday, personal use, like mail or

Web browsing. In such a situation, an operator must be aware that unexpected need for teleconsultation or downloading the library may cause rejection of lower priority connections. Telecommunication network operators are not yet ready or fully equipped in leasing fibre optic lines. In the foreseeable future such service may be available to customers [11].

Such an access connection technique is similar to leased lines (like xDSL or SDH trunks). Therefore security aspects seem to be no problem for both the administrator of the medical database and the client connecting to those resources. Point to point connections are mostly safe when the network operator performs special procedures and takes care of each user's trunks. The possibility of data leakage can be reduced when each participant uses separate accessories or access is restricted to a classified list of users (firewalls, gateways, etc.).

1.5 GSM

Global System for Mobile Communications (GSM) is the name of a land mobile pan-European digital cellular radiocommunications system. The GSM standard is currently used in the 900 MHz and 1800 MHz bands. GSM standard provides several data services. These services include SMS (Short Message Service), fax, paging service, and data transmission. GSM users can utilize data transmission, at rates up to 9600 b/s, to users on POTS (Plain Old Telephone Service), ISDN, Circuit Switched Public Data Networks, and Packet Switched Public Data Networks [7]. A modem is not required between the user and GSM network, because GSM is a digital network. A number of telemedical services can be offered using GSM networks. The most popular one is an electrocardiogram. Integrated systems and devices will play an increasingly important role in monitoring patients with debilitating conditions, such as heart disease and diabetes. Today, GSM data transmission is often used for measurements such as blood pressure, level of glucose in the blood etc.

Although there are numerous data transmission services, their main drawback is a slow data rate. Three solutions have been proposed to improve data transmission capabilities of the GSM system: more traditional approach called High-Speed Circuit-Switched Data Service (HSCSD), General Packet Radio Service (GPRS), and Enhanced Data Rate for Global Evolution (EDGE).

HSCSD operates across a GSM network, and therefore no extra hardware is required by a mobile communications operator to offer the service, just a network software upgrade. The main idea of HSCSD is the co-allocation of multiple full-rate channels in a single HSCSD link. The maximum data rate can then achieve 76.8 kb/s (8 time slots × 9.6 kb/s). However, in practice, the maximum data rate of 57.6 kb/s is received. This speed makes it comparable to many fixed-line telecommunications networks and will allow users to obtain more medical data services via a GSM network [20].

GPRS is a second extension of the standard GSM system to support higher data rates. It replaces the current circuit-switched services available on the second-generation GSM networks. GPRS eliminates the main disadvantages of HSCSD: long setup connection time and waste of resources while sending bursty and asymmetric data traffic. GPRS system users share the same physical channels and due to statistical multiplexing the system resources can be used more efficiently. Using all eight slots at once, a GPRS connection can achieve a data transfer rate of up to 171.2 kb/s (the maximum data rate highly depends on channel condition and the selected coding scheme). GPRS services should be much cheaper than circuit-switched connections, with the network only being used when data is being transmitted. The GPRS networks can be seen as subsets of the Internet, with the GPRS devices as hosts with their own IP addresses. In the GPRS system QoS profiles have been defined using parameters as priority of service, throughput, delay, and reliability.

EDGE is a high-speed mobile data standard, intended to enable second-generation GSM networks to transmit data at up to 384 kb/s. For GSM, EDGE is an evolution of GPRS to Enhanced GPRS (EGPRS), and HSCSD to Enhanced Circuit Switched Data (ECSD). The most important features of EDGE are: 8-PSK modulation, slow frequency hopping and link quality control. 8-PSK modulation automatically adapts to the radio conditions and offers up to 48 kb/s per channel, compared to 14 kb/s per channel with GPRS and 9.6 kb/s per channel for traditional GSM system. Slow frequency hopping has a substantial influence on the level of co-channel interference and overall system capacity. The link quality control uses mobile stations to inform the base station about the channel quality. This information is used to determine the modulation and channel coding to maximize the throughput. EDGE provides an evolutionary step to universal mobile telephone systems (UMTS), by implementing some of the changes expected in future third-generation systems. Relatively high data rates of the EDGE system allow for provisioning most of modern telemedical multimedia services (including high-quality video and audio transmission) as well as for teleconsultations and fast medical database access and Internet access.

1.6 WLAN

Wireless Local Area Networks are becoming increasingly popular due to their flexibility and convenience. Users can deploy WLANs to transmit data, voice and video within individual buildings, meeting rooms, warehouses, across campuses, metropolitan areas, etc. WLANs are being widely implemented in many venues from hospitals and airports to retail, manufacturing and corporate environments. These networks seem to be the alternative path for signal propagation where installation of fixed copper or fibreoptic wires is too expensive or too harmful to the environment [8]. WLANs may be very attractive to patients due to their harmless and almost invisible data transmission of specified measurements or to doctors willing to access hospital medical databases on their way to an accident victim or injured person. Using personal or business mobile phones (PDA, palmtop) one can easily and quickly get required information about previous injuries, other medical data or inform the hospital to prepare a surgery block. WLAN use over a wide-ranging medical party will facilitate the use of services and alleviate time-consuming activities. The WLAN technique utilizes bandwidths on the 2.4 GHz and 5 GHz bands, reserved only for industrial, medical and scientific handling [14]. Typical range of penetration of a single access point is restricted to 100–150 meters; but connecting several access points enables it to spann over larger distances. Wireless technology allows the network to go where wire cannot go. WLANs can also be used to provide point-to-point or point-to-multipoint wireless links between hospitals through a lack of suitable cable infrastructure. The maximum distances can reach up to 40 km using high-gain directional antennas. The present WLANs allow effective and immediate information sharing at highspeed. This technology offers the highest level of performance and features among others wireless solutions. IEEE 802.11b is a standard that has emerged for these networks and helped to promote their use. It provides 11 Mb/s in the 2.4-GHz band. IEEE 802.11a, the other major standard, uses Orthogonal Frequency Division Multiplexing (OFDM) modulation in the 5-GHz band providing bit rates in the range of 6 to 108 Mb/s [2]. WLANs can provide both secure and insecure traffic to and from a medical database or doctors.

1.7 Satellite Networks

An untypical method of access in telecare is the use of satellite links. This solution is required over hard-to-span areas, where users need to change its location and there is no way to use cellular networks. A typical example may be health monitoring of patients or sailors on ships at sea. Advantages are the unstoppable availability and relatively high throughput of transmitted data (1 Mb/s to 15 Mb/s), but there are also disadvantages. Enormous latency (several seconds) and cost of renting the channel and devices limit this technique to more affluent users or institutions. It is difficult to consider the use of satellite links by typical urban patients, doctors or students of medicine, because there are many alternative and cost-effective ways, but it is worth keeping in mind that in the future satellite mobile phones may have significant penetration.

When considering inter-medical party connections, satellite links gain more importance. If no fixed or mobile trunk may be leased, then this could be the ultimate way to transfer large amounts of data, in secure channels (more secure than fixed lines) and over large distances. If medical institutions (hospital, clinic or other) are willing to consult remotely or share the same database, they may use satellite links as a primary or secondary means of access.

1.8   xDSL Networks

One of the most promising wired technologies in recent years is Digital Subscriber Line (DSL) where customers can gain a fixed access to the Internet network. From the users' point of view it acts like a standard leased line, with a permanent connection and broadband access. Depending on the users' demand, a variety of connection throughputs might be selected, from 128 kb/s up to 2 Mb/s. The different throughput and signal transmission specifications result in different DSL techniques, so xDSL refers to a family of communication techniques [9]. Depending on the network operator and physical location (as well as on the subscribed throughput), the costs of using xDSL may be low or intermediate. Certainly it is more costly than a LAN, but might be less expensive than dial-up or fiberoptic access. Due to establishing a permanent fixed connection, with the selected network devices, customers may achieve a high degree of security, especially when implementing SSL or VPN techniques. Thus, combining average penetration on the market, decreasing installation and operational prices and high bandwidth with privacy, xDSL techniques seem to be a very promising area in modern telecare.

2   Emerging Solutions

Wireless networks are one of the youngest and most dynamically developed fields of telecommunication. This technology seems to be the most promising one over the next few years. It is not to be forgotten that investing in the healthcare sector is very difficult for companies developing emerging technologies due to strict regulations and conservatism of equipment buyers in hospitals. Many technical issues such as interference, power consumption, security, reliability, and interoperability have to be dealt with. There are a few new standards that are coming out and seem to be emerging solutions for telecare. Three that appear to be the most interesting are Bluetooth, UMTS, and LMDS.

2.1 Bluetooth

Bluetooth is a digital radio standard developed to economically and reliably allow devices to communicate wirelessly over short distances. This standard belongs to the Personal Area Networks (PANs) group. The Institute of Electrical and Electronic Engineers (IEEE) has developed and approved the 802.15.1 standard, which is fully compatible with Bluetooth [3]. It replaces the cables that connect one device to another with one universal short-range radio link (can form piconets and more complex scatternets). Each Bluetooth device can be a Master (device which initiates an exchange of data) or a Slave (device which responds to the Master) at any one time. A scatternet occurs when if we have more than one piconet and the Bluetooth device fulfills Master/Slave role at the same time or exists as a common Slave for two piconets. Bluetooth allows for point-to-multipoint voice and data transfer with maximum rate up to 1 Mb/s. Two different types of links were defined between any two devices: Synchronous Connection Oriented (SCO) links for voice transmission and Asynchronous Connectionless (ACL) links for data transmission. The SCO links operate at 64 kb/s, and it is possible to define up to three duplex voice links at once, or to mix voice and data. The ACL link can be set as symmetric (432 kb/s) or asymmetric (721/57 kb/s). Bluetooth provides a universal bridge to existing data networks as well as a mechanism to form small private ad hoc groups of connected devices away from fixed network infrastructures. Its nominal link range is from 10 cm to 10 m. It uses the frequency hopping technique (79 hops displaced by 1 MHz) in 2.4-GHz ISM band[10]. Bluetooth is not primarily meant for transferring great amounts of data as in the case of WLAN, but it is sufficient for telephony, fax, videoconference and limited LAN communication. Many popular and daily used devices such as cellular phones, notebook computers, PDAs and earphones are factory equipped with proper Bluetooth interfaces. The Bluetooth standard provides user protection and information privacy mechanisms. Authentication and encryption is implemented in each Bluetooth device. Advanced mechanisms defined in the standard save power (most devices are powered with limited power sources like batteries and accumulators). There are a number of medical devices that are currently integrated and tested with Bluetooth technology. This list includes: heart rate monitor, ambulance crew device, ultrasound imager, infusion pump, glucometer, ECG/respiration bedside monitor, hearing aid programmer, stethoscope, sleep monitor, epileptic brain monitor, and handheld patient record. Some hospitals currently use Bluetooth enabled handhelds to input patient data and retrieve information from their databases. In summary, there are three categories that seem to be promising for Bluetooth technology: hospital patient data management, telemedicine and patient life data monitors.

2.2 UMTS

Universal Mobile Telecommunications System (UMTS) is a third-generation mobile communication system able to support integrated digital wireless communications at data rates up to 2 Mb/s in the 2-GHz band. It is designed to continue the global success of the 2G GSM system. UMTS is comprised of the radio access network (mobile and base stations and radio interface between them) and the core network. The core network connects base stations as well as offers gateways to other networks. It is expected that ATM technology with its flexibility to carry different traffic types will be selected as a transport technique for UMTS in the core network. UMTS offers a variety of services. It defines different QoS classes for four types of traffic [4]:

- Conversational class (voice, videotelephony, video-gaming),
- Streaming class (multimedia, video on demand),
- Interactive class (Web browsing, network gaming, database access),
- Background class (email, SMS, downloading).

The UMTS system can also be considered a wireless extension of ISDN networks that supports basic ISDN access at a rate of 144 kb/s. It is possible to use the UMTS system with data transmission rates up to 2 Mb/s that allow for providing many modern multimedia services (simultaneous transfer of speech, data, text, pictures, audio and video). UMTS is built in a hierarchical way in layers of varying coverage. The maximum data rate and the maximum speed of the user are different in each hierarchical layer. The UMTS Terrestrial Radio Access (UTRA) is often called Wideband CDMA (WCDMA). It has two modes of duplex transmission: FDD and TDD. The operation in FDD mode is assigned for macro- and micro-cells; the operation in TDD mode is assigned for pico-cells and unlicensed cordless applications. The UMTS system assures a high level of security, not only for conventional telephony calls but also for tele-banking and e-commerce applications. UMTS provides alternative ways of billing (e.g. pay-per-bit, per session, asymmetric bandwidth, flat rate) as demanded by many emerging medical data services. UMTS is also designed to offer "data rate on demand", which, in combination with packet data, will make the system much cheaper. The variety of possibilities and the features of the UMTS systems make it very promising for many present and future medical applications. High transmission rates, mobility, security, handovers and strong QoS support are the strongest features of this new 3G system [17].

2.3 LMDS

Local multipoint distribution system (LMDS) is the broadband wireless technology used to deliver voice, data, Internet, and video services in the 25- to

40-GHz range (depending on the country's regulations). Its large bandwidth (hundreds of Mb/s) makes it suitable for "last mile" access technologies. The cell size for the LMDS system in general is limited to 15 km. The term "local" denotes that propagation characteristics of signals in this frequency range limit the potential coverage area. It is necessary to have a permanent line of sight between the LMDS transmitter and a receiver. "Multipoint" indicates that signals are transmitted in a point-to-multipoint or broadcast method. The term "distribution" defines the wide range of data that can be transmitted (from voice, data or video to Internet and video traffic) [5]. The last term de facto means "service" and represents the subscriber nature of the relationship between the operator and the customer. LMDS uses a significant amount of spectrum transmitted as milliwave signals within small cells. This allows for a realization of high-quality communication services transmitted with very high data rates. The LMDS network architecture consists of four parts: network operations centre (NOC), fibre-based infrastructure, base station and customer premises equipment (CPE). ATM and Internet protocol (IP) transport methodologies are considered for LMDS. As a transport system LMDS can be engineered to provide 99.999 % availability. Various access techniques are proposed for LMDS upstream link: TDMA, FDMA and CDMA. In the downstream direction from base station to customer, most companies supply Time Division Multiplexed (TDM) streams. The main advantages of LMDS are as follows [16]:

- provides support for high-bandwidth application,
- is cost effective,
- has very scalable architecture,
- network management and maintenance is relatively simple,
- a large part of investment is shifted to CPE (operator spends money only if a customer signs up).

The main disadvantages of LMDS are the reduced area of coverage of a single cell, impractical usage as a mobile wireless technology (LMDS should be considered only as a stationary system) and weather conditions can reduce transmission distance to 5 km. To sum up, LMDS promises a wireless alternative to fibre and coaxial cables. For example, it can be used to connect some hospitals wirelessly within a city.

3 Hospital – Hospital Scenario

Transmitting data between two medical parties reflects the need to share medical and confidential records when a teleconsultation or remote diagnosis is going to be made. The database could also contain educational material or even typical medical records of the patient's diseases. One has to be aware, that the "hospital" identifies any medical party involved in the process of providing healthcare to patients, not only hospitals.

Typical hospital-to-hospital connections require a wired and broadband link to provide transmission of a high amount of data at any moment. However, permanent wireless access is nowadays more commonly used. Whenever a hospital is willing to consult with medical specialists from another institution, connection must be established on both sides. This situation involves using stationary personal computers, so no mobility is required. Using permanent links facilitates high throughput and ease of installation. For long fixed duct and short line-of-sight distances, using wireless techniques is better, more economical, and even more secure.

For connections between two immobile locations, a set of services may be used. This includes both continuous (long term) and temporary (short term) applications, like online server access, videoconference, audioconference or even live coverage of medical operations. For the time being, not many educational activities can be found, but one of them might be "whiteboards" in the case of personnel training or videoconference.

Permanent linkage might also be used for public Internet access (WWW, mails, newsgroups) where medical staff can cooperate with remote partners, driving to establish some form of cooperation. If mail to be sent does not contain restricted medical data, no special security is needed. On the contrary, implementing safety rules, like secure protocols, coding algorithms or digital signature will highly decrease the probability of data leakage.

The typical Internet services don't care about confidentiality and security aspects, but during videoconsultation or when sending patient's personal details, there are obligations to apply high level of security. This means durability to overhearing, modifying or spoofing classified records, therefore fibreoptic cables and wideband but narrow-beam radio systems are better than wired lines.

Some occasional, singular connection scenarios may include mixed types of used techniques, e.g. wireless and mobile connections as well as establishing instant consultation from an ambulance or reserving and preparing the surgery room.

4 Hospital – Patient Scenario

Telemedicine, by definition, delivers some medical services at a distance via an underlying communications technology. Some of the possible scenarios of usage of access technologies in telemedicine are concerned with patient-hospital or patient-monitoring centre cases. Telehome care usually encompasses patient health monitoring. It covers skin temperature, user activity, heart disease (irregular heartbeat, pulse, arterial blood pressure), respiration, oximetry, spirometry or diabetes (level of glucose in the blood) in most cases. It could be used at home after discharging someone from a hospital. Of course, the database of detailed patient information, including medications, active diagnoses, lab results and therapies, is instantly available at the hospital to give the doctor full information about the patient's health. The pure measurements or measurement results obtained from medical devices in patients' homes that gather data on their condition can be sent to the hospital using one of the available access technologies. Usually, patients' monitoring devices enter basic physiological data at the beginning and answer some questions about their condition. All of the gathered data can be processed locally or filtered to remove noise and artifacts. Then, the medical data are sent to the hospital or monitoring centre to be analysed by monitoring centre staff, doctors or nurses, who check for early illness symptoms (if a measurement lies outside the predefined ranges for that patient). This allows them to react very quickly before hospitalisation is needed. If a patient has not transmitted data at the recommended time, monitoring centre personnel will make a phone call to remind the patient of the scheduled measurements. However, collecting numerous incoming medical data requires a dedicated workstation, links and human power. Thus, it might be even better to create a telemonitoring centre than use hospital power to deal with the problem. In this case "hospital" means not only a certified hospital party, but any medical party serving remote connection to and from the patient. The monitoring centre (a novice doctor or nurse practitioner) can also send the medical records of a patient to the specialist who is supposed to diagnose the problems and propose treatment if possible. On the other hand, supporting a live consultation with medical experts many tens or hundreds of kilometres distant seems to be a solution for people not served by local medical resources. The connection could be established during all measurement processes or only for a specified amount of time when the device is needed to send some collected medical data. Some of them might be sending once a week, once a day or 3 to 4 times a day. The monitoring devices usually generates small data rates (less than tens of kb/s), so the requirements for the telecommunication networks are relatively low. Modern telemonitoring applications assume increasing mobility of the people and thus the monitoring devices are portable, power management is ready, light and simple to use. The most popular access technologies used for telehome care are PSTN, ISDN, GSM or leased networks and WLAN radio links. Medical consultations by conventional phone are also possible.

5   Case Studies

Theoretical analysis is not always applied or implemented in real situations. There are many examples of using the above-described methods of access, but there are always discrepancies in an area, so two real case studies are given below.

5.1   ISDN Connection

After analysing different access techniques with all their advantages and disadvantages, remote hospitals decided that since the program was only a trial and testbed solution, the ISDN network is to be applied in the research. In this way, if the program fulfills medical requirements, they will introduce more advanced techniques in the future. The propagation, availability and prices of TP S.A.'s network supported the idea of connecting two exterior medical parties (in Kielce and Oświęcim).

It has been assumed that establishing connection is necessary only from time to time, for a specified period of time – when medical data will be transferred (e.g. during teleconsultation) and thus LAN PC devices must be used at the end node. This method is much cheaper than leased lines from network operator, which is a very important matter to hospitals and other medical parties.

Such scenarios are possible on any software platform and operating system (PC, Mac, OS/2, etc.) and at any distance. In this solution a TP S.A. leased line was applied: TP S.A.'s network exchange with two BRA lines was used. The architecture of this system is depicted in Figure 2-2.

Specific proposals suggest using additional PCs with Windows or Linux inside or an ISDN router. A router may already be running in the medical centre and will be accommodated for video connections only and IP traffic accompanied by them. Supplementary improvement is achieved in terms of management and configuration of this router. It is possible to configure services more precisely assuring better safety conditions than before. Unfortunately, higher cost of an ISDN router, when buying it for access to a digital video library, reduces the possibilities of using this system. The main benefit of a software router (on the PC) is reduction of costs, as one of the existing computers might be accommodated for medical access.

In this project the ISDN router with Windows workstations was chosen, putting stress on the quality and flexibility of an achieved streamlined communication, using owned OptiBase video encoding cards, and computers already running

Windows. The cost of installation of a single point of access to a medical video server with full capabilities (with camera and capture card) was acceptable.

The minimum bandwidth for a medicine specialist was set to 256 kb/s, and ISDN router ZyXel Prestige 480 was chosen. The second interface of the router LAN was Ethernet 100 Mb/s technology. Such a configuration worked out without significant problems or errors; a stable and secure connection was to be established on demand between two parties.

5.2 Single MAN Scenario

Another scenario of access to a medical database (see Figure 2-3) was based on the connections within the metropolitan computer network. The close co-operation between medical and technical partners, including the Academic Computer Centre supervising MAN in Krakow, resulted in establishing separate links for telemedical applications. A safe and almost separate network combined MDVL point-of-presence, academic computers and medical locations. Transfers up to 100 Mb/s were possible within this network, so operations on stored contents were carried out smoothly.

This scenario was used in the case of Oświęcim and Kielce locations. Two or three teleconsultations a week, involving the thoracoscopy and bronchoscopy areas, have been carried out in order to certify the diagnosis of exterior doctors.

The time of the teleconsultation was always set a day before, and the place was always the same, so the council could gather in the conference room to correspond. At first, the reaction of doctors was very restricted. They did not believe in the quality of the picture and sound, but after some adjustments and adaptation to new software, they were satisfied.

Still picture or moving frames have been carried bidirectionally through the routers and ISDN network, and the voice could be transmitted via the same network or eventually via telephone network. However, such situations emerged only twice, as a result of the network congestion which prevented real-time voice transmission.

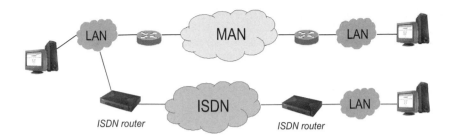

Figure 2-3 Possible accessing scenario using computer networks [19].

5.3 ISDN with MAN Scenario

The connections within the metropolitan area network assure fast and reliable data transmission in relation to medical resource access. However, a considerable number of medical institutions and health professionals are not able to use such links. ISDN network was chosen as the supplementary solution. Peripheral medical centres used the ISDN connections for a limited time to get access to the medical database or to provide telemedical consultations.

For optimal bandwidth connection to the telecare system or in the case of teleconsultations, two ISDN lines were leased, merging channels for a total throughput of up to 256 kb/s. One of the disadvantages of ISDN line use was the necessity of establishing a special router, splitting the entire video stream into a few basic B channels. This generated further problems, such as cooperation of video stream adaptation protocols and dynamic link bandwidth adaptation protocols (applied in the router). When applications required throughput of the stream based on available traffic, the router detected the required traffic and initialised the necessary number of channels.

Only specified users (login and password information) and from specified location (ISDN number) were able to connect and access any database.

5.4 Wireless Connection

A connection had been proposed between II Department of Interior Illness CM UJ and Bonifratów hospitals for teleconsultation. The first idea was to use leased lines and some modems but there were not enough free accessible lines at the moment. The next idea was to connect it wirelessly. Establishing a wireless local area network was considered. It was less expensive than hard-wired networks because it requires less hardware and is much easier to install and maintain. The products of D-Link manufacturer were installed which comply with the worldwide standard for wireless LANs - IEEE 802.11. Figure 2-4 presents the network architecture of the WLAN system installed between II Department of Interior Illness CM UJ and Bonifratów hospitals.

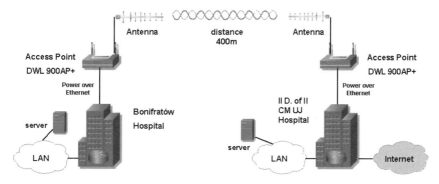

Figure 2-4 Point-to-point wireless link architecture between hospitals.

Simple stand-alone cell was used to create a point-to-point wireless link. The point-to-point link was created using D-Link DWL-900AP+ access points. To extend the range the external directional antennas have been used.

D-Link DWL-900AP+ delivers a fast rate of up to 22 Mb/s, with automatic fall-back to 11 Mb/s, 5.5 Mb/s, 2 Mb/s and 1 Mb/s when necessary. It is possible to provide such a high rate with the Packet Binary Convolutional Coding modulation technique (the maximum rate from the view of user application is usually less than 7 Mb/s). It also delivers unmatched range and coverage, providing reliable connectivity over distances in excess of 400 m in open spaces, and from 25 to 100 m in office environments.

DWL-900AP+ access point has been developed in compliance with the IEEE 802.11b+ wireless LAN standard. This product uses Direct Sequence Spread Spectrum radio that operates in the 2.4-GHz ISM band allowing license-free installations. The DWL-900AP+ can be configured to operate in any of five modes as an access point, as a wireless client, as a point-to-point bridge, as a point-to-multi-point bridge, or as a repeater. In our case it operates as a point-to-point bridge. Bridging allows wireless connection between two networks. This mode of operation is usually used for interconnecting networks, when a traditional wired solution is too costly or prohibitive [13].

The strong point of DWL-900AP+ is the encryption capability. It is possible to enable 256-bit WEP encryption for a high level of security. MAC address filters allow or deny wireless connection to access point and fill up the next level of security. An important feature is that this access point has an easy-to-use Web-based interface for managing and a configuration that is independent of the operating system. It is possible to connect an external antenna to the DWL-900AP+. It also has some LEDs for signalling and diagnostic of work.

It was necessary to use two external antennas because the link distance was about 400 m. Avaya directional antennas with 13 dBi gain were used to realize 22 Mb/s connection. Unfortunately, access points are not weatherproof, so they were located under the building's roofs. Additionally, some special connectors as well as low-loss cable were used to connect the access points with external antennas. The other problem was to provide power to the devices. It is a risk to install high-voltage power in the wooden attic, so Powerover Ethernet adapters were used to power the access points. Powerover Ethernet adapters deliver data and electrical power to access points using standard category 5 Ethernet cable. Power is transmitted on unused Ethernet pairs. The operational range is up to 100 m, which is a requirement of the fast Ethernet standard. This eliminates the need for electrical cable at each access point location as well as risk of fire. The power supply adapters are located in server rooms.

6   Summary

From the variety of fixed and mobile access techniques, according to assumed selection criteria, one can determine which technology to choose. Looking at both incumbent and emerging solutions, each medical party and patient may obtain as many benefits as necessary. When the scenario requires mobile telemetric of patients' health, GSM or WLAN connections might be chosen. When medical specialists have to perform videoconference or live surgery coverage, they may utilize broadband techniques like xDSL or IP networks (LAN/WAN).

7   Bibliography

[1] Bates R.: *Broadband Telecommunications Handbook*. McGraw-Hill 2002
[2] Bing B.: *Wireless Local Area Networks*. John Wiley & Sons 2002
[3] Bray J., Sturman C.: *Bluetooth – Connect Without Cables*. Prentice-Hall 2001
[4] Castro J.: *The UMTS Network and Radio Access Technology*. John Wiley & Sons 2001
[5] Clark M.: *Wireless Access Networks: Fixed Wireless Access and WLL Networks – Design and Operation*. John Wiley & Sons 2000
[6] Danda J., Łoziak K., Sikora M., Watza R.: *Access Techniques to the Telemedical Multimedia Resources*. Workshop on Multimedia Communications and Services, Kielce 23-25.04.2003
[7] Dubendorf V.: *Wireless Data Technologies*. John Wiley & Sons 2003
[8] Geier J.: *Wireless LANs*. Sams Publishing 2002

[9] Gorshe S., Papir Z.: *Topics in Broadband Access*, IEEE Communication Magazine, two times a year since 1995

[10] Held G.: *Data Over Wireless Networks: Bluetooth, WAP, and Wireless LANs*. McGraw-Hill 2001

[11] Jajszczyk A.: *What is the future of telecommunications networking?* IEEE Communications Magazine, vol. 37, no 6/1999

[12] Jajszczyk A.: *The ASON approach to the Control Plane for Optical Networks*. 6th ICTON 2004, Wroclaw, Poland, 4-8 July 2004

[13] Lin Y., Chlamtac I.: *Wireless and Mobile Network Architectures*. John Wiley & Sons 2001

[14] Natkaniec M., Pach A.: *Simulation analysis of multimedia streams transmission in IEEE 802.11 networks*. ISWC'99, June 1999, Victoria, Canada

[15] Peterson L., Davie B.: *Computer Networks – A Systems Approach*. Morgan Kaufmann Publishers 2003

[16] Prasad R., Munoz L.: *WLANs and WPANs towards 4G Wireless*. Artech House 2003

[17] Smith C., Collins D.: *3G Wireless Networks*. McGraw-Hill 2002

[18] Tanenbaum A.: *Computer Networks*. Prentice Hall 2003

[19] Watza R.: *Methods of accessing resources of medical libraries with support of fixed networks*. E-Health in Common Europe, Kraków 5-6.06.2003

[20] Wesołowski K.: *Mobile Communication Systems*. John Wiley & Sons 2002

3   Internet Technologies in Medical Systems

Jacek Cała[1], Łukasz Czekierda[1], Krzysztof Zieliński[1]

[1]   Department of Computer Science, AGH University of Science and Technology, Krakow, Poland

Combining medical sciences with technologies associated with the Internet results in an incredibly wide spectrum of new applications under the umbrella term *telemedicine*. As a developing domain, telemedicine appears more and more frequently in everyday life. The most important factors which propel its expansion include the need to reduce healthcare costs as well as the perceived improvement of patient care through easier dissemination of expert knowledge through medical portals, teleconsultation and telesurgery tools.

To fully appreciate all the benefits created through the synergy of medicine and Internet technologies it is necessary to recognize the requirements of medical systems which are to be hosted in the Internet environment and the benefits, which the Internet may offer for medical applications. Coming up with answers to these questions is not easy as the problem domain is very broad. Nevertheless, we will try to present some ideas in the following sections.

1   Requirements of Medical Systems in the Internet Environment

Internet technologies offer a wide range of facilities for medical systems including video and audio medical conferencing, virtually ubiquitous access to medical data, convenient user interfaces, and many others. However, in the case of patient care, modern Internet technologies should be applied only with considerable oversight and this requirement concerns nearly every aspect of system construction. Following are the most crucial demands to be fulfilled by medical systems implemented in the Internet environment:

- **privacy** and **security** – the most important factors in this environment, due to the confidential character of data processed by medical systems and the relative ease of violating privacy on the Internet. The level of security of a medical system could be compared with that of a banking system.
- **reliability** and **availability** – these two correlated factors are very important prerequisites, guaranteeing user confidence in services and comfort of usage. Moreover, both play a pivotal role in constant monitoring systems when reaction to an emergency situation must not be delayed.
- **quality of network service** – as interaction with the system relies on Internet links, quality of network service in terms of throughput, delay, etc. is also significant. This requirement mostly concerns such applications as telesurgery systems and teleconsultation tools, which require diagnostic quality of transferred images and real-time interaction between remote sites. In this case, both broadband and low-delay network connections are essential.
- **data integrity** – the growing popularity of Internet-based medical services calls for maintaining integrity of patient data; otherwise, they would dissolve into tangled fragments of health records, hardly improving overall patient care. Chapter 7 tackles this problem in more detail.

Apart from the above general requirements placed on Internet-based medical systems there are many functional requirements which depend mainly on the system application and include, among others:
- audio and video streaming – in teleconsultation and telesurgery systems there is a need to effectively transfer multimedia data between two or more participants. Existing teleconferencing solutions based on VoIP technologies may be easily adapted for medical teleconferences.
- consultation organization – besides transferring multimedia, organization of telemedical sessions in a virtual hospital environment is also a very important point. These problems seem not to have been fully handled yet.
- conformance to DICOM standard – this standard facilitates interoperability of medical devices by defining communication protocols as well as by providing vendor-independent data formats [14]. Conformance to the standard either by satisfying communication protocols or data formats or both requirements together is a must, considering the broad range of telemedical applications.
- means of digitalization of existing data – currently, many medical institutions do not fulfill requirements related to a paperless or filmless

organization; hence, systems should allow for integration of existing non-digital medical documentation by providing open interfaces supporting various types of data.

- diversity of user interfaces – systems should offer many different and convenient user interfaces depending on the client terminal used for access. Enabling access from a variety of end-user devices greatly improves the overall convenience of any system.

Currently, medical institutions are not prepared to satisfy all the presented requirements; mostly due to financial obstacles. On the other hand, not all technologies are mature enough to support medical systems demands, e.g. providing complete solutions to support different user interfaces is an open problem. Nevertheless, the above demands point existing medical research in the direction of state-of-the-art telemedical systems.

2   Internet Medical System Architectures

Proper design of a medical system is a very serious issue and should be preceded by detailed analysis and supported with knowledge and experience in the area of medical data representation, distributed systems, and computer networks. Software architectures and styles of computer systems programming are in continuous flux, thus it is highly desirable to follow the emerging trends in order to develop efficient applications, built with state-of-the-art technologies.

The analysis presented below is of a rather general significance but can be successfully applied to Internet-based medical systems, as they are, after all, computer systems and the requirements regarding architecture or implementation remain the same. On the other hand, however, they are usually mission-critical applications with very high requirements regarding reliability and accessibility, which should focus our attention on developing a proper software architecture.

In mainframe systems of yesteryear, programs were usually monoliths, using batch data processing. However, progress in the electronic industries has resulted in widespread adoption of personal computers, initially as standalone devices, but later as parts of distributed software systems communicating via a computer network. Client-server architectures in which clients are requestors of services, and servers are their providers, have been implemented in numerous ways, using various techniques and mechanisms. The clients software tends to become thinner and thinner in terms of business functionality, which, initially implemented on the client side, gradually migrates towards the server. Paradoxically, this movement, spurred mainly by management and maintenance considerations, has turned "thin" client architectures into something resembling their mainframe counterparts (Figure 3-1). The only major difference is in the methods of server/client and mainframe/terminal communication, respectively.

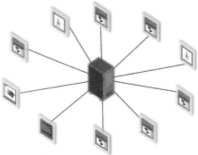

Figure 3-1 Communication in mainframe and thin client architectures.

Nevertheless, the current standard for designing software involves multi-tier client-server architectures supporting thin clients (Figure 3-2). Application logic is divided into components according to function, and the various application components that form such multi-tier systems may be distributed over several different machines depending on the tier they belong to [1]. The advantages of this architecture, resulting from its centralized management, are as follows: easier maintenance, smooth introduction of improvements, updates, error corrections, etc. All these activities are performed online and often remain invisible to the end user.

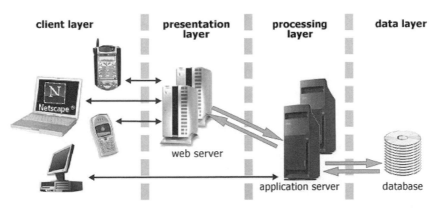

Figure 3-2 Multitiered applications built e.g. with the J2EE platform.

A novelty in designing computer software architectures is the Service-Oriented Architecture (SOA) paradigm. In this style, the main functional components of the software are packaged as separate loosely-coupled service implementations providing simple and well-known interfaces for use by other architectural components (Figure 3-3) [12]. SOA is an architectural style that formally separates services into two categories: services which *are* the functionality that a system can provide, and service consumers who *need* that functionality. This separation is accomplished by a mechanism known as service contract, which is coupled with a mechanism allowing providers to publish contracts and consumers to locate the contracts that provide the service they desire.

The functional components being developed are supported by special preexisting infrastructure components, providing a set of common, reusable services. They can, among other things, supply the programmer with remote communication between functional components (e.g. CORBA, J2EE, Web Services, COM/DCOM, JMX), data and event logging, security mechanisms, transactions support, thread management and user interfaces. Full exploitation of the rich scope of available services guarantees considerable speed-up in system development and increases code reusability.

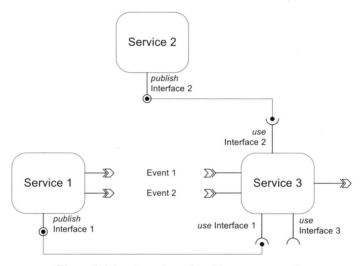

Figure 3-3 Service-oriented architecture example.

Still, the question remains: what to do with systems developed using old, so-called legacy software architectures? Being aware of the advantages of the SOA and component-based environments one could say the solution is to "adjust to new paradigms." Yet, initial enthusiasm is soon tempered by the costs counted in hundreds or even thousands of man-months – depending on the scale of the system. Modernization of nontrivial systems is usually such a complex undertaking that it is not performed unless there is a critically important reason. The stimulus which forces action is mainly the lack of some crucial feature, necessity of integration with other systems or porting to other platforms.

There are, however, other approaches than simply rewriting the system from scratch. Sometimes it may be sufficient to replace malfunctioning parts of the system or satisfy the required needs within the existing architecture. If the system is composed of loosely-coupled components with well-defined and well-documented functionality, such an undertaking can be relatively simple. Unfortunately, legacy systems are, often as not, elephantine monoliths, which complicates the problem considerably.

According to the authors' knowledge, most existing medical systems have been built using legacy architectures [11]. They are fairly monolithic in nature and thus very hard to enhance and modernize. This is certainly due to financial factors, but blame also rests on decisionmakers, who do not keep abreast of trends in computer science.

3 Internet-Based Telemedical Services

Telemedical services hosted in the Internet environment are created through a synergy of medical applications and Internet technologies [1]. This is done by adapting medical applications to a technologically new environment or by adapting existing, well-established Internet solutions for use in medical areas. It is often hard to ascertain the direction of information flow, but for better comprehension of these services and the benefits which they create it is good to divide the whole area into three major segments, focusing on different aspects of medical services hosted on the Internet [6]:

- content, services and community,
- connectivity and communications,
- e-commerce.

3.1 Content, Services and Community

Health portals belong to this category. They are organized medical sites that contain information connected with the functioning of medical centers and provide expert information to a wide range of recipients. Medical portals can act in a number of ways:

- they can provide community facilities such as moderated discussion forums, mailing lists, news, etc., and give patients the ability to discuss health problems, exchange best practices and search for medical information from scientific sources,
- they can improve the healthcare service level for patients allowing them e.g. to make appointments at hospitals or outpatient clinics,
- by personalization, more advanced solutions can provide users with direct access to their EHR or even allow for interaction with medical personnel or equipment tracking their health condition.

The role of this segment of healthcare systems is significant as they are often the first point of contact between patients and the medical community. By offering a variety of important information, they provide patients with a sense of security and comfort.

Currently, there are many sites offering medical content and basic services, and that number will keep increasing due to straightforward system design and diversity of technologies supporting Web-based portal solutions. Internet technologies in this area are mature enough to fulfill all the requirements placed on such services. The only problem in this case is supplying adequate, professional content: information available through any medical portal should be reliable and trustworthy [11].

3.2   Connectivity and Communications

The second area of applications involves streamlining of healthcare operations. Internet-capable applications are able to electronically deliver medical records, claims submissions, referrals, eligibility verifications, lab reports, prescriptions and other clinical and administrative data. Moreover, online remote consultations between medical centers either in well-known Web-based style or with the ability to conduct collaborative, interactive work on shared medical data can considerably diminish costs as well as provide great educational value.

In this area a new, promising application, namely telesurgery, may also be counted. Currently, remote surgery is inhibited by very high costs of such a service and deficiencies of specialized surgery devices which ought to be controlled remotely. Nevertheless, it is only a matter of time before these appliances acquire the proper level of accuracy and allow surgeons to work with no constraints at all.

3.3   E-commerce Applications

The e-commerce segment of the Internet health industry generates the greatest opportunity for revenue. Pharmaceutical companies have recognized the value of this alternative form of marketing and distribution channels. Health-related e-commerce also encompasses other products, including health insurance and business-to-business services.

4 Next-Generation Point-of-Care Information Systems

Over the last decade, progress in miniaturization techniques has enabled a new class of devices. Mobile Point-of-Care (POC) appliances focus on extending medical services to healthcare providers and their patients. Patients' POC terminals are specialized appliances worn by patients or even implanted on them and performing various tasks e.g. monitoring injections. Handheld or tablet computers typically serve as POC terminals for medical staff and professionals. The ubiquitous availability of wireless communication infrastructures allows the devices to work in virtually any place, even if it is required to stay online with continuous access to a remote service.

There exist a number of applications for POCs, some of which are enumerated below:

- **emergency healthcare**. Ambulance staff provided with suitable terminals able to communicate with hospital databases containing patients' EHR can, in many situations, provide rapid and effective help to victims. Mobile emergency access can also be needed inside hospitals since important decisions are sometimes taken on the run – in emergency wards, halls or lifts.
- **clinical and outside-hospital care**. Doctors and nurses visiting patients at their beds in hospitals or at their homes can have access to complete medical documentation of any patient and thus monitor their up-to-date health condition.
- **electronic prescription systems**. These can automate order entry, preparation and delivery, as well as check patient records for drug allergies and interactions.
- **constant patient monitoring**. Patients with serious illnesses requiring continuous monitoring of their health conditions can live and work normally, aware that an appliance worn by them supervises their state and will notify them in case of an emergency, and even call for help automatically. See Chapter 5 for details and a case study.

As can be seen from the above examples, the benefits of using POCs are numerous. Thanks to them, many patients are able to lead normal lives, and emergency healthcare becomes much faster and efficient. Diagnoses can be made more rapidly and accurately, medication errors can be reduced and patient safety improved. For medical managers this translates into better utilization of the available staff and a considerable reduction of costs.

Nevertheless, many problems have had to be overcome and many still remain unresolved. One of the most important organizational problems is the issue of standardization. Thanks to OSI/ISO and TCP/IP models, standardization has brought about interoperability among various systems in the area of traditional networking protocols. When considering telemedicine, however, such approaches are still in the early phases of development. Mobile POCs are expected to seamlessly cooperate with running Hospital and Laboratory Information Systems (HIS/LIS); unfortunately, deployment of incompatible, proprietary multi-vendor solutions inhibits the process of connecting POC devices to existing information systems. Lack of standards has resulted in unreasonable costs and must be seen as a significant barrier to the adoption of mobile solutions.

Important effort in the area has been exerted by the Connectivity Industry Consortium, founded in 2000 [7]. The organization was established by 49 healthcare institutions, POC diagnostic vendors, diagnostic test system vendors, and system integrators. A specification issued by the consortium provides the basis for seamless multi-vendor interoperability between POC devices and clinical information systems.

The specification describes the attributes of an access point called POCIS (Point-of-Care Information System) acting as a proxy between simple POC devices and sophisticated LIS/HIS systems. The core of the standard is a specification of communication aspects between POCIS and clinical information systems on one side, and POC devices on the other side. The Universal Connectivity Standard for Point of Care (POCCIC) specifies the protocols required to integrate POC devices with POCIS. The first two POCCIC standards define the low- and high-level network protocols for communication between POC and POCIS. The third standard defines XML-based message exchange between POCIS and LIS/HIS systems compatible with the HL7 specification. POCIS-LIS/HIS communication is often realized using Web Services technologies, which, being open and non-proprietary mechanisms of communication, are very promising from the interoperability point of view. Web Services will be described in more detail in the next section.

Some other issues which must be considered are the following:
- **efficient access methods**. The notorious "last mile" problem is also significant in the context of medical information systems. A number of wireless standards exist, however, and mobile wireless terminals owned by medical personnel should be able to operate in at least two of them. In Europe, open-area devices should be able to use the existing and available public networks — GPRS or UMTS — in a secure way. Once inside a hospital, cost-effectiveness demands that they switch to an

internal wireless local-area network (WLAN) making use of broadband secure connectivity.

- **provision of strong security**. Existing means of securing data transfers on the Internet by (among others) session encryption are secure enough, but introduce communication overhead, which may prove to be considerable.
- **provision of QoS**. The desired level of Quality of Service in terms of proper bandwidth, reliability and accessibility must be provided.

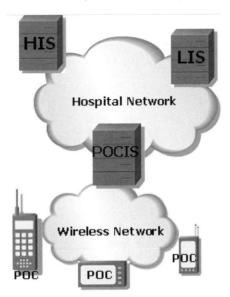

Figure 3-4 Integration of POCs with hospital systems.

Chapter 5 discusses the requirements of wireless connectivity for medical purposes in more detail.

5   Internet Access Technologies in Telecare

This section contains a description of several access technologies with application in healthcare. Since there are a variety of technologies which can be used for construction of telemedical services and since their architectures can vary considerably, this section should only be seen as an outline.

5.1   Web Services

Web Services [8] can be defined as a software construct that exposes business functionality over the Internet. Exposing in this context means identifying business processes, providing them in loosely-coupled, service-oriented interfaces and describing these interfaces in a standard way. Web Services-based applications are often built using the promising SOA approach described in the previous section. Loose coupling applied when constructing services allows for independent development of small, well-defined pieces of code and minor changes and enhancements in services do not usually require updates in other services (especially client applications). Web Services allow users to organize communication in various ways, best suited to the characteristics of each particular service: traditional request-response synchronous operation invocations and asynchronous or event-driven models, which are especially useful when considering long running transactions (LRT).

Web Services make extensive use of the XML language. Its advantages include simplicity of processing in any software environment, as well as portability – XML documents are strictly formatted text documents. Considerable overhead resulting from verbosity when compared with binary representations is perceived as a disadvantage of XML.

To describe business functionality, Web Services use Web Services Description Language (WSDL), an XML-based language presenting the interface of a service. To publish the interface, WSDL descriptions can be advertised in UDDI (Universal Description, Discovery and Integration) repositories.

Communication in the Web Services environment is performed using messages formatted according to the Simple Object Access Protocol (SOAP) which is an XML-based protocol. SOAP messages are usually sent via HTTP or HTTPS protocols. The benefit of using these particular protocols is that communication can easily pass through firewalls. Upon arriving at the destination, the original message is extracted from its SOAP envelope and delegated to the proper business protocol instance.

Systems built with various technologies such as CORBA, .NET, EJB may be accessible via Web Services interfaces. In this case, Web Services runtime components handle the reception of the message, translation of the XML to another format if necessary and invocation of the back-end business functionality. The advantages of this common approach coincide with Web Services advantages, but the introduced overhead may in some cases prove unacceptable.

The main elements of the Web Services architecture are presented in Figure 3-5.

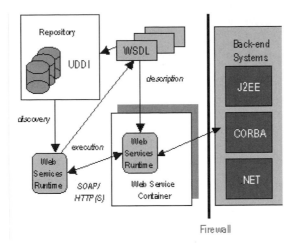

Figure 3-5 Web Services architecture.

Web Services are extensively used in medical environments. By hiding the details of implementation of Web Services, this loosely-coupled model helps healthcare information systems overcome integration challenges faced by POC devices, POCIS, LIS and HIS systems.

5.2 Portal Technologies

Many enterprise-scale systems are accessible for their users via portal interfaces. Portal platforms provide numerous ready-to-run mechanisms which enable managing access to the entire system in a convenient and consistent manner.

Portals are usually the main entry point to the enterprise, providing users with Web interfaces for virtually any exposable content and integrating their separate systems and functionality into one common interface. Portals can provide access to databases, various services, legacy systems, etc. In the context of e-health environments, access to LIS/HIS systems can be particularly important. Portals can have built-in mechanisms making integration with some systems almost automatic (e.g. with databases and Web Services).

By using portal solutions, access to resources can be efficiently secured — including authentication, authorization and encryption of data transfer with the HTTPS protocol. Portal platforms usually support a single sign-on (SSO) mechanism, not requiring multiple logins when requesting another portal resource within the same session. Users of portals can usually be divided into groups with different interests and permissions; portal technologies support this fact by providing granular authorization to portal content, according to users' roles or individual needs.

The users themselves can also have influence on the appearance of their workspace. They can customize both the content and the interface in the way they like — creating private workspaces. Moreover, portals are able to support different types of displays allowing users to access portal services from various kinds of devices, e.g. handheld appliances and desktop computers. In each case, the workspace is automatically arranged in such a way as to be properly adjusted to the display dimensions of the system the user logs in from.

There are many mature portal environments available on the market. The most popular ones include [9] the Oracle 9ias Portal, the Sun Java Enterprise Portal System, the IBM WebSphere Portal and Microsoft SharePoint.

Referring to medical systems, portal technologies efficiently facilitate creation of e-health solutions. They can be perceived as the perfect tool to provide modern medical services for medicine professionals and staff as well as for patients. The former group will be supported in everyday work and the latter one can seek information or advice, and can have access to personal data regarding health state.

5.3   Interactive and Multimedia Communication

Portal technologies allow users to access the content of the portal in a client-server manner. One side (typically a Web browser) is the requestor and the other side (portal system) acts as the service provider. As mentioned before, portals encompass various media types but sometimes this model of communication is not appropriate because the Web architecture is not well suited to interactivity. Yet, such communication is often necessary, especially in audio- and videoconferences (although the range of applications is much broader). In the medical context, interactive communication is required e.g. when remote surgery or distributed collaborative consultations take place. In such cases, specialized applications are the preferred solution.

Nowadays the Internet is becoming more and more accessible as a basic, cost-effective communications channel, even for real-time voice and video. Nevertheless, transferring interactive multimedia data (so-called streams) requires a completely different approach than e.g. for file transfer. For example, the preferred transport-level protocol is best-effort UDP instead of reliable TCP because overheads associated with the latter are unacceptable. Moreover, interactive communication is very demanding and many issues regarding it remain unresolved.

The Internet, as a network in which all data get equal treatment, is practically devoid of Quality of Service guarantees so when strong constraints are imposed, using dedicated connections or signing a Service-Level Agreement with an Internet service provider should be considered, particularly in the area of medical services.

6   Case Studies

The authors have developed a number of systems to address the issues of access to medical data through the Internet for the purpose of reviewing them. Several approaches have been used, although the idea behind all of them was to reduce costs and effort required to perform medical consultations.

In some difficult cases, there is a need to discuss patient documentation with specialists from a referential center. In the past, a physician who needed advice had to drive from their hospital to the center and wait for consultation. Moreover, it was difficult to assess whether the patient should come along with the doctor, or if a diagnosis could be made on the basis of existing medical documentation. Our applications have been positively reviewed and are being put to everyday use at several Polish hospitals.

6.1   Supporting Teleconsultations with TeleNegatoscope

TeleNegatoscope, one of the deliverables of the Krakow Centre for Telemedicine and Preventive Medicine (KCT) project, is a tool for interactive medical consultations [1]. The name of the tool is connected with its initial aim – remote access to a negatoscope – but it quickly turned out that TeleNegatoscope may be successfully used to transfer not just radiological images, but also other medical documentation, such as ECGs, scanned paper forms, etc. (see Figure 3-6).

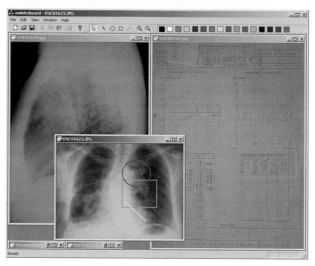

Figure 3-6 Sample TeleNegatoscope session.

The tool allows two sides, called peripheral and referential, to work on the same data at the same time and exchange opinions and comments with each other. The data utilized by the application consists of compressed digital images and annotations. The annotations are made using simple shapes: ellipses and rectangles shared between both sides. Consultation is also supported by common pointers, shared by participants, meaning that during consultation only small amounts of data are transferred, conserving network bandwidth.

As an efficient tool for peripheral medical centers with poor connection to the Internet, TeleNegatoscope is limited to medical documentation available in general-purpose graphical formats. Unfortunately, the quality of the acquired pictures is not sufficient for some types of examinations (especially CT or coronarography).

6.2   Konsul — an Efficient Solution for Non-interactive Consultations

Konsul, developed at the John Paul 2nd hospital in Krakow, is a prototype system providing medical teleconsultations for small peripheral hospitals. It allows professionals from a referential center to consult medical documentation using a Web browser once the data has been uploaded to a hospital server. Results are then sent back via e-mail or any other conventional means of communication. In case of a tentative diagnosis, the patient is directed to the referential center for detailed examinations.

As the idea behind Konsul met with wide acceptance and the system was installed at several hospitals, a complete rebuild has been performed to extend its functionality and provide a proper level of security urgently needed in such solutions [4]. A real advantage of the system is the ease of use and the possibility of combining DICOM files with other medical data in electronic form (e.g. Patient Information Card, raster image files, textual data) into one, consistent package.

The architectural model of the Konsul system is very simple and consists of three main components running in a client-server scheme. Each component is described below and their interactions are presented in Figure 3-7.

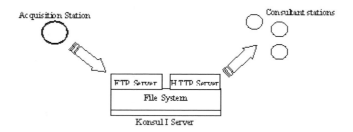

Figure 3-7 Architecture of the Konsul system.

- **The acquisition station** runs FPImage, one of many existing DICOM viewers, which can, among others, convert DICOM images to various general-purpose data formats. The main advantage of the tool, compared to other similar viewers, is the built-in simple proprietary scripting language which allows users to customize application behavior by writing their own programs. The language facilitates processing of loaded DICOM images, invoking operating system scripts and also contains an embedded FTP client. One of the scripts supplied with the FPImage distribution performs DICOM file conversion to AVI or JPEG formats, links converted files to generated HTML pages and uploads the resulting packages to selected FTP servers. By making several cosmetic changes, the script can be updated to perform data acquisition.
- **The Konsul system server** consists of an FTP server and an HTTP server. Patient examinations sent via FTP are stored in the file system, which is at the same time the interface used by the HTTP server. Finally, the HTTP server allows users to access data using Web browsers.
- **The consultant station** of the Konsul system is a simple Web browser. Doctors consulting the delivered cases use it to download and display files on their personal computers. Occasionally, phone calls to ordering hospitals are placed to provide the consulting specialists with additional

information regarding the discussed case. The computer used for consultations requires only a graphical Web browser and an AVI player, both of which are commonplace on ordinary PC computer systems.

Although the proposed model of consultation has been accepted by doctors and Konsul is performing well in practice, the requirements for interaction keep increasing. Even using Konsul, the consultee and the consulting team work independently and there is no communication between them during the diagnostic process. This leaves the physician from the peripheral hospital with no opportunity to take an active part in the consultation and describe the problem online. Generally speaking, the Web is not appropriate for interactive communications and hence another architecture must be proposed.

6.3 TeleDICOM — Collaborative Teleconsultation Environment

The idea behind TeleDICOM is based extensively on previous work in the areas of telemedicine and teleconsultations, performed by our group. The development of such environments has assured us that DICOM is the preferred format for integration of data and searching ease; however, medical documentation is often also stored in textual or graphical formats or in any other format, native to the device which generated the particular piece of data.

The experience gained in the development of the above applications has resulted in better understanding of real needs and constraints of telemedical environments. TeleDICOM integrates most of the features of such applications into one complex teleconsultation environment [4]. In fact, the system is a combination of a data storage and access system similar to Konsul and an interactive tool for medical remote consultations based on TeleNegatoscope. TeleDICOM can be used in two consultation modes: interactive and non-interactive. Whenever possible (i.e. if the intervening computer network provides a proper level of QoS), the interactive mode should be used. In less efficient environments, TeleDICOM offers the ability to perform non-interactive consultations using the same system.

TeleDICOM operates on the basis of so-called *sessions* (or *consultations*) tied to one particular patient. A session may consist of multiple *examinations*. Such an examination is usually a DICOM image, either static or animated, but it can also involve other graphical, textual or multimedia document. As yet, medical documentation often exists only in paper form and the fastest way to make it available to others via a computer network is to either scan it or simply take a picture of it with a digital camera. All these digital documents can be opened simultaneously and placed inside the application window.

Each of the images is then treated as a background and it is possible to operate on it in a mode analogous to whiteboard-like applications. TeleDICOM allows participants to draw basic geometric shapes such as lines, rectangles, circles, arrows as well as use specialized devices such as magnifying glasses or Hounsfield window adjustment tools. The shapes mark the region of interest and may be moved, modified or deleted by any of the participants depending on their access permissions. Together with the tools, they provide an intuitive and efficient means of performing remote consultations. An example of the interactive part of the TeleDICOM application in presented in Figure 3-8.

The interactive part of TeleDICOM system can also be seen as a specialized teleconferencing application, hence the features which are surely worth implementing include participant management: notifying about their appearance/disappearance and connecting/disconnecting. As mentioned before, it is desirable to integrate additional media with the TeleDICOM client application so as to improve user convenience. Support for live audio and text channels (i.e. chat) is crucial and video channels are also an option. Additional features, important in medical applications, are the following:

- **data anonymizing.** Beyond consultations between hospitals, the goal of TeleDICOM is to become a useful tool for educating medicine students. Students are offered the opportunity to witness medically-interesting cases and may be instructed by their supervisor. Each student has direct and convenient access to examination results from their personal computer. Such dedicated sessions would not differ from ordinary consulting sessions at all. In order to honor personal data protection principles, the medical documentation may be anonymized, with all personal data removed.

- **data filtering.** There are no contraindications for allowing students to participate in real consultations. This implies introducing a set of permissions for various participant roles e.g. clearing students for observation only. Data filtering mechanisms can easily be extended, since the bandwidth available for users may vary. Media filtering is also possible for users with less network throughput, either by completely disconnecting particular streams (e.g. video) or by downgrading their quality.

- **session logging.** Some sessions should be recorded for evidence reasons, or whenever one wants to interrupt a session and resume it at some later time.

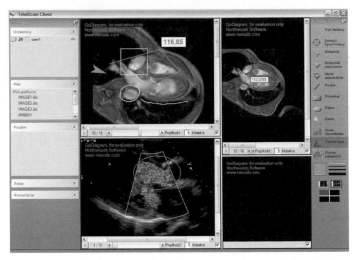

Figure 3-8 The TeleDICOM application during a sample session.

The examinations which are going to be used in consultations must first be uploaded to a central database, creating a patient file. From there, they are redistributed to session participants' computers whenever necessary (the same data can be used in many consultations). Since the volume of data earmarked for consultations can sometimes reach several hundreds of megabytes, it is desirable to be able to deliver it to participants' computers prior to actual meetings, e.g. overnight, when the available network bandwidth is better and cheaper. Of course, it is also possible to download any additional examinations during the session.

The resulting diagnosis and a record of the session are stored in the central server database as evidence and extensions of the patient's file.

In cases which do not require interactivity, consultations can be arranged in a Konsul-like style using only the central server providing data through a Web interface. Compared to the previous version of the system, main changes include reorganization of the architecture according to the SOA paradigm and extending functionality with some minor improvements.

7 Summary

Telemedical services have begun to play a more and more important role in our everyday life. As a discipline which unites medical and computer sciences, telemedicine is very demanding and telemedical applications need to be built with deep knowledge and understanding of both domains. The chapter depicted the most important requirements of such systems and emphasized the importance of choosing the proper architecture for them.

The chapter presented applications developed or co-developed at the Department of Computer Science within the confines of a few telemedical projects. They address the issue of remote access to medical information. Applications have been received with interest by the South Poland medical environment and participants of medical conferences showing that there is substantial acceptance and demand for such services.

8 Bibliography

[1] Armstrong E., et al.: *The J2EE 1.4 Tutorial, For Sun Java System Application Server.* http://java.sun.com/j2ee/1.4/docs/tutorial, August 2004

[2] Cała J.: *TeleNegatoscope – medical consultations for low-bandwidth networks (TeleNegatoskop – konsultacje medyczne w sieciach o niewielkiej przepustowości).* 6th Conference of Internet and Medical Telematics, Krakow 2002

[3] Cała J., Czekierda Ł.: *Teleconsultations - Synergy of Medicine and IT Technology.* TASK Quarterly, Scientific Bulletin of Academic Computer Centre in Gdańsk, vol. 8, no. 4, TASK Publishing, pp. 471-486, October 2004

[4] Cała J., Czekierda Ł.: *TeleDICOM - the environment for Collaborative medical consultations.* International Conference on e-Health in Common Europe, Krakow 5-6/06/2003

[5] Cała J., Czekierda Ł., Zieliński K.: *Migration Aspects of Telemedical Software Architectures.* 2nd International Conference on e-Health in Common Europe, Krakow 11-12/03/2004

[6] Cala J., Kwolek B., Laurentowski A., Rzepa P., Zielinski K.: *Architektury nowoczesnych systemów telemedycznych i telediagnostycznych.* In proceedings of PIONIER 2002 conference, Poznan April 2002

[7] DuBois A.J., et al.: *Connectivity Industry Consortium; Approved Standard,* ISBN-1-56238450-3. http://www.nccls.org/es/source/orders/free/poct1-a.pdf

[8] Frankel D.S.: *MDA, SOA and Technology Convergence,* MDA Journal, http://www.bptrends.com/publicationfiles, December 2003

[9] Kosińska J., Słowikowski P.: *Technical Aspects of Portal Technology Application for E-health Systems.* Proceedings of II International Conference on E-health in Common Europe, Krakow March 2004

[10] McGeady S.: *The Internet as Disruptive Force in Healthcare.* Internet Technologies in Healthcare, Industry Report, 1999

[11] Politis Communications: *Client/Server- vs. Internet-based Practice Management Systems: Why 'Net andWhy Now?* AdvancedMD Software, July 2004

[12] Wilkes L., Veryard R.: *Service-Oriented Architecture: Considerations for Agile Systems,* CBDI Forum, April 2004

[13] Woo-Ming M.: *Medical Information on the Internet: Ten Rules to Know.* WorldNetDaily, 2004

[14] *Digital Imaging and Communications in Medicine (DICOM).* http://medical.nema.org, National Electrical Manufacturers Association 2004

4 Security and Safety of Telemedical Systems

Paweł Słowikowski[1], Krzysztof Zieliński[1]

[1] Department of Computer Science, AGH University of Science and Technology, Krakow, Poland

Agencies and standards bodies within governments of several nations have developed evaluation criteria for computing technology security. In the United States, the relevant document has the designation "Trusted Computer System Security Evaluation Criteria," or TCSEC. The European Commission has published the Information Technology Security Evaluation Criteria, also known as ITSEC, and the Canadian government has published the Canadian Trusted Computer Product Evaluation Criteria, or CTCPEC. In 1996, these initiatives were officially combined into a document known as the Common Criteria [8]. In 1999 this document was approved as a standard [28], [27], [1] by the International Organization for Standardization. This initiative paves the way to worldwide mutual recognition of product evaluation results.

The need of the healthcare industry to reliably and confidentially exchange patient healthcare information in support of the portability of healthcare insurance and patients between employees, insurance companies and healthcare providers has resulted in creating a document called "The Health Insurance Portability and Accountability Act of 1996" (HIPAA)[17]. To support the confidential maintenance and exchange of electronic healthcare information, the Department of Health and Human Services in the US has developed regulations that support and enforce HIPAA privacy and security. These regulations prescribe care in handling paper records, as well as care in handling electronic records for protected health information. Protected information that is stored in distributed e-medical information systems is potentially subject to inappropriate access or modification, also known as an *attack*.

A similar security architecture, but with a wider scope, has been developed as part of the government's commitment to developing a corporate IT strategy. It has been prepared, for instance, by the UK Government [24]. This security architecture specifies framework policy, guidelines and implementation experience for UKonline services and market developments. This document is aimed at bodies engaged in procuring and providing e-Government services, including central government departments, non-departmental public sector bodies, local authorities and other local government bodies charged with the provision of e-Government services. It also encompasses regulatory bodies responsible for proper auditing and control of public assets and information. Other security architectures can be found, for example, in [3], [25].

This chapter shows how to secure an e-medical system using widely-available digital security technology and mechanisms.

1 E-medical Secure Environment Requirements

HIPPA security mandates the following security rule: "Ensure the confidentiality, integrity, and availability of all electronic protected health information (PHI) the covered entity creates, receives, maintains or transmits." The security system assumes reasonably anticipated threats or hazards and reasonably anticipated (unauthorized) uses or disclosures. Its general objectives are to:
- guarantee health insurance coverage of employees,
- reduce healthcare fraud and abuse,
- introduce/implement administrative simplifications in order to augment effectiveness and efficiency of the healthcare system in the United States,
- protect the health information of individuals against access without consent or authorization.

HIPAA presents a threefold challenge to device and software vendors:
1. incorporating necessary security technology into products to protect the privacy of the protected health information generated, managed and exchanged by the products at customer sites,
2. reevaluating and enhancing their own internal policies and training to ensure secure and confidential handling of protected health information exposed during testing, field services, product evaluation and research,
3. supporting their customers in the creation of HIPAA-compliant workflows that incorporate their products, while at the same time ensuring that those resulting product-enabled workflows do not impede clinical communications or negatively affect patient care.

Device and software vendors are typically not directly responsible for the organizational policies and procedures of their customers. However, their own policies and procedures must protect the confidentiality of information and their products can be developed to make it easier to comply with HIPAA. Specifically, HIPAA precisely specifies certain critical security policies and technologies, including:

- unique IDs for authorized users,
- automatic logoff,
- audit trails for access to specific types of protected information,
- encryption (optional),
- digital signatures (optional),
- virus checking procedures,
- backup/restore plans,
- disaster recovery plans,
- compliance auditing,
- testing programs,
- training programs.

It is necessary to note that security solutions require more than just a few pieces of technology. To be effective, technical security solutions must be complemented by training, physical security, appropriate best practices-derived security policies and proper configuration of operating systems and applications.

Physical security can range from simple locks on doors to high-tech biometric authentication scanners, to trusted human guards. The challenge is determining what level of physical security is necessary given the sensitivity of the information, the robustness of technical security, the accessibility of the computing environment and the trustworthiness of human staff.

Networks: Information being exchanged between distributed healthcare systems is exposed to potential discovery through various types of eavesdropping. Physical security of the networking components and communications media may be sufficient in small environments. In larger environments and whenever protected health information is to be exchanged across a public network, the privacy of that information must be maintained through cryptographic and security technology.

Computer Operating Systems: Most modern computer operating systems provide sufficient security for protecting medical records. However, that security needs to be properly configured based on best-practices security policies. Configuration must include deleting unused and unnecessary user accounts, as well as ensuring that all passwords meet modern security requirements. A properly secure operating system must include both proper configuration to remove security holes and proper policies to ensure the users themselves don't open new security holes.

Application Software: As with operating systems, most modern applications have the potential to be configured for secure use. However, as with operating systems, most applications are configured by default to have very weak or nonexistent security (e.g. DBMS systems with well-known default username/password pairs). Each application must be configured for secure use.

Data: Many types of information can be read by multiple applications (e.g. image files). Relying solely on application-based security to protect the privacy of information will fail if unauthorized users can simply turn to a different less-protective application to read the information. Access control must be applied at the most fundamental level (files, database, etc.) in which the information is stored. In addition, in the case of information stored in databases, security must be applied at a minimum at the level of individual records. In some cases, database information may also need to be protected through some form of access control on the individual fields within records.

2 System Architecture Modeling for Security

Common Criteria [8], [9], [10] provide a taxonomy for evaluating security functionality through a set of functional and assurance requirements. The Criteria include 11 functional classes of requirements: security audit, communication, cryptographic support, user data protection, identification and authentication, management of security functions, privacy, protection of security functions, resource utilization, component access, and trusted path or channel [14], [20], [25]. These 11 functional classes are further divided into 66 families, each containing a number of component criteria. There are approximately 130 component criteria currently documented, with the recognition that designers may add additional component criteria to a specific design. There is a formal process for adopting component criteria through the Common Criteria administrative body.

Governments and industry groups develop functional descriptions for security hardware and software using the Common Criteria. These documents [29], known as protection profiles, describe groupings of security functions that are appropriate for a given security component or technology. The underlying motivations for developing protection profiles include incentives for vendors to deliver standard functionality within security products and reduce risk in information technology procurement.

The classes and families within the Common Criteria represent an aggregation of requirements [7]. The aggregation is more reflective of abstract security themes, such as cryptographic operations and data protection, rather than security in the context of IT operational function. A summary mapping of CC classes to functional categories is provided in Table 4-1.

Table 4-1 Relations between Common Criteria classes and functional categories [8]

Functional Category	Common Criteria Functional Class
Audit	Audit, component protection, resource utilization
Access control	Data protection, component protection, security management, component access, cryptographic support, identification and authentication, communication, trusted path/channel
Flow control	Communication, cryptographic support, data protection, component protection, trusted path/channel, privacy
Identity/credentials	Communication, cryptographic support, data protection, component protection, trusted path/channel, privacy
Identity/credentials	Cryptographic support, data protection, component protection, identification and authentication, component access, security management, trusted path/channel
Solution integrity	Cryptographic support, data protection, component protection, resource utilization, security management

This structure supports the assertion that the five categories described in Table 4-1 represent a set of interrelated processes, or subsystems.

Security audit subsystem: A security audit subsystem is responsible for capturing, analyzing, reporting, archiving and retrieving records of events and conditions within a computing solution. From Common Criteria, security requirements for an audit subsystem would include:

- collection of security audit data, including capture of the appropriate data, trusted transfer of audit data, and synchronization of chronologies,
- protection of security audit data, including use of time stamps, signing events, and storage integrity to prevent loss of data,
- analysis of security audit data, including review, anomaly detection, violation analysis, and attack analysis using simple heuristics or complex heuristics,

- alarms for loss thresholds, warning conditions, and critical events.

Solution integrity subsystem: The purpose of the solution integrity subsystem in an IT solution is to address the requirement for reliable and correct operation of a computing solution in support of meeting the legal [6] and technical standard for its processes. From Common Criteria, the focus of a solution integrity subsystem could include:
- integrity and reliability of resources,
- physical protections for data objects, such as cryptographic keys, and physical components, such as cabling, hardware, etc.,
- continued operations including fault tolerance, failure recovery, and self-testing,
- storage mechanisms; cryptography and hardware security modules,
- accurate time source for time measurement and time stamps,
- prioritization of service via resource allocation or quotas,
- functional isolation using domain separation or a reference monitor,
- alarms and actions when a physical or passive attack is detected.

Access control subsystem: The purpose of an access control subsystem in an IT solution is to enforce security policies by gating access to, and execution of, processes and services within a computing solution via identification, authentication, and authorization processes, along with security mechanisms that use credentials and attributes. From Common Criteria, the functional requirements for an access control subsystem should include:
- access control enablement,
- access control monitoring and enforcement,
- identification and authentication mechanisms, including verification of secrets, cryptography (encryption and signing), and single- vs. multiple-use authentication mechanisms,
- authorization mechanisms, to include attributes, privileges, and permissions,
- access control mechanisms, to include attribute-based access control on subjects and objects and user-subject binding,
- enforcement mechanisms, including failure handling, bypass prevention, banners, timing and timeout, event capture, and decision and logging components.

Information flow control subsystem: The purpose of an information flow control subsystem in an IT solution is to enforce security policies [23] by gating the flow of information within a computing solution, affecting the visibility of information within a computing solution, and ensuring the integrity of information flowing within a computing solution. From Common Criteria, an information flow control subsystem may include the following functional requirements:

- flow permission or prevention,
- flow monitoring and enforcement,
- transfer services and environments: open or trusted channel, open or trusted path, media conversions, manual transfer, import to or export between domains,
- mechanisms observability: to block cryptography (encryption),
- storage mechanisms: cryptography and hardware security modules,
- enforcement mechanisms: asset and attribute binding, event capture, decision and logging components, stored data monitoring, rollback, residual information protection and destruction.

Identity or credential subsystem: The purpose of a credential subsystem in an IT solution is to generate, distribute, and manage the data objects that convey identity [6] and permissions across networks and among the platforms, the processes, and the security subsystems within a computing solution. From Common Criteria, a credential subsystem may include the following functional requirements:

- single-use vs. multiple-use mechanisms, either cryptographic or noncryptographic,
- generation and verification of secrets,
- identities and credentials to be used to protect security flows or business process flows,
- identities and credentials to be used in protection of assets: integrity or nonobservability,
- identities and credentials to be used in access control: identification, authentication, and access control for the purpose of user-subject binding,
- credentials to be used for purposes of identity in legally binding transactions,
- timing and duration of identification and authentication,
- life cycle of credentials,
- anonymity and pseudonymity mechanisms.

The security design objectives and the solution environment have a central role in the selection and enumeration of subsystems. Table 4-2 shows a possible mapping of the sample design objectives to security subsystems. It indicates where a subsystem may be required (R) or supplementary (S) in satisfying an individual security requirement. Actual subsystem selection requires documented rationale.

Table 4-2 Mapping design objectives to security subsystems [8]

Security Design Objectives	Audit	Integrity	Access Control	Flow Control	Credential Identity
Control access to systems/processes	S	S	R	S	S
Control access to information	S	S	S	R	R
Control the flow of information	S	S	S	R	S
Correct and reliable component operation	S	R	S	S	S
Prevent/mitigate attacks	R	R	R	R	S
Accountability through trusted identity	R	R	S	S	R
Prevent/mitigate fraud	R	R	R	R	R

3 Techniques for Making E-medical Systems Secure

The techniques for making e-medical systems secure [15], [22], [21], [2], [19], particularly as relates to subsystems, are depicted in Figure 4-1 and will be elaborated in more detail below. They address three major areas: Application and Data, System Infrastructure, and Networks.

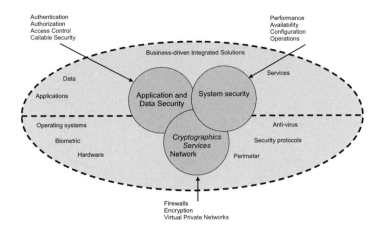

Figure 4-1 Range of various security-related technology applications.

Basic cryptography: The computer security services that are required to protect electronic information are based on technology called *cryptography*. Most of the security techniques are built upon either "secret key encryption" or "public key encryption" cryptography. Encryption can be implemented using either a single key to scramble and unscramble the text (symmetric or secret key encryption) or a pair of keys; one to scramble and a different key to unscramble the text (public key encryption) [11]. Each underlying technology requires a different set of supporting concepts and mechanisms.

Many security mechanisms are based on the consequences of digitally "signing" protected information using either secret key encryption or public key encryption. When a piece of information is "signed" using public key encryption, the signer uses their private half of the public/private key pair to encrypt the information. If anyone wishes to test that signed information (e.g. to validate the source of the information or integrity of the information), they use the public half of the key pair to decrypt the message. Digital Certificates are encrypted documents generated by a Certificate Authority, which confirms the identity of the owner of a public/private key pair.

Authentication of users: Authentication is the process of verifying the identity of a potential user of a system. Most authentication mechanisms are based on some combination of one or more "shared secrets" (e.g. password), security devices (e.g. access card) and/or physical characteristic (e.g. fingerprint). A common combination (sometimes called "two-factor authentication") is authentication based on something you *have* (e.g. your ATM card) and something you *know* (e.g. the ATM account PIN). At its simplest, authentication is performed through the verification of an access code or a username/password pair entered by the user at the time they wish access to the system. More sophisticated authentication mechanisms include the use of "smart cards" to store encrypted credentials and even biometric analysis of fingerprints, face scans or retina scans. Authentication on its own does not mean access to any information or services specific to the system; it only verifies, with some level of certainty, that you are who you claim to be.

Authorized access to protected information: Access control is sometimes also called *authorization*, particularly when referring to the process of determining whether a user is authorized to have access to a system or application. Access to a specific piece of information can only be granted to a properly authenticated, authorized user with appropriate levels of access (e.g. a physician may have complete access to their own patient's information, yet only have access to de-identified or statistical information about another physician's patients).

Accountability of changes to protected information: Users of protected health information are accountable for all access, modifications and distribution of that information. Any unauthorized access to protected health information should be reported. Audit logs are tools for logging the authorized and unauthorized use of the applications and/or services of a system, as well as access and/or changes to protected health information. Regular inspection of audit logs is critical to protecting the security of the system, the integrity of the protected information and the legal standing of the organization.

Integrity of protected information: Protected health information must be represented, stored and distributed in such a way that any attempt to alter the information (whether authorized or not) can be identified and tracked. Typically a system-independent mechanism bound tightly to the information (e.g. checksum, CRC, or digital signature) provides corroboration of the integrity of the information.

Non-repudiation of changes to protected information: Non-repudiation mechanisms provide non-refutable evidence of creation, deletion, modification or distribution of information. This ensures that not even an authorized user can access, change or share the information and then deny having accessed it.

Confidentiality of protected information: Data in a secure system, or data being exchanged across secure distributed systems must not be viewable by unauthorized users or systems. Privacy often must extend to any requests made with regard to the secure system. Unauthorized users can potentially obtain important information about data on the system simply by "overhearing" a request regarding such data.

Confidential information should never be stored in plain text on a non-secure system. If the physical or electronic security of a system is suspect, confidential information should be encrypted using keys that *are not* stored on the non-secure system. Depending on the nature of the information, it may be stored in an encrypted file, stored as a set of message digest records or stored as encrypted fields within a database.

Protecting the privacy of data that is being exchanged across a network requires encryption of that data. This encryption can happen at a number of different layers in the communications process:
1.   network layer encryption,
2.   session layer encryption,
3.   application layer encryption.

Network layer encryption is usually implemented between secure network routers based on the IETF IP sec standard. These routers encrypt all (IP payload) traffic sent between themselves and other mutually authenticated routers. If the sending and receiving local-area networks (LANs) and associated systems are secure, and the path between them is secure (e.g. configured as a virtual private network using network-level encryption), then session-level and application-level encryption is not necessary.

The challenge with network-layer encryption is that information is only encrypted between the edges of the LANs of each organization. The information will be in plain text within each LAN and on the end-systems of each organization. When you are unsure if the network between end-systems is secure, session-layer encryption can be used to secure the information being exchanged between end-systems independent of whether the network layer itself is encrypted. Session-layer encryption is often implemented using the secure socket layer (SSL) industry standard. SSL is used for secure transactions by Web, e-mail, and file transfer applications.

Monitoring access and modification of protected information: Each of the security mechanisms used to protect sensitive systems and information has the potential of being breached by an attacker. To maintain security and integrity of the protected information, discretion is required, not only in the selection of technology and implementation of policies, but also in monitoring the systems to identify attempted breaches as well as suspicious access trends, and track compliance with specified policies and procedures. Monitoring covers audit logs, trend analysis, alarms and event reporting.

4 Access Control Models

Access control is a very important instrument for implementing security policy in e-medical systems. It can be implemented with at least three levels of sophistication:

- user-based access control,
- role-based access control [4], [5], [12], [16],
- context-based or rules-based access control.

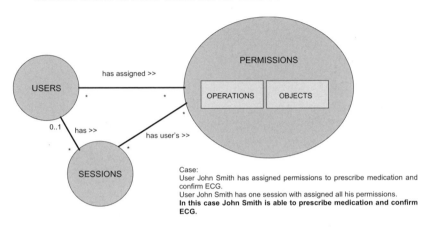

Figure 4-2 User-based access control (UBAC)

User-based access control is depicted in Figure 4-2. Implementing authorization policies can be as simple as maintaining and referring to a list that matches individual user identity and a specific access right for a given resource. These are usually implemented by a specific application on a specific system (e.g. a file system access control list (ACL)). The challenge with user-based access control is that it requires considerable system administration effort to maintain the access control lists for all users on all systems for each piece of protected information.

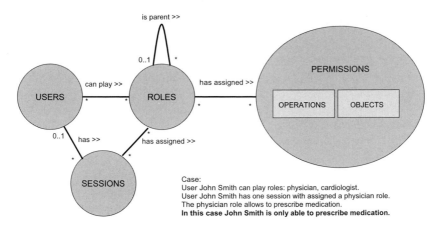

Figure 4-3 Role-based access Control (RBAC).

Role-based access control is presented in Figure 4-3. Since users often play specific roles (e.g. administrator, physician, covering physician, etc.), the administrative overhead of managing a protected system can be reduced by matching a user's role to a specific access right for a resource. However, this too becomes problematic when managing access rights across many different systems. In addition, individual user rights must still be granted for information owned by individuals and not accessible by other members of the user's groups.

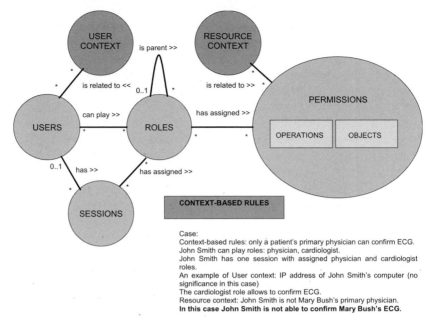

Figure 4-4 Context-based access aontrol (CBAC).

Context-based access vontrol is illustrated in Figure 4-4. Under normal circumstances, a user in a healthcare facility has limited access to patient information. Only those with a direct need-to-know are allowed access to detailed protected information. However, there are a number of situations in which healthcare professionals require access to information based on the current context:

- a covering physician must have access to patient information in a unit,
- a physician receiving a referral must access some subset of a patient's protected information,
- an emergency room nurse must access historical information while performing triage in a busy ER.

More sophisticated approaches to implementing context-based access control policy involve the use of policy and rules services for all of the resources within a system or a site. These access control services may support both static policy (e.g. applications that can be used, files that can be accessed, directories that can be viewed, access hours, storage quota, etc.) and dynamic rules based on real-time context (e.g. whether currently covering for another healthcare provider).

5   Service-Oriented Security Architecture

Service-oriented architecture (SOA) is a set of principles for designing extensible, federated, interoperable services [12]. SOA principles can (and should) be applied not only to the services that compose a service-oriented business architecture, but also to the services that compose a service-oriented security architecture (SOSA). SOSA, based on the set of Web Services Security (WS Security)-related standards recently proposed by IBM and Microsoft, is currently under development at the Organization for the Advancement of Structured Information Standards (OASIS). The fundamental goal of the emerging XML and WS Security standard is not to replace the diverse security infrastructures already deployed, but to enable them to interoperate in an end-to-end fashion.

For a service consumer to delegate responsibility for executing a process to a service provider, a policy of trust must underlie that delegation. For example, a consumer, before delegating responsibility for holding her savings to a medical database, must first trust the medical service. Thus, the ultimate goal of SOSA is to enable such trust by establishing and enforcing security policies defined by a trust model, without regard to specific enforcement mechanisms. Accordingly, SOSA is not based on any specific enforcement mechanism, but rather on a generic model of policy-based trust:

- **identifiers:** for consumers and services,
- **formats:** for tokens and policies,
- **protocols:** for exchanging tokens and policies.

In other words, SOSA should be defined in terms of generic protocols for exchanging generic (token) claims offered by service consumers and generic policy rules regarding such claims enforced by service providers. The interoperable formats of SOSA define a generic policy model, modularized into the following conceptual building blocks:

- **policy:** a set of policy assertions.
- **policy assertion:** a specific preference, requirement, capability, or other property. A more general and perhaps clearer definition of policy assertion is "rule that governs a choice in the behavior of a system".
- **security token:** a set of security claims. Security tokens can be either binary (e.g., X.509, Kerberos ticket) or XML (e.g., SAML, XrML). A certificate (e.g., X.509) or a ticket (e.g., Kerberos) is simply a signed security token. XML tokens can be signed as well; thus, certificates are also either binary or XML.
- **claim:** a policy-relevant statement made by or about a subject accessing a service.

The interoperable protocols of SOSA define a generic process model, modularized into the following subprocesses:

- generating and distributing service security policies via service definitions (e.g., WSDL) and service directories (e.g., UDDI),
- generating and distributing security tokens,
- presenting tokens in messages and service requests,
- evaluating whether presented tokens meet required policies.

Several standards embodying various aspects of this type of SOSA have been designed over the past several years. They are described in Table 4-3.

Table 4-3 Standards Embodying SOSA Principles

Acronym /Doc. No.	Full name of document
AAA	Authorization, Authentication, Accounting
XNS	Extensible Name System
XACML	Extensible Access Control Markup Language
PCIM	Policy Core Information Model
SAML	Security Assertion Markup Language
WSSM	Web Services Security Model
RFC 2753	A Framework for Policy-Based Admission Control

6   RAD Case Study

RAD (Resource Access Decision) is a mechanism of access control, i.e. limiting resource access to a group of authorized users. It has been implemented with the idea of protecting medical resources provided by a portal application and accessed via a Web browser. RAD is based on the Resource Access Decision Facility developed by the Object Management Group [18]. The goal of the Resource Access Decision Facility is to separate authorization logic from application-specific business logic and make the authorization service independent of the specific security models and policies. RAD is able to support, among other models, user-based access control, role-based access control, context-based access control and rules-based access control. The architecture and features of RAD make it a valuable addition to our Medical Portal.

The following case study illustrates how RAD is used to authorize access to patient examination results and how it can be used to authorize access to other medical resources. It refers to the scenario in which a patient comes to a hospital for an examination. Following examination, the results are stored in the hospital's IT system. Only the patient and authorized personnel are allowed to access these results. The case study focuses on providing examination results through the portal. We describe the authorization mechanism that was used in our solution. The authentication process is omitted, because RAD only addresses authorization.

RAD architecture: RAD architecture is derived from the Resource Access Decision Facility. The main difference between the original specification and our implementation is that the middleware which constitutes the basis of the solution is Java RMI, EJB and Web Services, whereas in the original specification it was CORBA. We have also made some additional minor changes in order to improve service performance. Nevertheless, the general architecture, presented in Figure 4-5, remained unchanged.

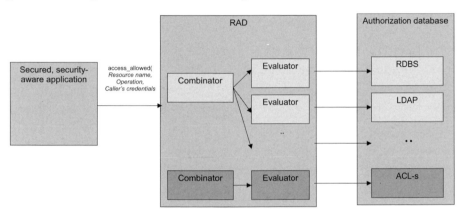

Figure 4-5 RAD architecture.

The main steps of the authorization process are [26]:
1. Whenever required, the secured, security-aware application checks if the user has been granted access to the requested resource. The application invokes the access_allowed method of the RAD interface, passing three arguments: resource name, operation to be executed on the resource and user's credentials.
2. RAD selects evaluators and a combinator based on the resource name. Evaluators are responsible for interpreting authorization policies that control access to the requested resource. In order to evaluate an access request, the evaluators refer to the authorization database. The combinator is responsible for combining results from evaluators according to the authorization policy. The result of the combinator, a Boolean value granting or denying access to the resource, is returned to the application.

3. The application grants or denies access to the resource on the basis of the result received from RAD.

RAD makes an access decision based on the user's credentials (user name, certificate, etc.), the operation to be performed on the resource and the resource name. User credentials, which are coeval with patient identity, are one of the results of the authentication process. The resource name identifies the patient's examination result. The operation is understood as the action associated with the resource (e.g. READ, WRITE).

RAD consists of two parts: an access control service and an access control administration module. The access control service provides its interface to secure-aware applications that require authorization. The interfaces are low-level and require adaptation of secured applications. In the case of the Medical Portal, such adaptation took place during the design phase of the application. The administration module is intended to be a tool for managing Medical Portal security.

RAD in Medical Portal: One of the essential security mechanisms for enforcing security policies is access control to resources. In our system, RAD was used to provide an authorization service. The Medical Portal was implemented as a J2EE (JSP/Servlets/EJB) application running on the JBoss application server. Communication between the Medical Portal and RAD was through Java RMI. Patient information, as well as the authorization database, were stored in a relational database management system (Oracle).

In order to combine RAD and the Medical Portal, some steps had to be taken: an authorization database had to be created (with defined users, groups, resources and permissions), a specific evaluator had to be implemented and calls to RAD had to be added in the code of the Medical Portal.

Figure 4-6 shows how RAD is used to authorize access to patient examination results provided by the Medical Portal.

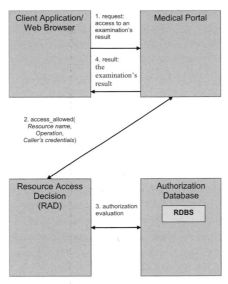

Figure 4-6 RAD in Medical Portal.

Access to examination result consists of the following steps:

1. Following authentication in the Medical Portal, the user requests an examination result.

2. The Medical Portal intercepts the request and extracts the user identifier (caller's credentials), the identifier of the examination result (resource name) and the operation to be performed on the examination result (READ). Next, the information is sent to RAD as parameters of the authorization method.

3. RAD chooses appropriate evaluators and combinators basing on the resource name. For the examination result, only one evaluator is required. RAD delegates the authorization request to the evaluator and after having received the result, makes an authorization decision using the combinator. In this step RAD accesses the authorization database which stores authorization information. The model of authorization is user-based access control extended with context-based rules.

4. If the authorization decision is positive, the examination result is provided to the user; otherwise an "unauthorized request" page is displayed.

Usage of RAD in the described manner ensures authorization of access to Medical Portal resources. In our case, access control is based on a very simple security policy; however, RAD can support much more sophisticated security policies without changes to the architecture of the whole system. It is only necessary to implement specific plug-ins called evaluators and to reconfigure

RAD. In this way, we can include support for time-dependent permissions, as well as context-based or role-based access control.

A comfortable GUI interface for RAD administration and management of the authorization database makes Medical Portal administration an easy task.

7 Summary

Telemedical systems contain and provide information that is extremely sensitive. Disclosing or damaging that information in an unauthorized way may be catastrophic both for organizations and patients. In order to assure the security of telemedical systems, suitable security policies, security architectures and security mechanisms must be applied. Additionally, a secure and safe working environment must be guaranteed. The rules for setting up such an environment are described (for example) in HIPPA.

Best-practice telemedical systems should satisfy such evaluation criteria as TCSEC or ITSEC. Conformity with these standards helps achieve a well-protected and secure system.

8 Bibliography

[1] P. B. Checkland, *Systems Thinking, Systems Practice*, John Wiley & Sons, Inc., New York (1981).
[2] W. R. Cheswick and S. M. Bellovin, *Firewalls and Internet Security: Repelling the Wily Hacker*, Addison-Wesley Publishing Co., Reading, MA (1994).
[3] Committee on Information Systems Trustworthiness, National Research Council, *Trust in Cyberspace*, National Academy Press, Washington, DC (1999).
[4] D. Ferraiolo, *Proposed NIST Standard for Role-Based Access Control*, ACM Transactions on Information and System Security, Vol. 4, No. 3 (August 2001), pp. 224–274.
[5] D. Ferraiolo, D. Kuhn, and R. Chandramouli, *Role-Based Access Control*, Artech House, Norwood, MA (2003).
[6] *Digital Signature Guidelines*, American Bar Association (1996), Section 1.35, available at http://www.abanet.org/scitech/ec/isc/dsgfree.html.
[7] *Guide for Development of Protection Profiles and Security Targets*, ISO/IEC PDTR 15446, available at http://csrc.nist.gov/cc/t4/wg3/27n2449.pdf, pp. 69–74.
[8] *Information Technology—Security Techniques—Evaluation Criteria for IT Security—Part 1: Introduction and General Model*, ISO/IEC 15408-1 (1999); available at

http://isotc.iso.ch/livelink/livelink/fetch/2000/2489/lttf_Home/PubliclyAvailableStandards.htm.

[9] *Information Technology—Security Techniques—Evaluation Criteria for IT Security—Part 2: Security Functional Requirements*, ISO/IEC 15408-2 (1999).

[10]*Information Technology—Security Techniques—Evaluation Criteria for IT Security—Part 3: Security Assurance Requirements*, ISO/IEC 15408-3 (1999).

[11]H. Johner, S. Fujiwara, A. S. Yeung, A. Stephanou, and J. Whitmore, *Deploying a Public Key Infrastructure*, Redbook SG24-5512-00, IBM Corporation, http://www.redbooks.ibm.co.

[12]N. Kall, *Service-Oriented Security Architecture: Part 1*, Metagroup, ZDNet (2003).

[13]A. Kumar, N. Karnik, and G. Chafle, *Context Sensitivity in Role Based Access Control*, ACM SIGOPS Operating Systems Review (July 2002), pp. 53-66.

[14]P. T. L. Lloyd and G. M. Galambos, *Technical Reference Architectures*, IBM Systems Journal 38, No. 1, 51–75 (1999); available at http://researchweb.watson.ibm.com/journal/sj/381/lloyd.html.

[15]S. McClure, J. Scambray, and G. Kurtz, *Hacking Exposed: Network Security Secrets & Solutions*, McGraw-Hill Publishing Company, Maidenhead, Berkshire (1999).

[16]M. Moyer and M. Ahamad, *Generalized Role-Based Access Control*, International Conference on Distributed Computing Systems (April 2001), pp. 391-398.

[17]NEMA -Privacy and Security Committee, Security and Privacy: An Introduction to HIPAA (April 10, 2001).

[18]OMG, *Resource Access Decision, Version 1.0.* (2001); available at http://www.omg.org/technology/documents/formal/resource_access_decision.htm.

[19]A. Patel and S. O. Ciardhuain, *The Impact of Forensic Computing on Telecommunications*, IEEE Communications Magazine 38, No. 11, 64–67 (November 2000).

[20]E. Rechtin, *Systems Architecting: Creating and Building Complex Systems*, Prentice Hall, New York (1991).

[21]RFC 1825, *Security Architecture for the Internet Protocol* (August 1995); available at http://www.ietf.org/rfc.html.

[22]RFC 2316, *Report of the IAB Security Architecture Workshop* (April 1998); available at http://www.ietf.org/rfc.html.

[23]F. B. Schneider, *Enforceable Security Policies*, ACM Transactions on Information and System Security 3, No. 1, 30–50 (February 2000).

[24]*Security Architecture, e-Government Strategy, Version 2.0* (September 2002).

[25]*Security Architecture for Open Systems Interconnection for CCITT Applications*, ITU-T Recommendation X.800/ISO 7498-2 (1991); available at http://www.itu.int/itudoc/itu-t/rec/x/x500up/x800.html.

[26] P. Slowikowski and M. Jarzab, *Security aspect of medical portals*, Proceedings, the International Conference on E-he@lth in Common Europe, Krakow, Poland (2003).

[27] D. Verton, *Common Ground Sought for IT Security Requirements*, *Computerworld* 35, No. 11, 8 (March 12, 2001).

[28] J. J. Whitmore, *Security and e-business: Is There a Prescription?* Proceedings, 21st National Information Systems Security Conference, Arlington, VA (October 6–9, 1998); available at http://csrc.nist.gov/nissc/1998/proceedings/paperD13.pdf.

[29] http://www.commoncriteria.org/protection_profiles/pp.html.

5 Wireless Systems in e-Health

Łukasz Czekierda[1], Jacek Dańda[2], Krzysztof Łoziak[2], Marek Sikora[2], Krzysztof Zieliński[1], Sławomir Zieliński[1]

[1]   Department of Computer Science, AGH University of Science and Technology, Krakow, Poland
[2]   Department of Telecommunications, AGH University of Science and Technology, Poland

There are several key factors motivating the move towards wireless technology. Increasing mobility of network users is certainly one of them, while another – even more important – is the need to have universal access to applications and information. Over the past few years a major increase in availability and capabilities of wireless technologies could have been observed. However, the contemporary level of service is still not at the "access information anytime, anywhere" point. First, the availability of wireless communications is great, but low network capabilities may render access unusable. When considering a medical application, it is easy to observe that even if the available bandwidth is sufficient to download large medical data sets (e.g. radiological images) in a timely manner, the level of security offered by the networks sometimes prevents the medical institutions from providing such a remote access service to their workers. On the other hand, from a technical point of view, there are technologies that could be used to provide a satisfactory level of security. This article discusses the problems related to working and foreseen medical applications of wireless networks in the context of state-of-the-art technologies.

1 An Overview of Wireless Communication Technologies

Further automatization of business processes, considered by many organizations a key benefit resulting from the introduction of wireless technologies, can be easily observed in medical institutions. Hospital staff frequently change their locations. Their data requirements also change rapidly. The introduction of data access technologies that support mobility could really improve their efficiency, while keeping the critical information centralized and easier to manage.

Wireless technology comprises many different components, including networks, service providers, protocols, devices and tools for network management and development of applications. There are three classes of wireless networks, as defined by their range[3]:

- personal area networks (PANs),
- wireless local-area networks (WLANs),
- wireless wide-area networks (WWANs).

Personal area networks (PANs) span very limited areas (the typical radius is 10 meters) and operate at 1 Mbps. These cable replacement networks serve as frequency-hopping radio links between wireless devices. The Bluetooth standard is considered the most important representative of PANs. Most cell phones and headsets already come fitted with a Bluetooth interface for wireless communication.

Wireless local-area networks (WLANs) are a popular alternative to wired LAN. The coverage of a single WLAN is typically measured in hundreds of meters. There are many IEEE 802.11 specifications for WLANs. The 802.11b standard is the most widely used, and sustains data rates of up to 11Mbps. However, its frequency is susceptible to potential interference from cordless phones, microwaves, etc. The 802.11a standard provides a faster data rate (up to 54 Mbps), but requires a hardware upgrade since it operates on a different frequency band (5 GHz) than that of 802.11b (2.4 Ghz). The 802.11g standard operates at up to 54 Mbps in the same frequency band as 802.11b. Contemporary WLAN adapters are frequently compatible with two (b and g) or all three standards.

Wireless wide-area networks (WWANs) span a relatively large geographical area and operate on many different networks at many different speeds. Service is frequently provided by cellular telephony operators. The majority of WWAN data rate ranges vary anywhere from 9.6 kbps to 2 Mbps. Some proprietary networks even offer speeds of up to 100 Mbps. Figure 5-1 shows the evolution of WWAN networks over the past six years.

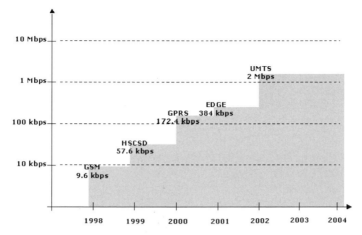

Figure 5-1 Evolution of wireless wide-area network services.

One of the key issues related to wireless technology is the need for mechanisms enabling interoperability between different types of communication networks. The most popular solution is offered by the wireless service providers' gateways, able to translate between different types of networks or applications. Wireless gateways enable mobile devices to access Internet Protocol (IP)-based applications over a wide range of wireless networks. Wireless gateways support both IP and non-IP wireless bearer networks [3]. Moreover, they usually support network-specific enhancements such as data compression, encryption, authentication, optimization, and retransmission.

Among networking standards governing the transmission and reception of data between devices and the Internet, the hypertext transfer protocol (HTTP) is the one used most often. Others include the wireless application protocol (WAP), a highly optimized XML-based method of displaying applications on constrained devices. Many institutions decide to provide access to their databases using Web interfaces. Even in the case of medical databases containing confidential information, Web-enabled clients are commonplace [21].

Support for all major networking protocols is not the only factor which should influence the selection of a handheld device. Processing power, battery life, screen size, and keypads are all key factors to contemplate when developing a wireless application. The three main types of mobile and wireless devices are cell phones, personal digital assistants (PDAs), and smart phones. Cell phones have poor user interfaces – such as small displays, no support for cookies and Java scripting, as well as URL length limitations. PDA devices are more powerful. The Compaq iPAQ depicted in Figure 5-2 is a representative of this class. Its latest version is equipped with WLAN and Bluetooth interfaces. It is also equipped with expansion slots, which can be used to attach extension cards such as a GPRS modem. The iPAQ provides an excellent color display, but its battery life suffers as a result.

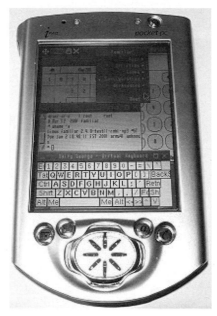

Figure 5-2 iPAQ PDA.

A smart phone is basically a cell phone merged with a PDA. Popular brands of smart phones include the Kyocera 7135, Microsoft Smartphone and the Palm Tungsten W.

Applying contemporary wireless communication technologies can turn the vision of mobile e-health services into a reality. The analysis of medical service scenarios [20] leads to identification of the following key mobile objects and mobility aspects: patient, patient's EHR, monitoring care center, medical staff and emergency teams. Each mobility category imposes characteristic requirements on applied telemedical solutions. The requirements may be divided into functional and technical groups. The most important functional requirements are as follows:

- access to patient's personal e-health environment on-line anytime and anywhere,
- ability to recognize medical conditions and patient's state and to notify a care center,
- localization of patient and automatic or semiautomatic selection of nearby medical services, such as monitoring care center or suitable hospital,

- transparent authorization and synchronization of patient personal medical e-health environment with medical equipment e.g. when the patient is taken over by an emergency team,
- on-demand access to a patient EHR at home or from a medical center and its automatic transfer to a nearby foreign care center,
- access to medical data from mobile devices.

Technical requirements are related to the process of making telemedical applications mobile. In order to enable telemedical application mobility it is necessary to overcome several challenges, including:
- determining the architectural approach,
- dealing with the current application environment,
- securing connected networks,
- managing user sessions,
- ensuring scalability of runtime environment,
- managing diverse content,
- handling and managing client devices,
- networking technologies diversity.

In the context of wireless e-health systems, the security aspect is particularly important.

2   Wireless System Security Aspects

Wireless systems are very sensitive to attacks and security violations. The following elements for security in wireless system implementations become apparent [4]:
- *Mutual authentication* – both the client and server must authenticate with each other in order to not only guarantee that the users allowed to access the network are authorized to do so, but also to help guard against spoofing access points and other wireless devices.
- *End-to-end encryption* – user data must never be allowed to appear in the clear on the network except at authorized end points.
- *Per-client keys* – keys must be unique for each authorized user. This prevents the compromising of security keys due to theft or otherwise unauthorized access and also provides for guaranteeing non-repudiation.
- *Secure automated key distribution* – a technique for central management of security keys is essential. Manual processes are both error-prone and subject to security violations.
- *Full support for mobility* – finally, any security implementation must take into account the fundamental nature of wireless LANs – that users can

move from access point to access point as they roam throughout a given facility, and even between facilities.

A wide variety of options for meeting the above exist. One of the most obvious is using services which operate at the OSI network layer or above. A popular technique is the use of a virtual private network (VPN), an approach based on "tunneling" encrypted traffic through a network. This has a number of benefits, such as centralized management, uniformity across media, and suitability for both in-building use and remote access. However, VPNs have not been standardized and may have implementation dependencies that can make them complex in operation. The Remote Authentication Dial-In User Service (RADIUS)[22] approach is also popular, and it can be effective for authentication of clients and servers. However, there is currently no support for mobility, no key distribution or support for key exchange, no inherent security features, and fundamental issues with latency that can interfere with roaming. Finally, there exists a range of proprietary techniques that have already been implemented, even by major vendors. The core common issues include lack of extensibility and compatibility with future WLAN products and standards. Though these approaches can be quite secure, their use may result in significant costs of introducing new network elements in the future. Clearly, an open, standards-based approach is the best.

Authentication ensures that only authorized users are allowed to access the network. Again, there are simple authorization techniques included in WLAN 802.11, such as the "SSID" which all clients must know in order to access the network. In some cases a simple mechanism for including or excluding a given wireless client from participation, such as an access control list, exists. However, as the entity being authenticated is a specific wireless network interface card (NIC) and not the human user, such approach results in creating a major security hole. More sophisticated authorization is required to ensure both network and data integrity. A single set of unified security techniques to manage both wired and wireless LANs is most desirable. The key to a successful security solution for a wireless LAN is meeting this requirement while supporting the key benefits of wireless access, most notably the users' ability to roam while remaining connected to the network [4].

Many encryption algorithms are currently used in IT, and the designers of the WLAN IEEE 802.11 standard included encryption in their original standard as released in 1997. Unfortunately, the "Wired Equivalent Privacy" (WEP) capability included in 802.11 has a number of weaknesses. Perhaps most notably, the key length in 802.11 is only 40 bits. This limit was included to meet export restrictions in place at the time 802.11 was ratified. A 40-bit key is quite easy to break given the inexpensive computer power available today. As a consequence, most vendors have implemented 128-bit or longer keys. While the 40-bit limitation in the standard will be removed in an update to 802.11, other problems remain. These include the lack of key distribution, key management (must be performed manually), key rotation (a security technique which changes security keys on a regular or irregular basis), and the fact that WEP only encrypts data over the wireless link, between an access point and a client. WEP also shares the same security keys among all WLAN users, creating a big opportunity for the WLAN to be compromised. In order to assure that data appears in clear text on authorized hosts, an end-to-end approach is required. Finally, it has recently been demonstrated that WEP (based on the RSA RC4 algorithm) can be broken in close-to-real time, and can no longer be relied upon when subject to a dedicated attack (such a passive attack is hardly observable in a wireless environment). Thus, WEP cannot be relied upon for complete security, and therefore network managers need to consider alternatives.

One of the most popular solutions is the reuse of the Kerberos [23] network authentication protocol, originally developed at MIT. As of version 5, Kerberos, being operating system- and application-independent, has been applied in a range of operating environments. Kerberos provides mutual authentication between a client and a server, and between servers before opening a network connection. Kerberos assumes that initial transactions take place on an open, insecure network, where packets can be monitored and even possibly modified at will. Such an assumption is accurate for today's Internet. What makes Kerberos particularly well-suited for WLAN is its low overhead. Its mutual authentication uses a technique that involves a *shared secret*, which works much like a password. Unlike many authorization techniques, including RADIUS, Kerberos does not send any keys or passwords in clear text – rather than sending the password, an encrypted key derived from the password is sent. This technique can be used to authenticate both sides of the communication. Once authentication takes place, all further traffic is encrypted, allowing even new encryption keys to be communicated securely. The aforementioned virtues of the Kerberos-based approach plus its independence from 802.11 technologies, makes it a valid choice for contemporary and future networks.

3   Wireless Radio Interference Issue

Introducing wireless technologies into medical environments presents a number of challenges.

Since wireless LANs use the same 2.4 GHz frequency band as medical appliances, radio interference in this spectrum should be carefully examined. This concern is often raised in relation to wireless LAN (WLAN) technology operation around medical devices [1].

The factors to be considered when deploying wireless networks in a medical environment include the location, frequency, and operating power of networking devices and the radio frequency immunity level of the medical devices. Radio devices using the 802.11b and 802.11g standards operate in frequency bands referred to as Industrial, Scientific, and Medical (ISM) which are allocated to these devices on a primary basis. Table 5-1 defines the frequency bands for ISM in comparison to the bands used by different standards of wireless networks, namely WLAN, the Unlicensed National Information Infrastructure – used in the USA and HyperLAN – used mainly in European countries.

Table 5-1 Comparisons of ISM and frequency bands used in different LAN standards [1]

Frequency	ISM	WLAN	UNII	HyperLAN
902-928 MHz	Yes	Yes		No
2400-2483.5 MHz	Yes	Yes		No
5150-5350 MHz	No	No	Yes	Yes
5470-5725 MHz	No	No	No	Yes
5725-5850 MHz	Yes	Yes	Yes	No

Wireless LAN radios operate at power levels five to six times lower than most cell phones or handheld radios, and on a non-interference basis. Non-interference means that they may not cause harmful interference but they must accept any harmful interference including even interference that may disrupt the service. Table 5-2 presents the frequencies and average values of effective isotropic radiated power (EIRP) for different types of devices.

Table 5-2 Wireless LAN Radios [1]

Transmitter	Frequency	Power output
Very high frequency (VHF) handheld radio	150 MHz	3 W EIRP
Cellular phone	900 MHz	3 W EIRP
WLAN PCMCIA card	2.4 GHz	100 mW EIRP

Interference between wireless networks and typical appliances such as hearing aids is very unlikely (although possible). For example, the feedback condition that may sometimes result from cordless and cellular phones used in close proximity to hearing aids is unlikely to occur with WLAN devices because they are not likely to come into direct contact with a user's body during normal operating conditions. Moreover, new medical appliances exhibit higher levels of radio frequency immunity than older models used to. Additionally, the interference was mostly caused by systems operating in the 900-MHz band.

Recommended Best Practices to minimize the potential of interference between medical equipment and WLAN infrastructure, defined in [23], are as follows:

1. Have a certified installer perform a professional site survey of the facility. This should include a comprehensive study of all devices operating in the radio frequency spectrum in the facility.
2. Have the system installed by qualified professionals.
3. Review the overall layout of the facility and determine areas containing devices prone to interference from wireless as well as various Internetwork status monitor (ISM) equipment. From this review, you can design antenna in which access point antennas are mounted several meters away from sensitive equipment to avoid possible problems.
4. Use only properly certified components for the system. This includes only using antennas certified for use with the radios.
5. Develop a frequency-management plan based on the spectrum survey to avoid interference from or with ISM and other onsite wireless equipment.
6. Consider reducing power or reorienting antennas if problems exist or appear. Consider performing some live tests based first on the ad hoc test methodology that is outlined in this document and then by conducting the more formal test procedure. We also recommend having either the manufacturer of the medical device in question or a third-party lab evaluate the system for operation in an environment with a WLAN. It is highly recommended that the ANSI C63.18 procedure be used.

Tests of WLAN equipment against medical devices are performed on an ongoing basis by a number of hospitals, medical device manufacturers, and even radio vendors.

4   Wireless Hospital Applications

In this section, typical applications of wireless technology in a modern hospital environment are considered. Particular attention is devoted to emphasizing advantages which mobility brings to standard medical procedures. The WLAN communication technology is the most frequently used one in this area of applications.

Computers and computer networks dominate our lives – and hospitals are no exception. In every modern hospital, a number of specialized systems operate. Three such systems will be presented shortly.

The goal of the **Hospital Information System** (HIS) is gathering, processing, and retrieving patient care and administrative information for all hospital activities. It also helps as a decision support system for the hospital authorities for developing comprehensive healthcare policies. The most important tasks of HIS systems [5], [8] can be divided into several groups:

- Storing patient data and monitoring their state:
  1. providing an accurate, electronically stored medical record of the patient, e.g. containing drug allergies,
  2. generating a visual or audible alert on workstation, CRT or printer at nurse station upon receipt of abnormal test results or other important data,
  3. specifying a time period during which no tests are permitted for a patient,
  4. processing data for statistical purposes and for research.
- Data flow and managing staff:
  5. supporting automatic transfer of patient data between outpatient and inpatient clinics,
  6. supporting the ability to display graphical, digitized diagnostic images from hospital digital imaging storage and retrieval systems,
  7. providing digital signatures to electronically approve orders,
  8. providing communication with Laboratory Information Systems (LIS),
  9. scheduling staff resources.
- Financial aspects:
  10. efficient administration of finance,
  11. monitoring of drug usage and ordering effectiveness,
  12. tracking and reporting on expected and actual treatment costs,
  13. automatically scheduling nurse staffing requirements,
  14. evaluating bed status and whole hospital performance.

Virtually all healthcare personnel in a hospital need to use a computer terminal in their everyday work. Cooperation and exchanging data via the Internet with external entities – other clinics, deliverers, etc. – is also a requirement placed on HIS systems. A popular scenario involves teleconsultations, when physicians consult their patients' cases with domain experts in other hospitals (see Section 6 for a case study).

Radiology Information Systems (RIS) specialize in management of radiology data. Their most important goals are as follows [7]:

- processing patient and film folder records,
- monitoring the status of patients, examinations, and examination resources,

- scheduling examinations,
- creating, formatting and storing diagnostic reports with digital signatures,
- performing profiling and statistical analysis.

Picture Archiving and Communication Systems (PACS) [6] have been designed to store digitally represented medical images in many so-called modalities (e.g. standard X-rays, CT, MRI, ultrasound and NMR) and allow images to be distributed electronically and interpreted on computer workstations. Thanks to digital representations, processing costs are reduced and patient healthcare is drastically improved. Patients and hospitals do not need to store film images any longer and instant simultaneous access to digitally-stored data from anywhere is possible immediately after processing and at any later time. PACS systems can be seen as a foundation of a totally digital hospital, with no film images, although for those situations, where films are still needed, the hospital will have the ability to print them.

When speaking of the influence of wireless systems on patient care and hospital operations, it has to be noted that mobile computer access can rationalize the functioning of virtually any large organization. Instant access to any piece of data from anywhere can make the enterprise less error-prone, faster and more efficient, leading to customer satisfaction. Nevertheless, one must be conscious of the fact that even the best wireless network is not able to help if the management computer system is not working correctly and suited to the enterprise's needs. This is why several of the above paragraphs have been devoted to HIS, RIS and PACS systems.

Adapting systems to a wireless reality can sometimes pose real problems. The issue is mainly in the limited resources (unless we consider laptop computers) of mobile devices. Tablet PCs, palmtops and other similar appliances are usually provided with small displays and have little in the way of memory, computing power, etc. This must be taken into consideration when expanding existing systems to include a wireless infrastructure. The case study presented at the end of this section partially addresses the issue in the context of a DICOM viewer running on a PDA device.

The advantages of using wireless networks in hospitals seen as enterprises, as mentioned above, are manifold. We will concentrate only on direct benefits for patients.

Patient care can be administered instantly. In hospitals, important decisions are often taken on the run – in halls or lifts. Thanks to a wireless infrastructure, the patient's complete Electronic Health Record (EHR) is accessible from anywhere. This seems to be especially important for patients requiring respiratory care, but even during routine visits at the patient's bed immediate access to EHR is desirable, since common practice used to involve a consulting team with files of paper charts, and sending nurses to collect missing documentation.

Sophisticated measurements and tests can be performed at the patient's bed with no necessity of taking him/her to a laboratory and the results can be immediately entered into EHR, thus eliminating the possibility of a mistake when copying data at a later time.

Specialized appliances – Point of Care (POC) terminals – can be attached to a patient, continuously monitoring his/her various vital functions depending on the illness or diagnosis. In an emergency, they are able to alert both nurses and doctors, who can be anywhere inside the hospital. In the future, so-called expert systems may try to automatically react on the alert and initiate appropriate procedures. In today's medical practice, POC terminals automatically administering the prescribed medicine doses are quite popular.

5 Case Study: Concept of an Environment for Mobile Medicine

Patients with chronic diseases require continuous care, but making them stay in hospitals would be very costly and would drastically lower their quality of life. In the case of patients with e.g. memory loss, expensive hospital care would be unreasonable. Today's preventive medicine is able to deliver long-term care to patients.

There exist a number of more or less advanced solutions allowing patients to feel safe at least at their homes, by being continuously monitored. They rely on PAN and WWAN wireless communication technology application. The simplest systems provide the patient with a remote alarm button in a watch (or similar appliance) which, when pressed in an emergency, connects the patient to an operator. A more sophisticated approach involves equipping the patient with devices, either implants or ones mounted externally, which monitor vital signs and can measure different quantities, such as glucose level, blood pressure, blood temperature or heart rate. (Sometimes they are even able to perform some actions, e.g. deliver insulin.) The quantities are then processed by a local monitoring system usually running on a PDA device or a home PC; exceeding the preselected threshold values triggers an alarm sent to an appropriate medical center. Reader interested in details of such solutions can consult [15], [17], or [18].

On the medical professionals' side, existing technology enables them to be equipped with small wireless computers allowing them to access patients' data or be notified by their monitoring systems whenever needed.

Current systems are based mainly on wireless personal area networks (PAN), thus overcoming the need to wire the patient's body. The standard used most commonly for communication in personal networks is Bluetooth [19]. Communication with a medical center is realized either by using a predefined static Internet connection, which limits the monitored area to patients' homes, or by using a wide-area GPRS connection.

The available wearable equipment is a basis for creating a personal medical environment, which can improve the quality of life of a chronically ill patient. It is important to distinguish the key components of such an environment, considering three different states of the chronically ill patient's life:

- stable state (e.g. the usual day of a diabetic) – in such a case, the personal environment may assist the patient in gathering and processing measurements of health-related parameters,
- dangerous state (e.g. reduction in blood sugar levels) – in such a case, the personal medical environment should start performing measurements more frequently and alert a medical center to pay attention to the patient,
- unstable state (e.g. loss of consciousness) – in such a case the personal medical environment should determine the location of the patient and alert a medical center to send an ambulance.

In order to perform the mentioned tasks, a personal medical environment should contain not only wearable sensors or implants, but some kind of an electronic agent able to process the measurements.

The e-soul concept. As proposed in our paper [20], the most innovative feature of this environment is the concept of an agent that is flexible enough to cooperate with many different sensors. Despite the diversity of places, environments and circumstances in which a patient may be situated, the agent should be able to pervade the medical environment in order to rescue the patient. That demanding task is taken on by the *e-soul*. The e-soul pervades the environment, i.e. gathers every piece of information from the patient monitoring sensors and – by "incarnating" into a hosting device – communicates the gathered results outside. Since there are many different types of devices (mobile phone, PDA, etc.) which the e-soul can use as means of communication, it needs to be able to utilize available network connections irrespective of their underlying technology.

Of course, there is no need to embed all of the above functionality into an e-soul. Some elements, such as network communication support, may be implemented in hosting devices; others – such as localization support – may be added as a wearable device (e.g. through wireless GPS-enabled devices) but all of them should be recognizable by an e-soul and taken into consideration when performing the required action. The key features of e-soul are as follows:

- Incarnates into hosting devices,
- Identifies and organizes a personal medical environment,
- Raises alerts,
- Operates autonomously.

Typically, a personal medical environment will consist only of a few sensors, but their number can increase dramatically when the patient changes his/her location (e.g. is transported to a hospital or is attached to many different sensors in an ambulance). The e-soul will contain the information needed by a hosting station to configure the patient's personal medical environment as well as to identify the patient. Moreover, it will perform some basic interpretation of the monitored parameters' values. It should be able to decide which data is important and should be stored and which can be discarded, and so forth. Moreover, the e-soul should be equipped with a set of rules needed for deciding whether to alert a medical center. Such a decision is taken by the e-soul without any support from outside. In that sense, the e-soul is an autonomous entity.

The e-soul can be understood as an immaterial entity which has only to interoperate with devices it incarnates into. However, the concept of an e-soul with functionality detailed above can be implemented by using a smart card. Using this "smart" piece of hardware, particular features may be implemented as follows:

- **incarnation into a hosting device** – the e-soul as software placed on a smart card is able to copy itself into and run on a hosting station; the functionality should be supported both by the e-soul and the host.
- **identification of a personal medical environment** – the software needed by wearable devices connected to the e-soul can be stored on a smart card and run immediately following incarnation or can be downloaded by using the hosting station's communication abilities.
- **authentication of a patient** – smart cards are equipped with specialized processors and memory for generating private/public key pairs and digital signing data. Along with certificates, this is the most straightforward solution for accomplishing the task of patient identification.
- **alerting** –specialized code performing this functionality may be stored on the smart card and run if needed.

- **autonomous activity** – smart cards offer memory space which may be used to store a critical subset of collected measurements. The code of the e-soul stored on a smart card can contain a set of pre-programmed decisions to be taken autonomously when it loses connection with the Internet (e.g. using hosting device's storage to save encrypted measurements).

Architecture of the system. In light of its importance, alerting a medical center is worthy of special note. The alerted center should have means of controlling the process of monitoring the patient (e.g. changing measurement sampling rate). Therefore, because of the diversity of monitoring centers and personal medical environments, the e-soul should expose some commonly understandable monitoring and management interface. That interface should be implemented by code transferred to a hosting station.

For remote medical support, the medical center carries all responsibility. Its importance has already been mentioned several times, earlier on. This section introduces its main functions. Figure 5-3 shows the key tasks of the center. The most essential one, called *Patient Remote Support*, means giving the patient a feeling of safety, and is performed in collaboration with the e-soul. The task consists of collecting measurements and alerts from the patient's personal medical environment. The alerts may result in *Case On-line Monitoring* in a dangerous state or even in *Emergency Action Initialization*, whenever the patient is in an unstable state. After an emergency team is sent to the patient, an important issue is *Emergency Action Guiding* — providing the ambulance with information on the patient's location and EHR, as well as recent measurements from his/her e-soul. All of the above may take place far from the patient's home monitoring center, in which case the *Patient EHR Localization* action occurs.

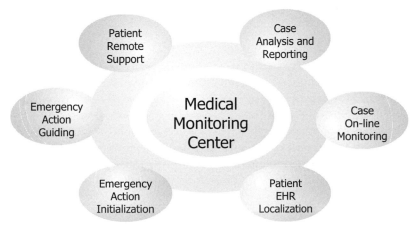

Figure 5-3 Roles of the Medical Monitoring Center.

As described, from the patient's point of view there is one **home monitoring center** and many possible **foreign monitoring centers**. As patients are mobile and may travel far from their original locations, it would be impossible to support them by their own monitoring centers, especially when an emergency team is to be sent. This task may instead be taken on by the nearest monitoring center.

The patient's home monitoring center should be distinguished for at least three reasons:

- it holds the patient's electronic health record (EHR),
- it is responsible for selecting the remote monitoring center to take care of a patient who is away,
- it is responsible for charging the mobile patient's insurance company.

All these tasks would certainly require formal agreements between medical sites. Moreover, to effectively support sharing EHR, the centers should implement a broker service operating continuously.

Irrespectively of the kind of monitoring center (home or foreign), it should be able to respond to an emergency signal either by starting continuous monitoring of the patient's state or – if needed – by sending an emergency team to the location indicated in the alert.

Handover between monitoring centers proceeds in the following way. The process is always controlled by the home monitoring center. In case of an emergency, the patient hosting station contacts the home center providing patient identity and localization and the reason for the alert. The home monitoring center localizes a remote monitoring center that is most suitable and closest to the current patient localization. In the next step, the selected center takes control over the patient.

The medical staff taking care of a patient who is monitored continuously should definitely be able to change locations. In some cases, a short textual information on a doctor's personal digital assistant (PDA) screen would be enough, unless a real emergency occurs. In a more complicated scenario, the doctor would need to download a part of the patient's EHR and e.g. review some X-ray scans. In general, the doctor changing locations should be able to "carry" a session containing some open files with him and continue to work on it in another place. For example, a doctor preparing for a surgical operation on a patient would like to transfer his notes to a screen installed in the operating room. From the system designer's point of view, there is a need to implement a mechanism for secure session transfer as well as a mechanism for adapting open sessions (that could contain various kinds of data) to the capabilities of end-user devices (varying from PDAs to diagnostic stations).

Scenario. To illustrate the usage of our conceptual system, let's imagine that John Smith, a 55-year-old scientist from Birmingham, has arrived in Krakow for a conference. Since he has undergone several serious surgical operations, including cardiosurgical ones, he must be continuously monitored. A few years before, he would surely have not decided upon such a journey. Fortunately, a new patient monitoring environment has been implemented all over Europe. Equipped with his three sensors and a mobile phone, John Smith feels safe. His personal e-soul, together with the hosting phone (or sometimes his pocket PC), continually process values acquired from sensors and, if the preset threshold is exceeded, it hands over control to the nearest center which begins monitoring Mr. Smith's state more accurately and prepares to help him immediately. The sole disadvantage for Mr. Smith is that he should remember to keep his phone charged and not forget to take it.

On the second day of his stay, Mr. Smith feels worse but his e-soul's hosting station does not indicate anything disturbing. He is tired and decides to take a walk in a nearby park, which is quite deserted, because evening is fast approaching. Suddenly he feels cold sweat and growing pain spreading through the upper body to the arms, neck and shoulders. His medical environment also realizes these worrying symptoms and initiates an alarm. Mr. Smith is unable to pick up the phone because he quickly loses consciousness. The alarmed monitoring center locates Mr. Smith's hosting station by means of GPS and hands over the treatment to the Krakow monitoring center, at the same time transferring part of his EHR. On the basis of the medical documentation and symptoms, one of Krakow cardiosurgical specialists is delegated to this case. His PDA device notifies him about the emergency just as he is on his way home. He comes back to the center and since there is no time to lose, he decides to look through the patent's documentation in the ambulance, which is ready to set off. In the meantime, the documentation is transferred to the ambulance where the doctor is acquainted with it. Thanks to GPS, finding Mr. Smith in a dark and empty park proves simple. From the documentation the doctor learns that Mr. Smith is allergic to a group of medicines and hence administers other medication. Help comes quickly enough to rescue Mr. Smith.

6 Case Study: Access to Radiology Database from Handheld Devices

Wireless handheld devices (PDAs) are become more and more advanced — not only capable of running simple local applications such as games and spreadsheets but also implementing applications which communicate over wireless networks and perform nontrivial data processing. These growing possibilities have allowed the authors to design and develop an application for remotely accessing DICOM images. A picture of the iPAQ device with the discussed DICOM viewer running is shown in Figure 5-4.

The application addresses the issue of home/street emergency access to a patient's medical radiology database over an IP network. In case of an emergency (e.g. a car accident) or during home visits, the medical personnel can review (but not change) the DICOM encoded radiology data and basic medical summary. In these scenarios, the hospital's data would be helpful when accessed as a reference. A small wireless appliance would be the most frequently used device, although, occasionally, laptop computers could be applied.

During the design phase, the idea of providing access through a Web browser was abandoned since the small sizes of PDA displays made the system hard to use. The final decision was to develop a standalone application. This helped organize the user interface optimally, with no overheads related to Web browsers and limitations of HTML access.

The layout of the application consists of several tabs devoted to different functions. The first of those tabs was designed for locating patients in the database; following ones are used for browsing through the chosen patient's data and, finally, viewing the selected image. The user interface has been constructed so as to be well suited to PDA requirements. Handheld devices usually come without a keyboard and so the virtual keyboard occupies a lot of area. This is why most actions can be performed with an easy-to-use touchstick.

The functional design of the viewer had to take into consideration its specified goals and limited resources. Nevertheless, the resulting functionality is quite rich and has been favourably accepted by radiology specialists from John Paul 2nd Hospital in Krakow. Several transformations can be performed on the downloaded DICOM image, including zooming and adjusting the Hounsfield window. Dynamic images can be animated. The user is also able to display the most important DICOM tags describing the patient and the examination associated with the image. The volume of radiology data could result in very large DICOM files, thus making bandwidth a critical issue. In order not to make the client very bandwidth-consuming (especially due to low bandwidth of GPRS networks), the database provides them with lower-quality (JPEG compressed) reference images useful for browsing.

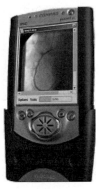

Figure 5-4 A view of an iPAQ device with DICOM viewer.

The application has been implemented in Java, making it fully platform-independent and capable of running on a number of devices. The only action required when porting is the reconfiguration of device display size and resolution. In the part responsible for DICOM file processing, the professional Java DICOM toolkit from Softlink (see http://www.softlink.be) has been used. Connections with the hospital database have been implemented using the next-generation IPv6 protocol, although traditional IP can also be used. Due to the fact that the system utilizes a public network, security mechanisms should be very strong. The user needs to be authenticated and verified (e.g. via a token or PKI), and the connection needs to be secure (i.e. encrypted). The transmission path encryption is assured by means of an HTTPS protocol suite performed by an HTTP server connected with the PACS system.

7 Case Study: GPRS Access to Database

In many cases it is impossible to assure the possibility of distant consulting for medical specialists who are away from the hospital area. Such a situation takes place when a quick medical consulting is essential for later medical treatment but should be done regardless of physician's current location and fixed access network availability. One and a very promising solution is the wireless access to the hospital systems. From among wireless networks especially the GSM system seems to be very interesting owing to the very good radio coverage and market penetration.

The GSM system offers a variety of different services to its subscribers. Besides a classic voice service, data transmission is a very important component of each GSM provider's commercial offer.

Until recently, GSM networks allowed the user to transmit data using one of the three basic services: CSD (Circuit Switched Data), HSCDS (High Speed Circuit

Switched Data) and GPRS (General Packet Radio Service). The first two of them are based on a circuit switched technique. It means that a data transmission in that mode requires a bi-directorial link reservation with constant data speed and delay in both directions, regardless of the amount of the transmitted data. GPRS is a typical packet switched technique.

In case of CSD or HSCSD, up to four time slots (of 8 for given frequency) within the TDMA frame is offered to the subscriber. Typically, the data transmission speed using one time slot is 9.6 kbps or 14.4 when no coding overhead is used and protection bits are replaced by the user's data. Depending on the coding scheme used, the data transmission speed in the HSCSD varies from 43.2 up to 57.6 kbps. Number of additional (more than one in CSD mode) time slots depends on current network load and the number of incoming calls within the BTS (Base Transceiver Station). The most important disadvantages of both circuit switched techniques are constant medium reservation, long connection negotiation phase before transmission and time based charging even when the user transmits no data.

The disadvantages of circuit switched transmission modes can be avoided in packet switched data transmission technique — GPRS. The most important innovations as compared with the techniques mentioned above are a permanent network connection, adaptive network resources sharing and a charging scheme based on the amount of data transmitted (sent and received). The GPRS offers the maximum throughput rate of 171.2 kbps. However, contemporary GPRS implementations and the terminal capabilities allow the user to achieve the transmission speed up to 57.6 kbps according to the current network load and the Coding Scheme (CS) used.

It is comparable to HSCSD but in fact the adaptive bandwidth allocation makes it more flexible. Depending on radio signal strength and link quality, a different number of bits can be allocated for protection and correction of the transmitted data. The higher the signal power level, the higher CS can be used. Commercial implementations of GPRS systems use the CS-1 and CS-2 schemes.

Nowadays the GSM providers offer more advanced third generation services such as: EDGE and UMTS. The main advantages of introducing EDGE and GPRS transmission supplemented with UMTS technology include the possibility of video calls and data transmission at the speed of up to 384 kbps.

A case study of GPRS service usage as a transmission bearer for accessing the telemedical system was performed. The researched system consists of two basic components: a server and several clients which connect to the server. The main idea of the system is to give physicians an access to a medical content, recorded and stored onto server as video sequences for the diagnosis purpose. The system architecture is shown in Figure 5-5.

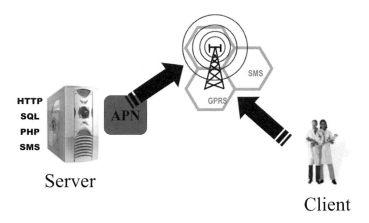

Figure 5-5 System architecture.

The main problem which was met during the trial phase was how to transmit multimedia content, especially video sequences, through a radio medium of limited bandwidth. The GPRS transmission channel, used during the connections, suffers from insufficient bandwidth. It results in long time delays which can be observed between the beginning of transmission and the displaying of first video frames at the client's terminal.

The other problem is that the radio channel characteristic varies in time even when the network load stays at the same level. Radio propagation phenomena result in bit errors, and consequently, packet retransmissions, as well as higher connection cost.

That is why the implementation of the content adjustment mechanism was expected to optimise the transmission as much as possible. The easiest way to improve transmission was the video sequences pre-processing.

Before a video sequence is recorded into the medical database, it is divided into smaller parts. Such a process, called an indexing mechanism, can be organised in two ways.

The first is based on the automatic splitting of a video sequence into smaller parts of equal size. The main advantage of such a solution is its full automation. The system operator sends recorded medical data onto server via a file transfer protocol. The stored data is extended with the id of the physician who would be responsible for the diagnosis and should be notified about a new stored record.

The next procedure is performed automatically by a specially designed application, run as a system daemon. Indexed video sequences are presented by a first video frame.

The other requires the medical specialist's support during the indexing process. The specialist selects only the most important parts of a video sequence and attaches text and voice comments. Such pre-processed data is then stored into the server database.

The following steps are identical for both types of indexing schemes. Right after the indexing procedure is done and the medical data is stored onto the system server the SMS (Short Message Service) module is run to notify the specified physician about the availability of a new record to be consulted on the server.

The SMS message about a new record to be consulted, which the physician receives, contains the medical record identification string and additional information about the priority of the record to determine the diagnosis urgency. The Physician connects his terminal to the medical server through the GPRS network and gateway – the APN (Access Point Node) of the hospital. After the connection is set up the physician's terminal is authorised by the hospital authentication centre.

Entering the distant diagnosis system as the first data of the patient, his personal data is shown, as well as his current medical state and previous diseases history. After that, the physician is granted the access to a medical video record containing the medical test result.

The visualisation panel allows the user to choose the most interesting parts of the whole video record and displays it on a mobile computer screen. The visualisation panel is shown in Figure 5-6.

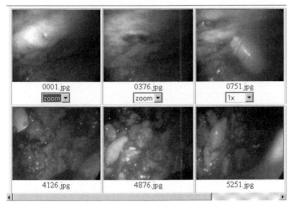

Figure 5-6 Visualisation panel.

The system user is able to choose the most proper quality of the video sequence displaying. The video sequence quality is strongly connected with displaying it in one of the three available resolutions. The higher the quality level and the resolution of the video frame, the longer a transmission delay via GPRS network. According to the tests performed during the system evaluation, GPRS transmission of a 30 second video of 300 kB size through the public GGSN (GPRS Support Node) lasts approximately two minutes.

The most important thing during the system development was to make it as little complicated and, at the same time, as flexible as possible. As a result of such an assumption, a typical web browser extended with a video sequences player plug-in was chosen as a client interface to the teleconsulting system. The video player plug-in is the Quick Time software from Apple characterized by a very high quality of compressed video and a quite small video file size.

All of dynamic layout formatting and the data processing are performed at the server's side. The server consists of the following components:
1. HTTP server daemon,
2. SQL compatible database,
3. and PHP script language interpreter,
4. SMS notifying module.

A typical internet browser as a client's interface allows for the seamless introducing of the system modifications without any reinstallations at the client's side. The server access is limited by server security mechanisms (i.e. transmission ciphering, users authentication) and mobile terminal authorised at the hospital APN.

The server needs to be maintained and managed by the system operator through the control panel. Typical system operator's activities are:
1. creation and management of the physician's system accounts,
2. contacts management (i.e. updating contacts to physicians),
3. emergency service schedule management,
4. video sequences processing and storing,
5. security configuring against non-authorised access.

During the system evaluation a public GGSN (GPRS Support Node) gateway was tested. Transmission scenarios based on freely available gateway result with frequent connection losses and long delays in packets delivery. Thus, real system implementation should be based on private APN which will extend the system security and eliminate packets delays.

8 Summary

The application of wireless systems in the e-health domain is very promising, although it is at the same time a very challenging task. Even though current modern mobile technologies are ready to fulfill any requirements of such systems, much has to be done on the medical side. The chapter shows that the implementation of a system similar to the one described in the conceptual part is desired not only on an experimental scale but at least all over the continent. Establishing such a network requires international effort and standardization of medical data exchange, medical procedures and legal agreements across the globe. Cost-effective environment construction is also a challenging requirement. While this seems to be a very long-term process, mobile medicine will definitely play a very important role in the future.

9 Bibliography

[1] IT Papers, *Wireless LAN Equipment in Medical Settings: Addressing Radio Interference Concerns*, http://www.itpapers.com
[2] Symbol – The Enterprise Mobility Company, *The Wireless Hospital Extending the Reach of Your Information System Directly to the Point of Activity*, http://www.symbol.com/products/whitepapers/whitepapers_wireless_hospital.html
[3] *Wireless Technology Overview* http://solutions.intergraph.com/core/white_papers/WirelessTech2004 3513A.pdf
[4] *Technology for a Secure Mobile Wireless LAN Environment: Evolution, Requirements, Options,* http://whitepapers.zdnet.co.uk/0,39025945,60026245p-39000582q,00.htm

[5] Online Consultant Software, *Hospital Information Systems,* http://olcsoft.com/HIS.htm

[6] The George Washington University Hospital, *Picture Archiving Communication System,* http://www.gwhospital.com

[7] Gannot I. *Hospital Information System,* http://www.eng.tau.ac.il/~gannot/

[8] Centre of Development of Advanced Computing, Sushrut, *A Hospital Information System,* http://www.cdacindia.com/html/his/sushrut.asp

[9] Flanagan D., Farley J., Crawford W., Magnusson K. *Java Enterprise in a Nutshell. First Edition.* O'Reilly, 1999

[10] Gabrick K., Weiss D. *J2EE and XML Development,* Manning Publications Co., 2002

[11] Gamma E., Helm R., Johnson R., Vlissides J. *Design Patterns. Elements of Reusable Object-Oriented Software.* Addison-Wesley, 1995

[12] Kwamura R., Stadler R. *Active Distributed Management for IP Networks,* IEEE Communication, Vol.38, No.4 April 2000

[13] MOBILEIP Working Group, Internet Engineering Task Force: http://www.ietf.org

[14] Leeper D. R. *A Long-Term View of Short-Range Wireless,* IEEE Computer, June 2001

[15] Zieliński K., Cała J., Czekierda Ł., Zieliński S. *Collaborative Teleradiology* Proceedings of 4th International Conference Computational Science - ICCS 2004, Springer LNCS 3039, p. 1172 ff, June 6-9, 2004, Krakow

[16] Digital Angel Corporation, http://www.wirelessrerc.gatech.edu/tutorial/digitalangel.html

[17] American Medical Alarms, http://www.americanmedicalalarms.com/

[18] Welch Allyn http://www.monitoring.welchallyn.com/

[19] The Official Bluetooth Membership Site, https://www.bluetooth.org/

[20] Zieliński K., Cała J., Czekierda Ł., Zieliński S. *A Concept of Environment for Mobile Medicine,* International Conference on e-Health in Common Europe, June 5-6, 2003, Krakow

[21] NetRAAD PACS, http://www.uhc.com.pl

[22] RFC 2865: *Remote Dial-In User Service: RADIUS,* http://www.faqs.org/rfcs/rfc2865.html

[23] *Kerberos: The Network Authentication Protocol,* http://www.mit.edu/kerberos/www/

[24] *Wireless LAN Equipment in Medical Settings: Addressing Radio Interference Concerns,* www.cisco.com

6 Relevance of Terminological Standards and Services in Telemedicine

Rolf Engelbrecht[1], Josef Ingenerf[2], Jörg Reiner[1]

[1] GSF National Research Center for Environment and Health, Institute for Medical Informatics, Munich-Neuherberg, Germany
[2] Medical University Lübeck, Institute for Medical Informatics, Lübeck, Germany

Efficient and effective delivery of healthcare requires accurate and relevant knowledge, patient-centred clinical data and medical information. While medical language is a useful means for human communication it has serious drawbacks when trying to make use of free text in terms of searching and evaluating data. This is because there are inherent phenomena like synonymy and ambiguity within every natural language. Either the data has to be analysed using linguistic algorithms or the data has to be entered in a structured and standardised way. Both approaches are dependent on the availability of terminological systems. There are many more reasons behind the need for knowledge such as "glaucoma *is an* eye disesase", "iris is a part of the eye" or "'Grüner Star' is synonymous with 'glaucoma'". The following Figure 6-1 gives an overview of the main reasons. First, there is a need for supporting the capturing of data – either by (dictated) free text, linguistic analysis and reconstruction of the semantics afterwards or by structured data entry and perhaps free-text generation afterwards. A terminological standardisation is needed for safe communication between humans, i.e. the communicated data has to be re-interpreted in other contexts. That is even more important when the data is communicated and interpreted by machines. Standardised terminology is important for searching and selectively presenting (through views) the data at different stages of patient care. All the so-called secondary usages of the data in Figure 6-1 are only possible if the once-entered primary data can be reused for that purpose. Therefore, the vocabularies should be as expressive as possible, to allow for generating arbitrary views and aggregations. For example the integrated linkage to online available literature or guidelines or the integration of knowledge-based systems is only possible if the patient data is based on standards, e.g. for a decision rule concerning contraindications of antibiotics, if the patient uses a medication called "penicillin" there is a need for knowing that "penicillin is an antibiotic". Furthermore, terminological standards are used for defining prospective payment systems. Finally, the entered data will be used for aggregation and statistical evaluation with respect to a defined population of patients. This usage depends fundamentally on the comparability of data collected. As we will see in the next section, so-called statistical classifications are used with clear definitions of classes in order to count every case uniquely, resulting in sound figures.

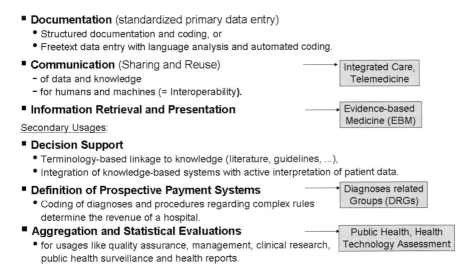

- **Documentation** (standardized primary data entry)
  - Structured documentation and coding, or
  - Freetext data entry with language analysis and automated coding.
- **Communication** (Sharing and Reuse) → Integrated Care, Telemedicine
  - of data and knowledge
  - for humans and machines (= Interoperability).
- **Information Retrieval and Presentation** → Evidence-based Medicine (EBM)

Secondary Usages:

- **Decision Support**
  - Terminology-based linkage to knowledge (literature, guidelines, ...),
  - Integration of knowledge-based systems with active interpretation of patient data.
- **Definition of Prospective Payment Systems** → Diagnoses related Groups (DRGs)
  - Coding of diagnoses and procedures regarding complex rules determine the revenue of a hospital.
- **Aggregation and Statistical Evaluations** → Public Health, Health Technology Assessment
  - for usages like quality assurance, management, clinical research, public health surveillance and health reports.

Figure 6-1 Reasons and targets for the use of standardised terminology in healthcare.

Figure 6-1 mentions associated special disciplines that are "hot topics" in the field of healthcare. They have a somewhat catalytic effect on the importance of the usage of standardised terminology in related healthcare applications. Besides evidence-based medicine with its impact on the topic of "providing relevant, actual and sound knowledge at the point of care", diagnosis-related groups and the interrelation between the quality of coding diagnoses and procedures with accounting and public health (with its focus on cost-benefit assessment of different healthcare components like instruments, therapies or care plans) we want to focus on the first topic, i.e. "integrated care" or "shared care" and "telemedicine". The main challenge is the interoperation of humans and especially computer-supported applications between several institutions.

The target for interoperability is to offer an exchange of clinical data between computer-based applications; e.g. for multicountry communication a chip card can be considered as a transparent device for all healthcare users regardless of card technology or contents. The information necessary to treat the patient as well as security functions will have to be available in the preferred language of the health professional. Under strict security conditions, authorized healthcare personnel will be able to read and write information locally or remotely.

The interoperability of health information systems is therefore defined as follows:

"Interoperability of computer-based health information systems is the ability to access, use and update computer-readable data issued by any health information system, healthcare organization, and healthcare facilities to the extent that accessing, managing and processing this data is possible for those healthcare facilities and healthcare professionals that are legally authorised."

Interoperability has to be seen on four levels:
- data, a common definition of the content;
- technical, enabling the use of different environments;
- data presentation, in order to integrate the different applications;
- security, to ensure a trustful environment.

1   Terminology

Terminology is defined as a collection of terms used in specific (scientific) fields. Collecting a terminology, defining and hierarchically organizing concepts as well as providing synonymous terms and codes as concept names are the basic steps for building classification and nomenclatures, as the intermediate step to coding[9]. There are different approaches for standardising terminology on several levels of granularity depending on its purposes. In Figure 6-2 those approaches are characterised and described along with their intended usages.

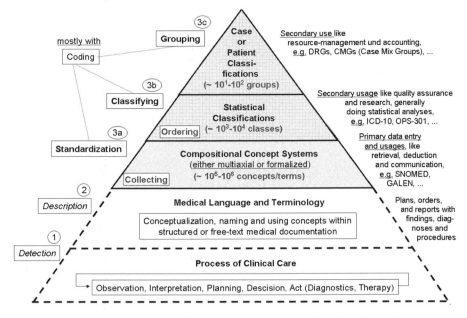

Figure 6-2 Terminological standardisation on several levels of granularity.

Already at the bottom level, within the process of clinical care, there is a selective iterative process of observing and interpreting phenomena in order to come to a decision in terms of examinations and other acts, that again produces data that has to be interpreted. Determining a diagnosis is also a judgement, that condenses real-world phenomena on a more abstract level. On the next level, all the produced data has to be expressed in a medical language and terminology. Otherwise, the observed and interpreted facts would be impossible to document and communicate. In order to standardise free text, data composition concept systems are used. It should be as expressible as possible for a standardised representation of the millions of terms that are necessary in medical language. Multiaxial systems like the one used within the SNOMED nomenclature or formal concept systems like the one developed in the GALEN project should be used for primary data entry. Otherwise, once-entered data would be impossible to reuse for other "secondary" usages as mentioned in Figure 6-1. Next, on level 3b there is another perspective on standardisation: not the patient-specific aspects but the population-specific aspects are of interest for supporting statistical evaluations of comparable data sets. For that reason statistical classifications like ICD-10 are used, in order to provide disjoint and exhaustive classes that are less expressive (for instance, ICD-10 entails about 12,000 classes). These classifications are used e.g. for quality assurance or clinical research. They are also used for defining prospective payment systems on the next level. Here, at the top of the pyramid, reside patient classification systems

(PCS) which, like DRGs, provide statistical classifications, called groupings, that are even less expressible. There are several hundred groups that are comparable with respect to the economical expense of cases. DRGs are used for calculating case expenses and, after that, for accounting.

Consequently, there seems to be a trade-off between losing information and improving order. However, the expressive concept systems on level 3a should be used for primary data entry, and the statistical classifications on level 3b should be aggregated on top of that for specific secondary purposes. Without level 3a the entered data cannot be reused successfully for purposes not known in advance (due to loss of information).

1.1 Existing Classifications and Nomenclatures

In the following sections we present some details of the most important standardised terminologies in terms of classifications, nomenclatures and thesauri.

1.1.1 The International Statistical Classification of Diseases and Related Health Problems, 10th revision — ICD10

The ICD is a classification system developed collaboratively by the World Health Organization (WHO) and ten international centers.

The Tenth Revision of the International Statistical Classification of Diseases and Related Health Problems is the latest in a series that was formalised in 1893 as the Bertillon Classification or the International List of Causes of Death. While the title has been amended to make clearer the content and purpose and to reflect the progressive extension of the scope of the classification beyond diseases and injuries, the familiar abbreviation "ICD" has been retained. The ICD-10 was approved by the World Health Organization in 1990 and has been available for implementation since 1993.

ICD-10 classifies diseases, injuries and causes of death, as well as external causes of injury and poisoning. The classification has 21 chapters with alphanumeric categories and subcategories. ICD-10 contains about 8,000 categories that are valid causes of death. ICD-10 uses 4-digit alphanumeric codes compared with 4-digit numeric codes in ICD-9. ICD-10 has an alphanumeric format with a code size ranging from 3 to 5 characters. Valid ICD-10 disease codes include three-, four- and five-character codes e.g. R11 Nausea and vomiting, J20.6 Acute bronchitis due to rhinovirus, M08.00 Juvenile Rheumatoid Arthritis. The range of ICD-10 codes is A00.00 to Z99.99. The Morphology code range is M0000/0 to M9999/9 [14], [7]. ICD-10 is published in three volumes.

Volume 1 — Tabular List:

The first volume, which runs well over 1,000 pages, contains the classification at the three- and four-character levels, the classification of the morphology of neoplasms, special tabulation lists for mortality and morbidity, definitions and the nomenclature regulations.

Volume 2 — Instruction Manual:

The second volume consolidates notes on certification and classification formerly included in Volume 1, supplemented by a great deal of new background information, instructions and guidelines for users of the tabular list.

Volume 3 — Alphabetical Index:

The final volume presents the detailed alphabetical index [24].

Overview of ICD-10 Chapters and Code Ranges [3]:
I   Certain infectious and parasitic diseases (A00-B99)
II   Neoplasm (C00-D49)
III   Diseases of the blood and blood-forming organs and certain disorders involving the immune mechanism (D50-D99)
IV   Endocrine, nutritional and metabolic disease (E00-E99)
V   Mental and behavioural disorders (F00-F99)
VI   Diseases of the nervous system (G00-G99)
VII   Diseases of the eye and adnexa (H00-H49)
VIII Diseases of the ear and mastoid process (H50-H99)
IX   Diseases of the circulatory system (I00-I99)
X   Diseases of the respiratory system (J00-J99)
XI   Diseases of the digestive system (K00-K99)
XII   Diseases of the skin and subcutaneous tissue (L00-L99)
XIII Diseases of the musculoskeletal system and connective tissue (M00-M99)
XIV Diseases of the genital urinary system (N00-N99)
XV   Pregnancy, childbirth and the puerperium (O00-O99)
XVI Certain conditions originating in the perinatal period (P00-P99)
XVII Congenital malformations, deformations and chromosomal abnormalities (Q00-Q99)
XVIII Symptoms, signs and abnormal clinical and laboratory findings not classified elsewhere (R00-R99)
XIX Injury, poisoning and certain other consequences of external causes (S00-T99)
XX Eternal causes of morbidity and mortality (V00-Y99)

XXI Factors influencing health status and contact with health services (Z00-Z99)

1.1.2 ICPM International Classification of Procedures in Medicine

The German ICPM (International Classification of Procedures in Medicine) is a classification of clinical procedures, describing diagnostic, surgical or other conservative procedures. The ICPM serves scientific statements, quality assurance and the representation of insurance claims and is an obliging basis of procedure documentation.

The ICPM is the German translation, adaptation and extension of the ICPM-DE (International Classification of Procedures in Medicine, Dutch Extension), based on the ICPM-WHO. The Friedrich-Wingert-Foundation is responsible for the maintenance, development and extension of the ICPM. Since 1994 Version 1.0 has been used by hospitals for routine applications of classifications. In further developments of the ICPM, the SNOMED nomenclature will be incorporated.

The main chapters of the ICPM cover:
- Diagnostic procedures,
- Prophylactic procedures,
- Surgical procedures,
- Other therapeutic procedures,
- Additional procedures.

Drugs, laboratory and radiological procedures are not included in the German version.

The concepts are arranged in a hierarchy. Each concept has a six-character alphanumeric code. The nomenclature is organized into six levels of hierarchy.

The following is a sample of the six-level hierarchy:
- Chapter: e.g. 5 — surgical procedures,
- Group: e.g. 5-010 to 5-049 — surgical procedures on the nervous system,
- Category: e.g. 5-01 — incision and excision on the skull, brain and meninges,
- Subcategory: e.g. 5-010 — cranial puncture,
- Five- or six-character extension: e.g. 5-010.0 — cisternal puncture.

The groups are ordered by the type of procedure. An exception is made in the chapter "surgical procedures". Here a topographic-anatomical order by organs and body systems is used. The German version of the ICPM is available as a book or in three different CD-ROM versions [10]. The ICPM version 2.1 (Operationenschlüssel nach Paragraph 301 Sozialgesetzbuch V (OPS-301)) provided by DIMDI — the German Institute for Medical Documentation and Information — is available online [5]. Unfortunately, in order to modify the German procedure classification OPS with respect to the needs of the German DRG-system (G-DRGs), the newer versions of the OPS and the ICPM are no longer compatible.

1.1.3   SNOMED Systematized Nomenclature of Human and Veterinary Medicine

The SNOMED Systematized Nomenclature of Human and Veterinary Medicine is a broad-based, comprehensive clinical terminology and knowledge base, developed and maintained by SNOMED International, a non-profit division of the College of American Pathologists.

SNOMED is a structured nomenclature and classification system created for indexing the entire medical record, including signs and symptoms, diagnoses and procedures. The terms are placed into natural hierarchies, each represented by a six-digit alphanumeric termcode. SNOMED International is updated annually; version 3.5, released in 1998, contains more than 150,000 terms. Additionally the ICD-9 terms and codes are incorporated, mostly along the Disease/Diagnosis axis. SNOMED International contains 11 axes:

- Topography (anatomy): A functional anatomy for human and veterinary medicine (13,165 records),
- Morphology: Terms used to name and describe structural changes in disease and abnormal development (5,898 records),
- Function: Terms used to describe the physiology and pathophysiology of disease processes (19,355 records),
- Disease/diagnosis: A classification of the recognised clinical conditions encountered in human and veterinary medicine (41,494 records),
- Procedures: A classification of healthcare procedures (30,796 records),
- Occupations: Developed by, and used with permission from, the International Labour Office in Geneva, Switzerland (1,949 records),
- Living organisms: Living organisms of etiological significance in human and animal disease (24,821 records),
- Chemicals, drugs and biological products: Including pharmaceutical manufacturers (14,859 records),

- Physical agents, forces and activities: A compilation of physical activities, physical hazards and forces of nature (1,601 records),
- Social context: Social conditions and relationships of importance to medicine (1,070 records),
- General linkage modifiers: Linkages, descriptors and qualifiers to link or modify terms from each module (1,594 records).

Of particular note is the systematised, multiaxial and controlled vocabulary.

Terms in SNOMED are all arranged in a hierarchy, represented by an alphanumeric term code where each digit represents a specific location in the hierarchy. For example, T-20000 represents the respiratory system; T-28000 the lungs; and T-28010 the alveoli. Multiaxial refers to the ability of the nomenclature to express the meaning of a concept across several axes. For example Tuberculosis (D-0188) affects the lung (T-28000), is caused by M. Tuberculosis (E-2001), appears as Granuloma (M-44060) and causes Fever (F-03003).

A controlled vocabulary allows the user to record data in the patient's record using any one of a variety of synonyms, but references it back to a single primary concept. For example the preferred term Atopic dermatitis, NOS (D0-10130) has the synonyms Allergic eczema, Besnier's prurigo, Atopic neurodermatitis, Allergic dermatitis, Prurigo of Besnier and disseminated neurodermatitis [13].

SNOMED International is rapidly being accepted worldwide. The American Veterinary Medical Association and the American Dental Association have adopted/endorsed SNOMED for their use. The American College of Radiology/National Equipment Manufacturers Association will be using a subset of SNOMED in their Digital Imaging Communication Standard (DICOM). SNOMED Clinical Terms will be a medical terminology resource that combines the content of SNOMED RT with the United Kingdom's Clinical Terms Version 3 (formerly known as the Read Codes V3) [23].

1.1.4   Medical Subject Headings MeSH

The Medical Subject Headings, published by the National Library of Medicine, consists of a controlled vocabulary used for indexing articles, for cataloguing books and other holdings and for searching MeSH-indexed databases, including MEDLINE. The MeSH vocabulary is continually updated by subject specialists in various areas.

There are more than 19,000 main headings in MeSH. In addition to these headings, there are 103,500 headings called Supplementary Concept Records (formerly Supplementary Chemical Records) within a separate chemical thesaurus. There are also thousands of cross-references that assist in finding the most appropriate MeSH heading, for example, "Vitamin C - see Ascorbic Acid". MeSH consists of a set of terms or subject headings that are arranged in both alphabetic and hierarchical structures. MeSH is a principal component vocabulary of the Unified Medical Language System (UMLS®) [15].

The Medical Subjects Heading is divided into two sections: Alphabetic List and Tree Structures. The Alphabetic List section contains the subject headings arranged in alphabetic order with cross-references. The tree structure is a list in which the subject headings are divided into categories. Most categories are further divided into subcategories, identified by an alphanumeric designation. The terms in each subcategory are arranged hierarchically, in up to seven levels, from the most general to the most specific.

MeSH Categories:
- Analytical, Diagnostic and Therapeutic Techniques and Equipment Category E,
- Anatomy Category A,
- Anthropology, Education, Sociology and Social Phenomena Category I,
- Biological Sciences Category G,
- Chemicals and Drugs Category D,
- Diseases Category C,
- Geographical Locations Category Z,
- Healthcare Category N,
- Humanities Category K,
- Information Science Category L,
- Organisms Category B,
- Persons Category M,
- Physical Sciences Category H,
- Psychiatry and Psychology Category F,
- Technology and Food and Beverages Category J [19].

1.2   Unified Medical Language System (UMLS)

The Unified Medical Language System (UMLS) is a product of the U.S. National Library of Medicine, published since 1986. The UMLS is meant to be consulted and used by application programs to interpret and refine user queries, to map the user's terms to appropriate controlled vocabularies and classification schemes and to assist in structured data creation. UMLS shows the source vocabularies with the properties of structure and contents transparent on the level of concepts. This view brings the vocabulary-inherent relationships and relations together on the level of concepts. Therefore UMLS is a complex and quantitative comprehensive collection of concepts, terms, strings and relations between them, originating from the included standard vocabularies [17].

UMLS consists of four main components: Metathesaurus, Semantic Network, Information Source-Map and the Specialist Lexicon.

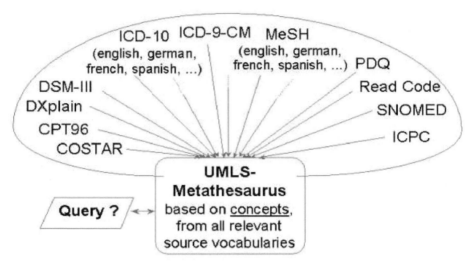

Figure 6-3 UMLS-metathesaurus integrating most relevant medical vocabularies, taken from [12].

The Metathesaurus is the central vocabulary component of the UMLS, based on hierarchies and associations, which are inherited from the source vocabularies and attached to the unique UMLS concept. The purpose is to link alternative names and views of the same concept together and to identify useful relationships between different concepts. Each concept or meaning in the Metathesaurus has a unique concept identifier (CUI). The Metathesaurus is built from most of the relevant medical vocabularies like ICD-9, ICD-10, SNOMED, MeSH, Read Code and COSTAR.

The 2001 edition of the Metathesaurus includes about 800,000 concepts and 1.9 million concept names in different source vocabularies. New in the 2001 Metathesaurus are: DDB00, Malcolm Duncan's Diseases Database 2000; ICD10AM, the Australian Modification of ICD10; ICPC2E, International Classification of Primary Care 2nd Edition Electronic Version; ICPC2P, International Classification of Primary Care, Version 2-Plus, Australian

Modification; and MTHICD9, NLM-generated entry terms for ICD-9-CM. The Semantic Network is a network of the general categories or semantic types to which all concepts in the Metathesaurus have been assigned. Through the Semantic Network the concepts are associated with the generic types (disease or syndrome) or relations (is_a, associated_with, etc.) [11].

The Information Source map contains meta-information concerning medical online-resources. The Specialist Lexicon contains linguistic information (e.g. Diabetes) about medical terms. Syntactic, morphologic and spelling information, necessary for natural language processing, is also included [21], [18].

1.3 Related Standards: HL7 and RIM

HL7 is a communication standard based on the needs described in level 7 of the ISO reference model. However, the new version 3 [9] "represents a significant departure from 'business as usual' for HL7. Offering lots of optionality and thus flexibility, the V2.x series of messages were widely implemented and very successful. These messages evolved over several years using a 'bottom-up' approach that has addressed individual needs through an evolving ad-hoc methodology."

HL7 version 3 addresses several issues by using a well-defined methodology based on a reference information (i.e., data) model (RIM). It will be the most definitive standard to date and is already the basis for several ongoing developments. The German health telematics architecture will use it for all levels of care. Version 3 creates messages using RIM in an object-oriented development methodology. RIM provides an explicit representation of the semantic and lexical connections that exist among the data carried in the fields of HL7 messages and constitutes a single model of healthcare information requirements. It uses XML encoding.

The RIM consists of six classes modelled in UML:

Act
represents the actions that are executed and must be documented as healthcare is managed and provided. Subclasses include "observation" (i.e. examination), "procedure" describing treatment, but also administrative ones, such as "FinancialTransaction".

ActRelationship
describes the relationship of "acts" e.g. between an order entry and its results/reports.

Entity
represents all beings (humans, animals) and objects in the healthcare system. A sample subclass is "LivingSubject" which again contains the subclass "person".

Participation
describes the context in which an "act" is performed: who performed it, where it was performed, etc.

Role
describes the roles of entities engaged in "acts". Important subclasses are "patient" and "employee".

RoleLink
describes relationships between the various roles.

The classes are linked either by a set of association relationships, identified by unique role names, or by generalization relationships. Each of these elements includes a textual definition. The appearance of attributes and associations is controlled by cardinality and related constraints applied to the attributes and to the roles that link the associations to the classes.

The HL7 Vocabulary Domain Values table is organized alphabetically by domain table name or domain name and includes a mnemonic code, concept identifier, print name and definition/description for each coded value (abstract domains are not assigned codes).

The External Domains table is organized alphabetically by domain table name and includes the domain name, concept identifier, the source code system, a defining expression for extracting the domain from the source system, and a description.

The HL7 Domain Tables and Coded Attributes Cross-reference Tables are organized alphabetically by domain table name in column one, and lists the coded RIM attribute(s) and/or the data type components that are supported by that vocabulary domain. For RIM attributes, the data types and assigned coding strengths are also shown. Both the RIM attributes and the data type components are hyper-linked to definitions in their respective documents.

2 The TOSCA Project

2.1 Terminological Standardization within TOSCA

A system has been developed within the TOSCA project to establish a common terminology. As an example in the next paragraph a solution for glaucoma is described. The terminology system enables the integration of different systems and services with patient data management systems and provides a basis for structured documentation and reports. The terminology module provides terms and definitions for medical concepts that are in accordance with international standards (ICD, SNOMED, MeSH, etc.). It also provides the functionality necessary for maintaining the consistency of medical contents and other components.

2.1.1   Terms for Glaucoma

Terms concerning glaucoma relevant for the TOSCA project have been collected according to the structure used for diabetic retinopathy. As no prior experience and sources could be derived from the OPHTEL project, the terms for glaucoma were collected from the following sources:

- The American Academy of Ophthalmology, Preferred Practice Pattern: Primary open-angle glaucoma suspect, 1995,
- The American Academy of Ophthalmology, Preferred Practice Pattern: Primary open-angle glaucoma, 1996,
- The American Academy of Ophthalmology, Preferred Practice Pattern: Primary angle-closure glaucoma, 1996,
- Duane's Ophthalmology on CD-ROM, Lippincott-Raven Publishers, 1996
- European Glaucoma Society: Terminology and guidelines for glaucoma, 1998,
- Shields, M.B., Krieglstein, G.K.: Glaukom, Springer Verlag, 1993,
- Hoskins, D., Kass, M.: Diagnosis and Therapy of the Glaucomas, The C.V.Mosby Company, 1989.

The terminology version for Glaucoma contains ca. 470 terms assigned to the following groups: patient data, anamnesis, finding, examination, laboratory finding, diagnosis, differential diagnosis, disease, treatment, medical treatment, organ part, organ function, risk factor, hormone, healthcare activity, therapeutic or preventive procedure, substance.

Each term is described by the following identifiers:

- TOSCA Concept Identifier (TCP);
- Semantic Type: e.g. Findings, Diagnosis;
- Preferred Term: Preferred term of the UMLS Metathesaurus. In case the medical concept could not be referenced by one of the vocabularies of the UMLS the preferred term corresponded with the term used in the medical source;
- Synonyms: Synonyms and abbreviations;
- German translation of the concept;

- Parent concepts: The terms are ordered in a hierarchical structure. Each medical concept belongs to a parent concept;
- Description: If available, a short definition out of the medical source was included to specify the concept;
- Description of the UMLS: If available, additional the semantic type and the definition from the UMLS Metathesaurus was added;
- CUI: Unique identifier for the Metathesaurus concept from the UMLS to which a term and string are linked.

The following coding systems were used as resources to identify the project-relevant concepts, terms and codes:
- ICD_10 Code: International Statistical Classification of Diseases and Related Health Problems (ICD-10). 10th revision. Geneva: World Health Organization, 1998,
- SNMI98: Code of the Systematized Nomenclature of Human and Veterinary Medicine: SNOMED, International. Version 3.5. Northfield: College of American Pathologists; Schaumburg: American Veterinary Association, 1998,
- RCD99: Clinical Terms Version 3 (Read Codes). England: National Health Service Centre for Coding and Classification, March, 1999,
- MSH2001: Medical Subject Headings (MeSH). Bethesda: National Library of Medicine, 2001,
- ICPM code: Codes of the International Classification of Procedures in Medicine, Version 1.1,
- ICPM-International Classification of Procedures in Medicine, Version 1.1 from 29.09.1995, published by DIMDI (German Institute of Medical Documentation and Information),
- ICPM, International Classification of Procedures in Medicine, Friedrich-Wingert-Stiftung, Version 1.0. Blackwell, 1994.

For identification, the following systems were used:
- MUSTANG-Terminology Server, MEDWIS-Arbeitskreis "Terminologie", Client Tool: UMLS-Accessibility Tool of MUSTANG (ORACLE-DBSystem mit UMLS-Daten; Web-Server zur Visualisierung), http://mustang.gsf.de/. MUSTANG provides access to various UMLS-based coding systems, especially to the vocabularies used in this project (ICD, SNOMED, Read Code, MeSH, ICPM),
- UMLS Knowledge Source Server, Metathesaurus; https://umlsks.nlm.nih.gov/.

2.1.2   Data Dictionary for Glaucoma

A central data dictionary is a prerequisite for the integration of systems and subsystems. It defines the syntax and semantics of data. The data dictionary contains definitions of parameters, including data types, value sets, units, etc., that are used for the documentation of data. The Data Dictionary for Glaucoma is based on the TOSCA Glaucoma screening data model. About 40 datasets are described as follows:

- Preferred term: The preferred term from the terminology system;
- TCP: TOSCA Concept Identifier from the terminology system;
- Name of Parameter: Name used in the screening data model;
- Unit: e.g. year, mm Hg;
- Datatype: Enumeration single (only one value can be selected from a list), Enumeration multiple (selecting more than one value is allowed), Date, Boolean (yes or no), Integer (value with comma), Real (value without comma), String (text);
- Value Set: Concept identifiers were also assigned to each value set;
- Title/Tooltip: Name for the user interface;
- Description for the documentation;
- Comments.

2.2   MUSTANG Terminology Server

The MUSTANG terminology server (Medical UMLS-based Terminology Server for Authoring, Navigating and Guiding the Retrieval to heterogeneous Knowledge Sources) is being developed to support indexing and data-recall facilities. MUSTANG, a CORBAmed-based central multilingual terminology server, provides the semantic foundation for a repository of XML-document forms. MUSTANG delivers terminological services to applications by standardized interfaces and provides access to terminology resource related to the Unified Medical Language System (UMLS). In addition, MUSTANG provides functions to retrieve medical information from Internet knowledge sources (e.g. PubMed) via MeSH-based queries. MUSTANG is implemented on a Windows platform using the ORACLE database management and development software [11], [12], [22].

The terminology, together with forms and IP protocols, represents the pivotal element for communication of patient-related data between sites and services. The terminology service is a basic feature of future infrastructures. One of the major drawbacks in communications between different medical systems in the past (at the information exchange level) was the use of different terminologies. Descriptive definitions and terminologies vary between countries and even between physicians in the same country. To achieve data integration on a semantic level, TOSCA has worked to build a standardized terminology.

Numerous coding systems (e.g. SNOMED nomenclature, MeSH thesaurus, ICD-10 and ICPM classification) can be used as a possible basis for standardization. However, these key systems are standalone vocabularies and are inadequately maintained as far as software engineering is concerned. With the aim of creating an "ophthalmology platform" health service, a suitable architecture of terminological services with a clearly defined server has been established. This server communicates with the information broker and subsystems as well. All TOSCA applications rely on a telemedical infrastructure for communication, based on established and new technical standards, such as XML for data transfer via networks, DICOM for image transfer and HTTPS for the interaction of different application systems within the telemedical communications infrastructure. All sensitive patient-related data is transferred according to European safety standards. The communication platform includes brokering services, telescreening, image processing, a reference image database and a monitoring system.

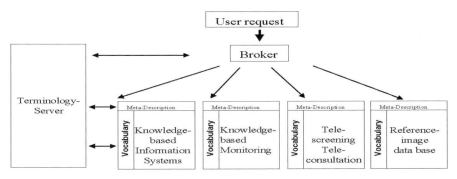

Figure 6-4 The architecture of the MUSTANG Terminology Server.

To enable integration of different systems and services, developed within the TOSCA project, as well as of patient data management systems, a standardized ophthalmological terminology for Glaucoma and Diabetic Retinopathy has been developed. Selected medical terms have been adopted from previous and current European projects (e.g. OPHTEL, MUSTANG) and adjusted for the TOSCA project. New terms relevant for TOSCA have been added to the terminological component.

The terminological component is the basis for structured documentation and reports. Descriptive definitions, hierarchical relations among concepts and language-specific terms of a common terminology for Diabetic Retinopathy and Glaucoma are provided. The terms and definitions for the medical concepts are in accordance with international standards (ICD, SNOMED, MeSH, etc.) The terminology also provides the functionality necessary for maintaining the consistency of medical contents and other components.

A central data dictionary is a prerequisite for integration of systems and subsystems. It defines the syntax and semantics of data. The data dictionary contains definitions of parameters, including data types, value sets, units, etc., that are used for documenting data. The basic resources of an evaluated TOSCA terminology are various coding systems and vocabularies that are relevant to the project. These extensive resources have to be managed by a special information system (for usability reasons). In TOSCA two such systems are used within this task: the MUSTANG Terminology Server and the KAMATO® terminology management module.

2.2.1   TOSCA Terminology in KAMATO

The terminological concepts for diabetic retinopathy and glaucoma are also stored in a KAMATO terminology module. KAMATO stands for Knowledge Acquisition and Management Tool, a system developed by AdaKoS GmbH. The Terminology Component of KAMATO ensures terminological control of knowledge bases and enables access to Internet knowledge sources (e.g. PubMed) via MeSH-based queries.

With the aid of a special search function, terminological concepts available in the UMLS Metathesaurus are automatically imported into KAMATO from the MUSTANG server. The preferred term, synonyms, source codes and (if available) semantic types and descriptions are added as well. KAMATO supports the following coding systems: UMLS-CUI, ICD-9, ICD-10, MeSH, Read Code, SNOMED 2, SNOMED Int 3.5, HL7 Terminology, WHOART, ICPM, ULMER and BLS. Further coding systems can be added on request.

The concepts are arranged in a hierarchical order, in parent–child concepts. Figure 6-5 presents the parent concepts of the TOSCA terminology project. Figure 6-6 shows the hierarchical order of the "Eye disease" concept.

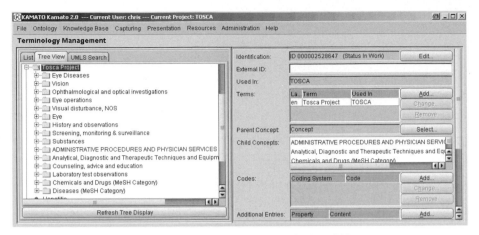

Figure 6-5 Terminology module of KAMATO.

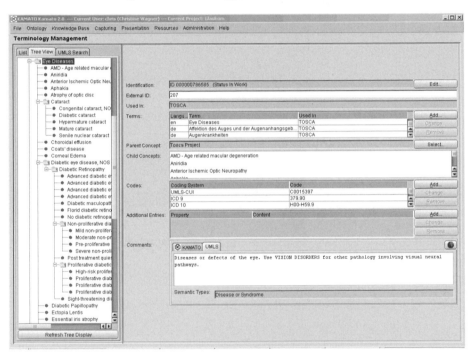

Figure 6-6 Terminology module of KAMATO: Hierarchical order of the "Eye disease" concept.

With the terminology module of KAMATO, the ophthalmological concepts for diabetic retinopathy and glaucoma can be presented in structured hierarchical order. The MUSTANG terminology server allows new concepts, based on UMLS, to be imported automatically. The structured order and the clear user interface allow easy and fast maintenance of the terminological concepts as well as multilingual usage.

Within the TOSCA project, the terminological concepts in KAMATO are used for the "Patient-centred Knowledge-based Information System for Glaucoma". The concepts provide the basis for indexing documents and contents of the knowledge base. Indexing enables terminological control of the knowledge base and accurate retrieval of documents and knowledge contents (Figure 6-7).

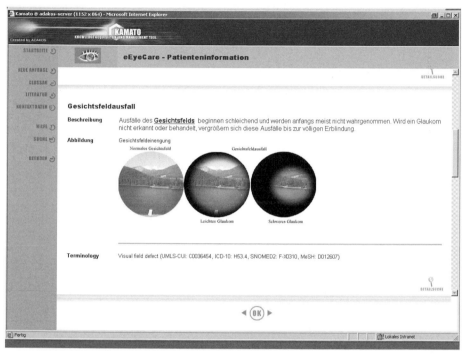

Figure 6-7 Patient-centred Knowledge-based Information System for Glaucoma:
preferred term and code set for "Visual field defect".

The terminology module of KAMATO also enables access to Internet knowledge sources (e.g. PubMed) via MeSH-based queries (Figure 6-8).

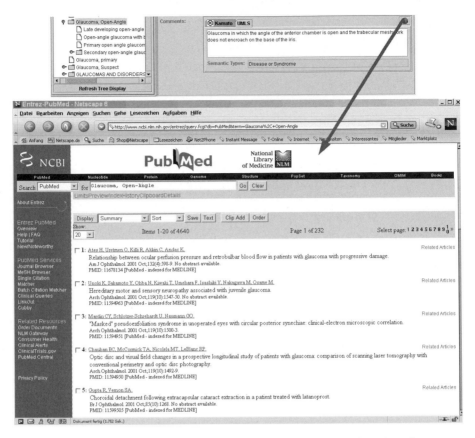

Figure 6-8 Access to PubMed via KAMATO: Publications on the selected term
"Glaucoma, open-angle".

2.2.2   Data Sets

Terminologies and data sets are closely related. Within the GALEN project the
DIABCARD data set has been used as a basis for a terminology server which
was then applied for developing a medical information system. It turned out
that additional effort is needed to harmonize data sets and terminology with the
goal of implementing interoperable EHRs.

The EFMI Special Topic Conference 2003 was held in Rome, under the heading
"The content of the Electronic Health Record: Clinical datasets for continuity
of care and pathology networks". Its working hypothesis was as follows: *Clinical
Dataset describes the set of predefined data Entries stored, shared or presented as a unit within
clinical applications, messages and EHR systems. A Clinical Dataset is able to describe a*

particular aspect of the patient's status, of a procedure, of a clinical document in relation to a given health issue or task, across heterogeneous contexts.

A set of recommendations was developed on the basis of the current situation in healthcare telematics:
- standardization efforts on the HER,
- need for sharing and aggregating clinical information,
- need for clinical datasets to improve the coherence of HER contents,
- a gradual process of convergence on clinical datasets.

The participating experts agreed on 20 recommendations, which were grouped under the following headers:
1. create a network of organizations interested in clinical datasets, within the context of the ongoing actions on HER;
2. stimulate the production and systematization of clinical entries (a kind of archetype) and clinical datasets (a kind of template),
3. define the role of the responsible organizations and produce the guidelines for accurate documentation on packages of clinical datasets,
4. set up a repository of templates, based on a standard processable formalism,
5. set up a gradual process of convergence, assisted by the repository of templates.

Group 4 is of particular interest in the context of terminology:
- Production, retrieval, distribution, implementation, comparison and systematization of clinical datasets should be facilitated by setting up a suitable repository of templates – with an appropriate version control – and by stimulating the production of authoring tools;
- The upload and download of the descriptions of clinical datasets to and from the repository of templates, as well as their usage, should be free of charge;
- Several organizations have already developed their own clinical datasets, according to a specific local formalism. It is expected that suitable software tools will be able to assist in the semiautomatic translation and refinement of the existing clinical datasets into a unique standard formalism, possibly passing through a set of intermediate formalisms convenient for developers and users of each particular type of clinical data set.

The collection of data sets has just started. Initial results will be discussed at a continuation workshop in October 2004 and will be available on the EFMI web pages (www.EFMI.org).

3 Summary

Specialist terminology has always been used in the medical field for communication between professionals. In early days it was Greek- and Latin-based and not to be understood by others, especially the patient. Coding was used for the analysis and description of diseases and the healthcare system. Structured documentation for better communication and easy data entry has been a step forward in exchanging clinical data between professionals, based on classifications.

The Internet is changing existing habits. More than 60% of adults in some countries have access and 75% of them use the Internet to look for healthcare information[14]. This fact is influencing the decisions of patients regarding treatment etc. Terminology has to be adapted to the consumers' clinical and mental models of diseases and their treatment. This will be a challenge for the coming years and it has to take into account the fact that health professionals also have to be knowledgeable about health consumers and their communication profiles. Health telematics stands a chance of benefiting all participants in the healthcare setting; first, however, it needs to organize the communication, storage and retrieval of data and knowledge as well as the structuring of information in a global healthcare system.

4 Bibliography

[1] Baud, R., *Natural language processing in the EHR context*, in: Contribution of Medical Informatics to Health, Blobel, B., Gell, G., Hildebrand, C., Engelbrecht, R. (eds.), AKA, 2004, 85.

[2] Beolchi, L., *Telemedicine Glossary 5th edition*, EC, 2003.

[3] Canadian Institute for Health Information (CIHI), ICD-10, *CCI and Implementation Information*, July 2004; http://secure.cihi.ca/cihiweb/dispPage.jsp?cw_page=codingclass_e.

[4] *Clinical terminology, NHS Information Authority*, July 2004; http://www.nhsia.nhs.uk/snomed/pages/ct_general.asp.

[5] Deutsches Institut für medizinische Dokumentation und Information – DIMDI: *Operationenschlüssel nach Paragraph 301 SGB V*, Internationale Klassifikation der Prozeduren in der Medizin, ICPM - Version 2.1 vom 2004; http://www.dimdi.de/de/klassi/prozeduren/ops301/.

[6] Diekmann, D., Peters, C., Diekmann, F., *The role of terminology in European HIS*, in: Contribution of Medical Informatics to Health, Blobel, B., Gell, G., Hildebrand, C., Engelbrecht, R. (eds.), AKA, 2004, 22-23.

[7] Duke University Medical Center, *Links to coding systems*; July 2004; http://nestor.duhs.duke.edu/DHTS/web.nsf/resources.

[8] Hasman, A., *Education and training in health informatics: the IT-EDUCTRA project*; International Journal of Medical Informatics, 50(1-3), 1998, 179-185.

[9] Health Level Seven (HL7), http://www.HL7.org.

[10] *ICPM Internationale Klassifikationen der Prozeduren in der Medizin*, Friedrich-Wingert-Stiftung, Blackwell Wissenschaft, Berlin, 1994.

[11] Ingenerf, J., Reiner, J., Seik, B., *Standardized Terminological Services enabling Semantic Interoperabilitiy between Distributed and Heterogeneous Systems*, International Journal of Medical Informatics, 64, 2001, 223-240.

[12] Ingenerf, J., Reiner, J., MUSTANG: *Wiederverwendbare UMLS-basierte terminologische Dienste*, Proc. Medical Informatics Europe MIE 2000, Hannover, 77 (2000): 685-690.

[13] Kudla, K.M., Rollins, M.C., SNOMED: *A Controlled Vocabulary for Computer-based Patient Records*, Journal of AHIMA; 1998 American Health Information Management Association; http://www.ahima.org/journal/features/feature.9805.2.html (last accessed 2001).

[14] National Center for Health Statistics, Centers for Disease Control and Prevention, *A guide to state implementation of ICD-10 for mortality*, July 1998.

[15] *National Library of Medicine; Medical Subject Headings*, July 2004; http://www.nlm.nih.gov/pubs/factsheets/mesh.html.

[16] *National Library of Medicine; UMLS Knowledge Sources, 12th Edition*, January 2001.

[17] *National Library of Medicine; UMLS Knowledge Sources, 14th Edition*, November 2003.

[18] *National Library of Medicine; UMLS Unified Medical Language System*, July 2004; http://www.nlm.nih.gov/research/umls.

[19] *National Library of Medicne, MeSH Medical Subject Headings; Supplement to Index Medicus*, Vol. 31, 1990.

[20] Reference Information Model, HL7 RIM Version 2.02, HL7 2004, http://www.hl7.org.

[21] Reiner, J., *Information-Retrieval medizinischer Daten mit Unterstützung durch einen Terminologie-Server*, GSF-Medis Institut, 1999.

[22] Reiner, J., Ingenerf, J., Glander-Höbel, C., *Terminologie-Server und Informationsbeschaffung als eine exemplarische Anwendung*, 43. Jahrestagung der GMDS, Bremen, MMV Medien & Medizin Verlag, 1998, 239-242.

[23] SNOMED International; http://www.snomed.org/.

[24] The International Statistical Classification of Diseases and Related Health Problems, tenth revision - ICD10, 2004, WHO; http://www.who.int/whosis/icd10/descript.htm.

[25] The Read Codes, CAMS Computer Aided Medical Systems, 1999.

[26]Zeng, Q., Kogan, S., Ash, N., Greenes, R. A. A., Boxwala, A., Characteristics of Consumer Terminology for Health Information Retrieval, Methods Inf Med, 41, 2002, 289-298

7   Electronic Health Records

Dipak Kalra[1], David Ingram[1]

[1]   Centre for Health Informatics and Multiprofessional Education, UCL, London, UK

Clinical care increasingly requires healthcare professionals to access patient record information that may be distributed across multiple sites, held in a variety of paper and electronic formats, and represented as mixtures of narrative, structured, coded and multimedia entries. A longitudinal person-centred electronic health record (EHR) is a much-anticipated solution to this problem, but the challenge of providing clinicians of any profession or speciality with an integrated view of the complete health and healthcare history of each patient under their care has so far proved difficult to meet. This need is now widely recognised to be a major obstacle to the safe and effective delivery of health services, by clinical professions, by health service organisations and by governments internationally.

From an academic vision in the late 1980s the EHR has evolved to become centre stage in the national health informatics strategies of most European countries, and internationally. Health services and vendors are now actively establishing national infrastructures to enable the communication of high volumes of clinical information, and incorporating the necessary security features to protect these data.

International research has highlighted the clinical, ethical and technical requirements that need to be met in order to effect this transition. There is a need for interoperability standards that can permit clinical computer systems to share health record data whilst preserving faithfully the clinical meaning of the individual authored contributions within it. Concerns about protecting the confidentiality of sensitive personal information must also be addressed if consumer confidence is to be maintained when EHRs are widely accessible.

There are many challenges and cultural changes facing the safe and effective delivery of contemporary healthcare services:

- the requirement to limit healthcare costs and to optimise resource utilization,
- the shift of care from specialist centres to community settings,
- the requirement to deliver evidence-based and quality-assured care,
- the growth of consumerism and patient active participation in health care,
- equity of access and public involvement in priority setting,
- an increasing complexity of healthcare provision,
- an increasingly distributed and mobile clinical workforce,
- changes in the working patterns and accountability of healthcare professionals,
- the overwhelming growth of medical knowledge,
- a critical reliance upon comprehensive patient records,
- increasing concerns about the confidentiality of patient records.

Smith suggests [62] that traditional models of healthcare services have been associated with inefficient and inequitable healthcare, favouring expensive specialised interventions over some more useful measures to provide support for patients and families at home. Information technology may enable a more patient-centred approach to healthcare: quality measures focused on individual patients' needs and experiences of care; services actively involving each patient in their self-management and providing care close to each patient's home and community.

Such a model depends on the capacity of information technology to support people, communications and workflow in highly distributed teams. It also requires a change of emphasis from the top-down specification of data collection serving a contractual model of healthcare delivery to the facilitation of data collection supporting the seamless flow of each patient between care providers and the continuity of their care over a lifetime.

The application of information technology to modernise health services has progressively become a key political issue. In his 1997 State of the Union address, President Clinton declared that "we should connect every hospital to the Internet, so that doctors can instantly share data about their patients with the best specialists in the field" [14]. This promise has recently been translated at the Presidential level into a US national strategic plan [24].

The UK Government has made promises of NHS modernisation. Realising the EHR is a core target of, for example, the UK National Health Service IM&T strategy [11]. Health Secretary Alan Milburn has pledged that every adult will soon be able to access his or her own at-a-glance electronic healthcare record

[21]. There is now a recognised urgency for a National Health Service longitudinal care record, for example to reduce the frequency of inappropriate and unsafe prescribing, to facilitate adherence to guidelines of best practice across enterprise boundaries and to increase consumer choice [16]. The National Programme for IT (NPfIT) has embarked on a ten-year plan, and currently committed £6.2 billion, to create a fully integrated electronic care record for the whole of England [15].

The NHS "big bang" approach, which is the largest current IT procurement programme on the planet, is in stark contrast to equivalent projects in, for example, Canada's Infoway [2] and Australia's HealthConnect [4] projects. In those countries the intention is to foster a network of regional projects, encouraged towards strategic alignment and interoperability through national co-ordinators and selected key infrastructure elements. In many countries there is also a recognition that a national solution will not in itself prove sufficient for our increasingly global society – international standards are needed to help ensure that patients and healthcare workers can experience a joined-up health service across national borders.

There is now an international momentum to establish the standards by which patient health record information can be shared between healthcare providers and follow patients as they move between them. Ilias Iakovidis, Project Officer for the European Commission's Health Telematics programme, identified that an important challenge for realising successful EHR implementations at a national or regional level includes "the storage, maintenance, communication and retrieval of multimedia information on heterogeneous and geographically distributed database systems" [32]. Rogers, in reviewing the report "Enabling Mechanisms for Global Health Networks" for the G7, suggests that the main challenges to realising a global health information society include data meanings, structures and database navigation [54].

1   Challenges Facing Clinical Care

Much is changing at the core of clinical practice, and the health record is today facing challenges for which paper systems are not adequate. Healthcare professionals need to document increasing volumes of information, as patients receive more complex and data-intensive care. More detailed records are also needed to demonstrate competence, to cover the increasing risk of litigation and to justify use of healthcare resources [65], [64], [66], [50], [22].

The delivery of safe and effective (i.e. evidence based) healthcare is a challenge for all clinicians, particularly as the extent of medical errors is becoming apparent. The US Institute of Medicine report "To Err is Human" has estimated that 100,000 US citizens die each year through medical errors [37]. These possibly rank as the eighth leading cause of death in the US, and contribute 4% ($37.6 billion) to the cost of US healthcare [3]. Surprisingly high rates of missing or erroneous information have been confirmed in a number of studies [68], [25], [71]. The widescale use of decision support and alerting systems that interact with patient records is considered an essential informatics solution to the prevention of errors [7], [72], [56].

Healthcare professionals need to share healthcare information with a growing range of professional colleagues, often on multiple sites. Patients are often under the care of more than one team or speciality at the same time: for example, a diabetic patient may be under a diabetologist, an ophthalmologist, a nephrologist, a dietician, a wheelchair clinic, their GP and a District Nurse. The National Health Service in England alone handles 1 million admissions and 37 million outpatient attendances per annum, requiring high quality and efficient communications between 2,500 hospitals and 10,000 general practices. Records also need to be efficiently transferred when a patient moves and seeks care at a new institution.

However, significant problems can arise in continuity of care if salient information is not communicated. Figure 7-1 shows the situations of high clinical risk regarded by east London GPs as requiring urgent communication from hospital [41]. East London GPs were asked to indicate the clinical situations in which they perceived their ability to care for a patient safely would be compromised by a delay in receiving notification from hospital. In these circumstances most GPs indicated that the relevant hospital doctor should personally notify them by telephone rather than rely on fax or letter.

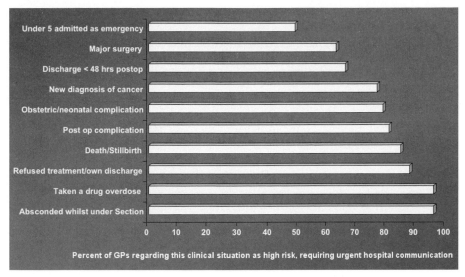

Figure 7-1 High-risk clinical situations requiring urgent communication from hospital to GPs.

The clinical requirements for which information technology solutions are needed are in the areas of [48]:

- improving multi-professional partnerships and clinical decision-making through ethically and legally acceptable access to patient record information and enhanced communication systems,
- developing an integrated knowledge environment that delivers evidence about best practice, clinical guidelines and educational materials directly to the clinical "coal face",
- promoting systematic clinical practice, for example through data templates, clinical protocols and integrated care pathways, embedded within patient records,
- providing patients with relevant education and support to enable good practice in their own self-management,
- enhancing clinical performance by collecting feedback from patients on the various aspects of their care,
- stimulating a culture of evidence-based practice by linking results from clinical audit with professional educational programmes and resources.

Patient care increasingly requires clinical practitioners to access detailed and complete health records in order to manage the safe and effective delivery of complex and knowledge-intensive healthcare, and to share this information within and between care teams. Patients nowadays also require access to their own EHR to an extent that permits them to play an active role in their health management. These requirements are becoming more urgent as the focus of healthcare delivery shifts progressively from specialist centres to community settings and to the patient's personal environment.

However, much of the fine-grained clinical information on which future care depends is still captured into paper records or within isolated clinical databases. Even very modern computerised health information systems limit the ability of users to extract clinical details in a form that can be communicated to other such systems, and few products can import clinical information received from external systems.

The main way in which integrated healthcare has been managed up to now, apart from via paper-based letters and reports, has been through defined sets of electronic messages, transmitted for example using EDIFACT or HL7. Most national health services have adopted a suite of these messages to support purchaser–provider communications, organisation and service administration, billing, and to communicate healthcare interventions for public health purposes. However, few such messages have been developed to support the clinical shared care process itself and, where they have been, these tend to be condition-specific such as for the management of diabetes or for antenatal care.

Present-day computerised systems have hitherto mainly been used to collect easily structured data, such as the reasons for encounters, chronic disease reviews and physiological measurements. Where such information has been entered methodically it provides a valuable resource for audit and for population analyses. Clinical governance activities require a more detailed analysis of clinical findings and actions than has hitherto been recorded in most computer systems, to present and compare performance and outcomes in ways that are readily understood by a wide range of professionals and by patients. Although the traditional approach of specifying audit data sets can support the evaluation of quality in individual clinical areas, this approach does not scale to the wide range of healthcare services that good practice now requires to be monitored. The process really needs to be underpinned by a comprehensive and longitudinal EHR.

Integrated care pathways (ICPs) combine medical knowledge, workflow guidance and a multi-professional record within one convenient tool. The EHR needs to be able to represent the workflow processes that have given rise to the care acts being documented, and to permit workflow systems to interrogate the EHR from a care pathway perspective. Although ICPs are gaining in popularity as they integrate the records of multiple professions, they also isolate the information gathered about each clinical problem within individual ICPs. They can therefore still fail to provide an integrated health record centred on the patient.

In the US Medical Records Institute's Survey of EHR Trends and Usage [69] over 70% of respondents regarded the need to share patient record information between different healthcare sites as the major clinical driver for EHRs. This, and much other research, would suggest that interoperability and faithful communication should be key requirements underpinning the specification of an EHR, in addition to data quality and clinical service governance.

The problem is complex because much of clinical meaning is derived not from individual data values themselves but the way in which they are linked together as compound clinical concepts, grouped under headings or problems or associated with preceding healthcare events during the act of data entry or data extraction. The medico-legal nature and accountability of healthcare delivery places additional requirements on the rigour with which health record entries are attributed, represented and managed. The ability to communicate this information efficiently in a mutually comprehensible way is crucial to achieving progress towards shared care, improved quality of care and effective resource management.

In 1998 Shortliffe wrote [60]:

> "System integration has emerged as a key element in the reinvention of environments for patient data management and health promotion. The ability to achieve the future vision of integrated health records depends in part on current research initiatives related to the role of the global information infrastructure in supporting health and health care.... Health care provides some of the most complex organizational structures in society, and it is simplistic to assume that off-the-shelf products will be smoothly introduced into a new institution without major analysis, redesign, and cooperative joint-development efforts."

His views remain pertinent today.

2 Visions of a Comprehensive EHR

There are many perceived benefits of using EHR systems to acquire, organise and view health record data. Duplicate data entry can be avoided if information is captured, maintained and communicated securely and consistently, in line with clinical needs. The same information can be displayed and viewed in a variety of ways, for example by problem or episode or through summaries, as well as in the traditional chronological order. Standard data sets and templates to assist in their capture and communication can be defined and adapted as practice evolves. A patient record may be accessed from any terminal on a network (even by multiple users simultaneously), and communicated electronically to support seamless shared care. Systems can deliver real-time alerts and decision support on the basis of medical knowledge and information previously documented about each patient.

In 1991 the US Institute of Medicine committee on improving the patient record published a classic report that powerfully endorsed these potential benefits and has shaped US and international thinking about the computer-based patient record (CPR) [17]. This report defined the CPR as

> "an electronic patient record that resides in a system specifically designed to support users through availability of complete and accurate data, practitioner reminders and alerts, clinical decision support systems, links to bodies of medical knowledge, and other aids."

The report proposed the above view of the CPR as the standard for electronic medical records. Its key recommendations were that the CPR:

- contains a problem list,
- supports measurement of health status,
- states the logical basis for decisions,
- can provide a lifelong record of events,
- addresses patient data confidentiality,
- is accessible for use in a timely way at any and all times by authorised professionals,
- allows selective retrieval and formatting of information,
- can be linked to both local and remote knowledge, literature, bibliographic and administrative databases,
- can assist in the process of clinical problem solving,
- supports structured data collection,
- can help individual practitioners and healthcare providers to manage and evaluate the quality and cost of care,
- is sufficiently flexible and expandable not only to support today's basic information but also the evolving needs of each clinical specialty and subspecialty.

In [70] Waegemann defined five levels of Electronic Health Record, of which Level 5 extends the vision of the Electronic Medical Record of the CPRI.

"The more comprehensive term "electronic health record" includes wellness information and other information that is not part of the traditional health care delivery process. Wellness information can include lifestyle and behavioural information captured personally by the individual or by a clinician, parent, or other caregiver".

The health record is an important tool supporting quality in clinical care. It is today used by personnel trained in different disciplines, working in different settings, on different sites and in different languages. These include:

- patients themselves and their appointed carers,
- clinicians, in therapeutic or anticipatory care roles,
- groups of clinicians working in primary or secondary care,
- paramedical colleagues working with the patient,
- clinicians and clerical or research staff undertaking clinical audit or quality assurance,
- hospital and general practice managers and healthcare purchasers (health authorities or insurers) undertaking quality assurance,
- healthcare planners at hospital, practice, district region or national level,
- legal advisors for the patient or the clinician,
- clinical researchers,
- medical students and medical teachers,
- commercial product developers for market research (e.g. the pharmaceutical industry),
- insurance companies for determining payment, or assessing risk,
- politicians, health economists, and journalists.

Just as there will be many different parties by whom it is accessed, the record can play many roles in the provision of care to individuals and to populations. The following list of roles for the EHR is a consolidated set derived from [6], [36], [26], [49] and collated by Heard et al. [28].

Table 7-1 Roles for the electronic health record

Supports consumer involvement
Protects personal privacy and reinforces confidentiality
Provides a consumer view of information
Accommodates consumer decision support and self-care
Ensures accountability of health professionals
Accesses information for the consumer
Supports consumer healthcare

Forms the basis of a historical account
Anticipates future health problems and actions
Describes preventative measures
Identifies deviations from expected trends
Accommodates decision support
Supports communication
Supports continuing, collaborative care and case management
Accesses medical knowledge databases
Allows automatic reports
Supports email generation and electronic data interchange (EDI)
Enables record transfer
Enables record access when and where required
Supports selective retrieval of information
Supports management and quality improvement
Enhances the efficiency of healthcare professionals
Supports continuing professional assessment
Facilitates management tasks and reduces routine reporting
Demonstrates and improves cost-effective practice
Accommodates future developments
Provides a legal account of events
Provides justification for actions and diagnoses
Supports population healthcare
Supports policy development
Provides evidence for development and evaluation of programs
Supports enquiry and learning
Supports clinical research
Assists with clinical audit
Supports medical education

This list of roles contains many possible conflicts of interest, for example those that would favour a narrative over a structured entry to retain expressiveness. EHR systems will need to support the creation of and access to health records for a wide range of information requirement contexts, whilst prioritising those of direct benefit to individual patients and to the immediate processes supporting their clinical care [36].

The EHR needs to represent responsibilities and intentions within the shared care process in order to support effective clinical workflow and to recognise the differing culture of nurses and doctors in the way information is used, even if the information itself is held in common.

Telemedicine is a major and expanding means of supporting distributed clinical decision making, for example by delivering expertise from centres of excellence to peripheral/community settings. This field of informatics poses requirements for the EHR to capture the substance of a tele-consultation, including the clear accountability for conclusions reached, for determining a clinical management strategy and for confirming the roles and responsibilities for effecting that strategy [1].

Remote monitoring systems (tele-monitoring) permit clinicians to assess their patients' condition on a frequent basis without the need for the patient to journey to a hospital or GP surgery, offering a new means of communication between patients and clinicians. They can also provide a valuable means to empower patients to play an active role in tailoring their own healthcare, provided that feedback on the acquired data is offered to them. A major drawback to contemporary tele-monitoring devices and systems is their use of a specific data structure to represent the acquired data, and often a specific exchange format for their communication back to a repository server or processing system. Patients frequently have multiple health problems, and it would be a pity if efforts on harmonising their health record information between enterprises were confounded by a diversity of incompatible information resources around their very person.

Computers offer tremendous opportunities to place patients in control of their own healthcare [61], and see them as informed partners in decisions about their own healthcare and in service priority setting [53], [10], [51]. Patients can acquire considerable expertise in managing their own health if they are given useful and appropriate material with which to educate themselves [12], [46], [38], [5]. A third of US home Internet users seek online health advice before calling their physicians [13].

Analyses of the utilisation of healthcare resources to investigate cost-effectiveness or equity of care are often limited by the lack of clinical detail to explain the individual circumstances behind a patient management decision. For cxample GP consultation rates, the admission rates to hospital and length of stay are all influenced by a wide range of socio-economic and health factors other than the patient's primary diagnosis. EHR systems need to be able to identify relevant patient characteristics to inform commissioning decisions and to reduce inequalities in access to service. For public health surveillance purposes, these kinds of analyses across population health records are needed in real time.

3 Characteristics of a Good EHR

Good health records are not just a scattered accumulation of health-related data about individuals. Entries are made as formal contributions to a growing and evolving story, through which the authors are accountable for healthcare actions performed or not performed. At any point in time a patient's health record provides the information basis against which new findings are interpreted, and its integrity, completeness and accessibility are of paramount importance. EHR systems need to offer a flexible framework for recording the consultation process, and accommodate the individuality of the clinician as well as the patient. When migrating to electronic health records, it is important to acknowledge how readily the tremendous richness of a clinical dialogue can be expressed on paper (see Figure 7-2).

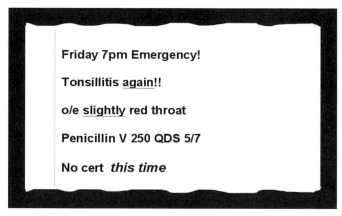

Friday 7pm Emergency!

Tonsillitis <u>again</u>!!

o/e <u>slightly</u> red throat

Penicillin V 250 QDS 5/7

No cert *this time*

Figure 7-2 An example narrative record entry, showing the richness that can succinctly be expressed but is full of ambiguity.

In this example, often found useful by the author for teaching, the reader can rapidly deduce:

- that the doctor was not pleased to see this patient, at least at that time of day,
- that the "tonsillitis" is a recurrent reason for attendance,
- that the physical findings are minimal, and not commensurate with that diagnosis,
- that an antibiotic has been prescribed with little or no sound clinical indication,

- that some change in the "usual" consultation for this recurrence has been introduced, by not providing a sickness certificate, with an implication that these have previously been given.

This kind of entry, rich in direct and indirect meaning, might have taken 15-20 seconds to write on paper, whilst an equivalent computerised system might require 1-2 minutes of data entry time. However, it should be noted that the lack of explicit structure has permitted the recording of a consultation in a way that is far from "objective", and the recording system (paper) has passively accepted both a diagnosis and a treatment that are not supported by the clinical evidence. EHR adoption, if it is to meet future challenges, will require a greater clinical attention to data quality.

Whether using terminologies or free text, clinical practice requires a rich and varied vocabulary to express the diversity and complexity of each patient encounter. An EHR system must be underpinned by a common terminology to express clinical content that can accommodate such freedom of expression, whilst supporting the need for structured and semi-structured interpretation of each entry.

The structural organisation of the EHR needs to be appropriate to the needs of clinicians [73]. Flexibility of data entry and support of narratives are major reasons for the retention of paper records by many clinicians [67]. Achieving the optimum balance between structured, systematised record-keeping and holistic narrative is difficult, and the EHR must not be prescriptive about this: it needs to accommodate both.

The way in which individual clinical statements are hierarchically nested within a record confers an important context for their interpretation. A comprehensive EHR system must enable statements to be grouped together under headings and sub-headings in a clinically meaningful way. Aspects of certainty, severity and the absence of findings must be capable of rigorous and unambiguous representation. For example, a patient with a family history of diabetes or in whom diabetes has been excluded must not erroneously be retrieved in a database search for diabetic patients.

Many contemporary systems lack both detail and uniformity to enable the consistent retrieval of good outcome data across providers [19]. Dolin argues that standards for the information model of an electronic health record are important, and that clinical data can be complex.

> "Data can be nested to varying degrees (e.g. a data table storing laboratory results must accommodate urine cultures growing one or more than one organism, each with its own set of antibiotic

sensitivities). Data can be highly interrelated (e.g., a provider may wish to specify that a patient's renal insufficiency is due both to diabetes mellitus and to hypertension, and is also related to the patient's polyuria and malaise). Data can be heterogeneous (e.g., test results can be strictly numeric, alpha-numeric, or composed of digital images and signals) ... a computerized health record must be able to accommodate unforeseen data."

Increasingly clinicians of all disciplines and professions wish to document the rationale behind their decisions, and to share this information with colleagues. Electronic health records must be medico-legally acceptable, for example as legal evidence, with a rigorous audit trail of authorship and amendments. They must be implemented within a formal security and access framework that ensures only the appropriate persons connected with the care of the patient can retrieve and edit their record, and within a secure communications infrastructure that allows for the seamless integration of existing (legacy) and new-generation computer systems.

In a teaching setting, it must be possible for medical, nursing and other healthcare students to have access to and to contribute to health records, such that their student status is explicit. Patients (and possibly their families) must themselves be valid authors of record entries to allow them to contribute their own impressions of health status and needs.

The medical record needs to be *faithful* [52], which implies that it needs to be:
- attributable,
- permanent (entries can be logically deleted or linked to a corrective comment, but never erased),
- authentic,
- allowing negative and uncertain statements,
- allowing conflicting statements.

Information with considerable sociological and clinical complexity may need to be captured within a health record. Much international research has highlighted the importance of incorporating the context surrounding the authorship of individual EHR entries. The medical record is not (nor intended to be) a faithful reflection of the life and health of the patient, but is authored by professionals working in an institution whose task is to manage the treatment or prevention of illness [47]. Their perspective will influence what is recorded and how it is expressed.

Berg points out that the medical record is not an accurate mirror of the consultation nor an actuarial document, but itself provides a means for organising ideas and contributes to the work of communicating, decision making and sharing with patients [9]. Records contain much reiteration, not because facts are not found elsewhere but to summarise the current focus of thinking. Many entries are brief, concise, and are understood by those who are familiar with the context of that recording, including a familiarity with the author and the clinical setting. Such entries often only note exceptions and emphasised information, and may even omit the routine. Such brevity allows the record to highlight what needs to be known rather than to document all that is known.

4 Research into Representing the Generic EHR

The increasing limitations of paper-based records, the potential benefits of electronic health records and the acknowledged challenges of delivering these in practice have stimulated a considerable investment in research and development over the past decade. Between 1991 and 1998 the European Union provided 47 Million Euro of direct funding support to research projects whose budgets totalled 76 Million Euro [31].

Realising the electronic health record has been at the heart of the European Union's Third, Fourth and Fifth Health Telematics Framework Programmes. Considerable research has been undertaken over the past twelve years to explore the user requirements for adopting EHRs (for example, published by the Good European Health Record Project [36], [33], [34], [35], [27] and the EHCR Support Action [18]). These have formed the basis of architecture formalisms to represent and communicate personal health data comprehensively and in a manner which is medico-legally rigorous and preserves the clinical meaning intended by the original data author (e.g. the GEHR architecture [44], and the CEN standards ENV 12265 [30] and ENV 13606 [43]). These results have at their heart the recognition that personal health data is often very sensitive and always to be regarded as confidential.

Other research has identified the additional requirements to support the communication of EHRs within federated communities of healthcare enterprises to support shared patient care across sites (the Synapses project [23]) and middleware architectures to integrate across R&D projects (SynEx [62]). EHR demonstrators have been established in many European countries, through these R&D projects and subsequently through national programmes, as the strategic importance of EHRs has grown. For example, University College London has been developing, evaluating and refining an implementation of the

EHR service architecture based on the results of these European projects and relevant CEN standards, with a principal demonstrator in cardiology [39].

In Australia a successor to the Good European Health Record, the Good Electronic Health Record project, has enabled various federal government-funded projects to establish demonstrators of an EHR server as an integrator of clinical information to support diabetes shared care and for laboratory test results [8] [58].

These research projects, standards and demonstrators have played a strong role internationally in defining the widely-accepted requirements for and information architecture characteristics of EHR systems, as reflected throughout this chapter, and in [42]. They have also provided the primary input for work internationally on EHR communication standards, and the *open*EHR Foundation, both described in later sections of this chapter.

Ongoing research continues to explore the optimal design of EHR system components, and tackle new informatics challenges such as clinical genomics and Grid computing and their consequent ethical issues [40].

5 Requirements for Representing the EHR

There is now a wealth of published clinical and ethico-legal requirements for the information architecture of an EHR if it is to be realised through the interconnection (federation) of diverse clinical systems. These requirements build on the work of the author and colleagues as part of a series of EU projects, literature reviews, empirical observations and interactions with many healthcare settings across Europe. These requirements have been distilled and analysed by expert groups, mainly within Europe, in order to identify the basic information that must be accommodated within an EHR information architecture to:

- capture faithfully the original meaning intended by the author of a record entry or set of entries,
- provide a framework appropriate to the needs of professionals and enterprises to analyse and interpret EHRs on an individual or population basis,
- incorporate the necessary medico-legal constructs to support the safe and relevant communication of EHR entries between professionals working on the same or different sites.

These requirements have recently been consolidated on the international stage within an ISO draft Technical Specification, ISO TS 18308 [57].

Joining up diverse and sometimes discipline-specific and culturally specific kinds of clinical information to compose a whole-person EHR that can safely, legally and useably replace paper records is a complex challenge. Research on the requirements for representing health record information has drawn attention to the essential nature of contextual information captured alongside the individual clinical entries at the time of recording. (A health record entry is considered here to be a quantum of information that is entered into a record, usually constituting a single fact, observation or statement.) These contexts can perhaps best be illustrated by an example: the entry in a health record of a diagnosis of supra-ventricular tachycardia (SVT). This entry could be associated with several kinds of context within an EHR, illustrated in Figure 7-3.

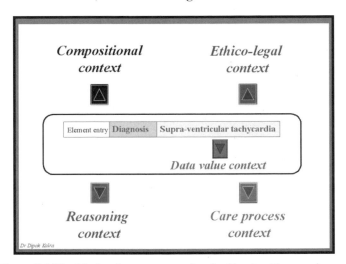

Figure 7-3 The kinds of context associated with a health record entry.

In the absence of these sets of contextual information the reader of this health record entry could not tell if this is a new diagnosis or a longstanding problem, nor the certainty with which it has been made. He or she could not be sure even if this diagnosis had been made on the patient or on a relative, recorded as part of a family history.

5.1 Compositional Context

This context refers to the way in which the diagnostic entry of SVT relates to other information entered along with that finding (the history and examination findings), and the higher level of those entries within the health record of that patient.

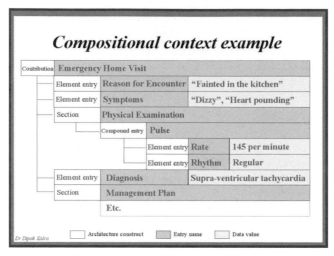

Figure 7-4 Illustration of the compositional context.

From the information in Figure 7-4 the reader can infer that the consultation has taken place in fairly rushed circumstances, with the patient possibly quite distressed about having fainted. The diagnosis has been made without the benefit of an ECG, but perhaps on reasonable clinical grounds. It would appear to be a brand new diagnosis for this patient. By naming the entry *Diagnosis* the reader is able to ascertain that this is a condition that has now been ascribed to the patient by the author; were it an entry of one or more named *Differential diagnoses* a different inference would be made. There are several facets to this context.

- Every record entry must be able to have a name that provides a label for each data value.
- Record entries can be:
  15. an element e.g. for Weight,
  16. or a compound e.g. for Blood Pressure.
- A formal record structure hierarchy must preserve the way in which entries were originally ordered and grouped by the author.
- The record architecture must define the minimum medico-legally acceptable cohort of data from which EHRs must be constructed.

5.2   Data Value Context

This context refers to the fine details associated with the chosen value itself. In this case, a term has been chosen from the Read code term set that is commonly used within GP systems in the UK.

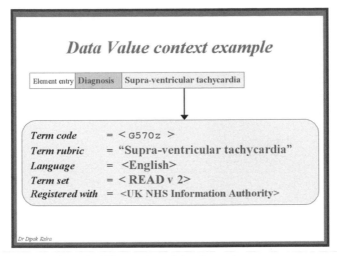

Figure 7-5 Illustration of the data value context.

The EHR clearly needs to be able faithfully to represent a comprehensive range of data types, including:

- text, quantities, time, persons, multimedia,
- names of term sets, versions and registering agencies,
- natural language used in a recording,
- accuracy, precision and units for quantities,
- normal ranges.

5.3 Ethico-legal Context

The ethical and legal requirements of good clinical care emphasise the importance of documenting, for example, the authorship and dates and times associated with each record entry. The EHR must be able to represent these data faithfully.

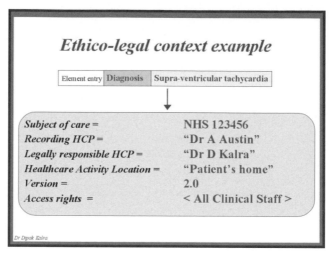

Figure 7-6 Illustration of the ethico-legal context.

In this example the reader can determine that this entry is a revision of an original version, implying that an error of recording had been made that has now been corrected. (Access to that original version might be more restricted than to the current version.) This kind of context may include:

- identifying authorship, authorising agents and those with legal responsibility for the documented healthcare,
- identifying the subject of care, and the subject of the information within each entry,
- dates and times of record authorship, care delivery and of the events being recorded,
- version control,
- access rights, amendment rights.

5.4   Reasoning Context

This context refers to information that might be associated with the entry to explain how or why it applies to the patient in this particular instance.

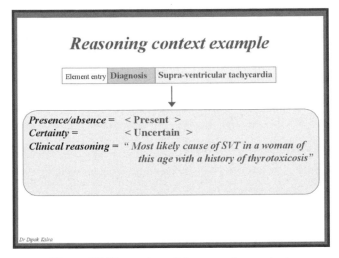

Figure 7-7 Illustration of the reasoning context.

In this case, the reader can see that the author has acknowledged uncertainty in the diagnosis, but has also provided some explanation of the clinical reasoning. In the future it may become commonplace for such reasoning to refer explicitly to an external source of medical knowledge, as illustrated in Figure 7-8.

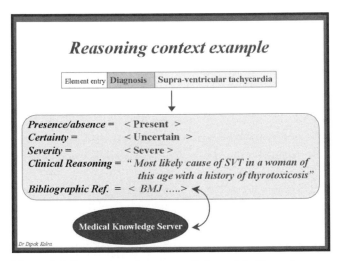

Figure 7-8 Illustration of a context link to a Medline reference.

The authors are aware only of a few pioneering centres where such linkage is presently implemented within clinical systems. The reasoning context might include:

- presence/absence,

- certainty,
- prevailing clinical circumstances (e.g. standing, fasting),
- supplementary comments made by the author,
- emphasis of exceptional or abnormal observations,
- justification or clinical reasoning,
- knowledge reference (e.g. Medline).

5.5 Care Process Context

Clinical entries are rarely isolated in the longitudinal evolution of health problems and of care delivery. This context relates to the sets of links and pointers that help to represent the non-chronological organisation of health records.

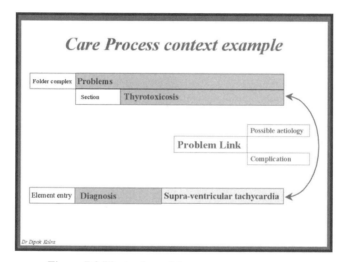

Figure 7-9 Illustration of the care process context.

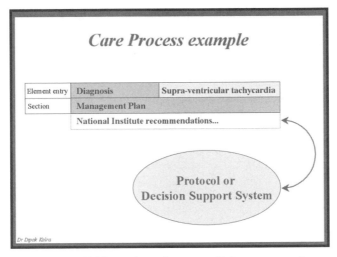

Figure 7-10 Illustration of a context link to a protocol.

The potential links and pointers to other parts of the record that might need to be represented in a health record include:

- cause and effect,
- request and result,
- process (act) status (e.g. a test that is requested and subsequently cancelled),
- to a defined problem,
- to an episode of care,
- to a stage in a protocol,
- to a decision support system.

If the EHR is to be capable of representing a comprehensive lifetime record of a patient, and support interoperability, it needs to be able to retain all of these aspects of context in a consistent and rigorous way to ensure that any future requesting clinical system can interpret the individual observations safely. The research and standards work on EHR information architectures, described in the chapter, has precisely this goal.

6 Scope of the EHR

The principal set of software components that would be deployed in a health setting to deliver a functional EHR are drawn in Figure 7-11. The services that directly implement the core EHR are shown in green, middleware services that support the EHR are shown in yellow, and the end-user facing applications are shown in pink. When clinicians and purchasers conceptualise an EHR system, they commonly consider the pink zone and assume the existence of the other components. Health informatics research and standards on the generic EHR has concentrated upon the green zone. It is this core EHR that absolutely must be interoperable internationally in order to support a whole-person EHR. Applications developed in the pink zone will probably always exhibit diversity across health systems and specialities.

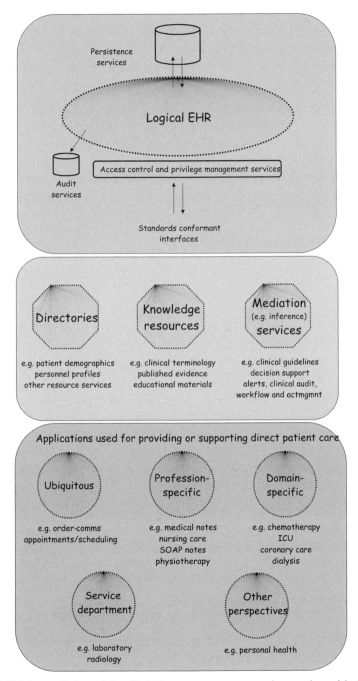

Figure 7-11 A layered view of the clinical system components interacting with the HER.

A vast number of requirements relate to the applications and systems that will capture EHR data from clinicians, carry out processing on that data including decision support, recalls and reminders, and deliver integrated or detailed views of EHR data back to clinicians. It is widely recognised that this vast field of clinical system design is broader than the EHR concept, which is limited in scope to the faithful and interoperable representation of EHR data itself. The full treatment of EHR clinical systems is therefore beyond the scope of this chapter.

7 Adopting an Architectural Approach to Representing the EHR

7.1 The Federation Approach

A comprehensive, multi-enterprise and longitudinal EHR will inevitably be realised through the joining up of the specific clinical applications, databases (and increasingly devices) that are each tailored to the needs of individual conditions, specialties or enterprises rather than by a single monolithic system that has to be used by all. The question that remains open is whether this joining up takes place in real time, logically, or physically through the creation of a large dedicated EHR repository which these distributed clinical systems all feed on a frequent basis.

The federation approach, as demonstrated by the Synapses project (1996-8), is a validated mechanism for realising a distributed EHR service, which can be physical or logical. The individual contributing systems, known as feeder systems, retain their autonomy by continuing to be accessed locally through their own applications and by electing which parts of their local database are to be accessed by the federation as a whole. In a healthcare setting this might be realised as a hospital federating a set of departmental clinical databases or as a regional healthcare network federating the set of hospital, GP and community systems within its geographical area. A national health care network might practically be delivered as a super-federation of such regional federated health records.

The federation can exist either as a logical integration, with the information required to meet a request extracted from the relevant feeder systems on demand, or using a physical store to cache in advance the desired common data from all participating feeder systems. In practice it is likely that any federation will employ a mixture of these to suit local requirements, taking into account the characteristics of the various feeder systems. There are strengths and weaknesses associated with each approach: live federation places considerable demands upon network and server performance and requires the constant and reliable availability of all participating feeder systems; a caching mechanism places a reliance upon potentially large repositories and upon regular version checking to ensure that updates to each feeder system are forwarded to the cache repository in real time to avoid the risk of a requesting client receiving out of date or incorrect information.

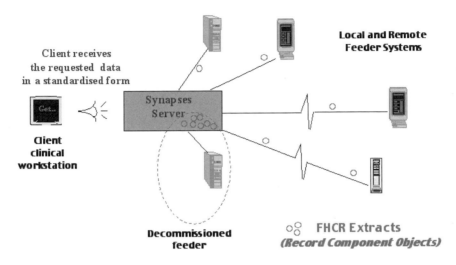

Figure 7-12 Distributed access to record components within a Synapses Federated Healthcare Record (FHCR) federation.

A key component in developing a database federation is specifying the federation schema: the unifying information model to which the diverse feeder system schemata are mapped. This requires a single mapping exercise to be performed for each feeder system, and avoids the alternative combinatorial explosion of mappings that are required were each feeder to develop a direct communication to all other relevant feeders. However, it requires that the federation schema is sufficiently generic and rich to represent faithfully the underlying information that could be extracted from any possible contributing feeder system.

This schema, in a health care context, is an information model that can represent any conceivable health record entry or a partial or complete EHR that might be contributed by any clinical database or EHR feeder system, now or in the future.

The strength of the approach taken internationally on the EHR architecture has been the development of a rigorous generic representation suitable for all kinds of entries, and the requirement for all labelling information to be an integral part of each construct. Provided that the core architecture is common to both a sending and a receiving information system, any health record extract will contain all of the structure and names required for it to be interpreted faithfully on receipt even if its organisation and the nature of the clinical content have not been "agreed" in advance.

7.2   The Two-Level Modelling Approach

The challenge addressed by the two-level (dual-model) approach to the design of the EHR information architecture has been to devise a scalable model for representing any conceivable health record entry. This needs to cater for records arising from any profession, speciality or service, whilst recognising that the clinical data sets, value sets, templates etc. required by different health care domains will be diverse, complex and will change frequently as clinical practice and medical knowledge advance. The two-level approach distinguishes a *Reference Model,* used to represent the generic properties of health record information, and *Archetypes* (conforming to an *Archetype Model*), which are meta-data used to represent the specific characteristics of the various kinds of clinical data that might need to be represented to meet the requirements of each particular profession, speciality or service.

The **Reference Model** represents the global characteristics of health record entries, how they are aggregated, and the context information required to meet ethical, legal and provenance requirements. This model defines the set of classes that form the generic building blocks of the EHR. It reflects the stable characteristics of an electronic health record.

Such a very generic information model for the EHR needs to be complemented by a formal method of communicating and sharing the named hierarchical structures within EHRs, the data types and value ranges that actual record entries may take, and other constraints, in order to ensure interoperability, data consistency and data quality.

Archetypes each define (and effectively constrain) legal combinations of the building-block classes defined in the Reference Model for particular clinical domains or organisations by specifying particular record entry names, data-types and may constrain values to particular value ranges. Archetypes express the rules by which useful clinical templates can be constructed from the Reference Model in *consistent and interoperable ways*. Archetype instances themselves conform to a formal model, known as an Archetype Model (which is related to the Reference Model) and can be optimally expressed in archetype description language (ADL), developed by the *open*EHR Foundation (see later in this chapter). Although the ADL and Archetype Model are stable, individual archetype instances can be revised or succeeded by others as clinical practice evolves. Version control ensures that new revisions do not invalidate data created with previous revisions.

Archetype Repositories. In each enterprise or region there is a diversity of health information stored on paper and in legacy feeder systems. The range of archetypes required within a shared EHR community is presently unknown. The potential sources of knowledge for developing such archetype definitions will include:

- health information which is used for semantic processing within current systems;
- health information used in secondary data collections;
- the clinical data schemata (models) of existing systems;
- the layout of computer screen forms used by these systems for data entry and for the display of analyses performed;
- data-entry templates, pop-up lists and look-up tables used by these systems;
- shared-care data sets, messages and reports used locally and nationally;
- the structure of templates and forms used for the documentation of clinical consultations or summaries within paper records;
- the pre-co-ordinated terms in terminology systems.

However, in order to realise the full benefits of a local or national federation, enterprises ideally should progressively agree on common definitions that they could use to exchange clinical information. By conforming to a common Reference Model and Archetype Model the individual libraries of archetype definitions held in each repository (however implemented) can be exchanged (e.g. via XML) in order to facilitate this progressive convergence across sites or regions.

In the longer term, it is anticipated that the involvement of national health services, academic organisations and professional bodies in the development of such definitions will enable this approach to contribute to the pursuit of quality evidence-based clinical practice. In the future regional or national public domain libraries of archetype definitions might be accessed via the Internet, and downloaded for local use within EHR systems.

The value of the approach described here is that diverse health and healthcare information can be represented and communicated in a standardised way that is also scalable and maintainable. The combination of the Reference Model and the use of Archetypes (as the EHR information architecture) preserves faithfully the set of contexts relating to a health record entry, to ensure the intended clinical meaning of the original author is preserved within the generic representation.

For example, if a user chooses to record a high blood pressure reading alongside (or linked to) an entry describing a recent bereavement, this associated information would not routinely be extracted when composing a table or graph of blood pressures over time. The bereavement might, however, have influenced a clinician not to respond to the raised blood pressure on that occasion. It is not possible to prevent users from requesting such graphs, nor is it possible to deny users the ability to compose links of this nature. However, the EHR architecture ensures that users curious about an unusually high blood pressure on a graph would always have access to the consultation in which it was recorded and therefore the ability to uncover the clinical context in which it was taken.

The instantiation of record entries conforming to specific archetypes must be formally managed by the EHR service in accordance with the overall archetype schema. This ensures that, for example, health record entries containing a *Diagnosis* can be identified from within a range of groupings such as a *Summary*, an *Outpatient Consultation*, or a *Referral Letter*. However, the risk of extracting all entries containing a diagnosis from a record is that the result may also include entries under headings such as *Family History*, *Possible Diagnosis* or *Patient's Concerns*; none of these would establish that the patient actually had those conditions. This is why key attributes in the Reference Model specifically record the subject of the information, degree of certainty and direct applicability of the information to the patent. This makes it possible safely to document *independently of the heading used* that the subject of the information is a relative, that a finding is uncertain or that the patient is at risk of having a condition rather than actually having it. This approach for certain key "modifiers" reduces the risk of misinterpretation given that clinical practice does not yet have a consistent approach to the labels or headings used within health records.

A potential strength of the approach lies in its ability to enable the sharing and analysis of health record data even if the original records do not share a single common archetype structure. However, there is also an opportunity to use the perspective of a shared library of archetypes to encourage clinical convergence on the organisational structure of health records. Once clinical teams are able to share records and to benefit directly from a consistent federated record framework they will naturally and deliberately seek convergence. It is the experience of the author through medical audit projects that this bottom-up approach to convergence is generally more successful, albeit slower, than a top-down imposition of standardised data sets.

The two-level approach described here is being adopted in three areas of work:

- the design of the *open*EHR information architecture specifications,
- as an input to the EHRcom Task Force charged with revising ENV 13606, and led by one of the authors (DK),
- as an input to the development of HL7 Templates specification.

Each of these three activities is summarised in the rest of this chapter.

8 EHR Interoperability Standards

8.1 European (CEN) EHR Interoperability Standards

CEN is the principal legislative standardisation body for Europe; Technical Committee 251 has responsibility for health informatics (interoperability) standards. Since 1990 CEN TC/251 has regarded the Electronic Healthcare Record as one of the most important and most urgent areas for the establishment of European standards.

A pre-standard ENV 12265, outlining the key architectural features of an EHR, was first published in 1995 [30], and followed in 1999 by a more comprehensive four-part pre-standard ENV 13606. This defined the logical model of an EHR [43], and a message model derived from it [45], a set of access control measures that ought to be applied to the process of EHR sharing [29] and a set of vocabularies to support the overall EHR model [55].

These standards drew on the results of successive EU-funded research projects, summarised in Section 8.4 of this chapter). Since 1999 several demonstrator projects and a few suppliers have elected to use ENV 13606 in an adapted form as their means of EHR interoperability between systems and enterprises. Regrettably the adaptations made to ENV 13606 have been rather *ad hoc*, so the exchange of EHR information between demonstrators or systems has not been possible, unfortunately largely defeating the object of such a standard.

Task Force 13606: EHRcom. In December 2001 CEN TC/251 confirmed a new Task Force, known as "EHRcom", to review and revise the 1999 four-part pre-standard ENV 13606 relating to Electronic Healthcare Record Communications. The intention of this work is to propose a revision that could be adopted by CEN as a formal standard (EN) during 2005. One of the authors (DK) is leading this Task Force, which has set out to base the revision of ENV 13606 on the practical experience that has been gained through commercial systems and demonstrator pilots in the communication of whole or part of patients' EHRs. Its overall mission is to produce a rigorous and durable information architecture for representing the EHR, in order to support the interoperability of systems and components that need to interact with EHR services:

- as discrete systems or as middleware components,
- to access, transfer, add or modify health record entries,
- via electronic messages or distributed objects,
- preserving the original clinical meaning intended by the author,
- reflecting the confidentiality of that data as intended by the author and patient.

The main provisions of this draft standard have already been widely reviewed within Europe, and internationally. The final draft is expected to be published in 2005. When published, it will be the most comprehensive standard specifically targeted at supporting electronic health record interoperability, and possibly the best-underpinned by research and implementation experience.

8.2   HL7 Standards Relevant to the EHR

The Health Level Seven (HL7) organisation was formed in the United States in March 1987. It arose initially to tackle the growing diversity of messages developed within the US health insurance industry. The HL7 protocol is a collection of standard formats that specify the interfaces for electronic data exchange in healthcare environments between computer applications from different vendors. The focus of the HL7 organisation, and its practical experience base, has historically been the interface requirements of large healthcare enterprises. Version 2 is presently the most deployed health messaging standard internationally.

However, despite its wide uptake, the problems of inconsistent implementations of Version 2 and the unsystematic growth of message segment definitions have limited the realisation of interoperability. A key feature of Version 3 is the Reference Information Model (RIM): a means of specifying the information content of messages through an information model that clarifies the definitions and ensures that they are used consistently. Message definitions are created via an incremental refinement process beginning with the RIM, and passing through various intermediate models, including Restricted Message Information Models (RMIMs) and Hierarchical Message Definitions (HMDs).

The **HL7 Clinical Document Architecture (CDA)** is a generic RIM-derived structure for the communication of clinical documents, and has sometimes been regarded as the HL7 equivalent of a record architecture, although it is designed as a single-document *transfer* mechanism. Level One of the CDA 1.0 is a formal

American standard, and is primarily intended to represent narrative-style documents plus some basic header information in a structured form [20]. CDA Release Two is a draft specification, approaching final standardisation, for the structural organisation of fine-grained information inside a document. In this regard it is close in scope to that of the inner hierarchies of an EHR architecture, and work is ongoing between CEN and HL7 to enable best fit (and cross-mapping) between the EHRcom standard and the CDA, since both will undoubtedly be used to exchange clinical information in different settings.

The **HL7 Template Special Interest Group** is actively developing a specification for constraints to be applied to RIM-derived message models. This work is drawing upon the *open*EHR archetype approach, and it is expected that some parts of the *open*EHR Archetype Definition Language will form part of this future HL7 standard.

The **HL7 EHR Technical Committee** has released an EHR System Functional Model as a draft standard for trial use. This standard describes an inclusive set of functions that might be available in EHR systems in particular (profiled) settings – now and in the future. This set of functions provides a standardised way to describe EHR systems and their capability, as an aid to system comparison and procurement.

8.3   International (ISO) EHR Interoperability Standards

The ISO Technical Committee 215 (Health Informatics) was formed in late 1999 to support the compatibility and interoperability of Information and Communication Technology (ICT) systems in healthcare. There are presently five Working Groups:

- WG 1 Health records and modelling co-ordination
- WG 2 Messaging and communication
- WG 3 Health concept representation
- WG 4 Security
- WG 5 Health cards

This ISO forum, bringing together a diverse international set of informatics and health service stakeholders, will progressively define standards for the EHR. Working Group 1 has published a set of requirements [57] referred to earlier in this chapter, and is presently defining the overall scope of the EHR. It has provisionally approved a process of reviewing the CEN EHRcom draft standard (draft of EN 13606) with a hope of accepting it as a full international standard in due course.

8.4 Standards for Images

The Digital Imaging and Communications in Medicine (DICOM) standard arose out of a precursor standard for images (ACR-NEMA) that was first published in 1985 by the American College of Radiology (ACR) and the National Electrical Manufacturers Association (NEMA). The DICOM standard is the most widely used common data representation internationally for the various medical images acquired and communicated. It has addressed many of the issues of vendor-independent data formats and data transfers for digital medical images. It is presently in version 3, with 14 chapters each relating to a different kind of image or signal data type or to a communication type. CEN and ANSI have adopted DICOM by reference in their imaging standards.

8.5 IHE

Integrating the Health Environment (IHE) is a recently-formed industry-sponsored organisation seeking to promote interoperability between systems within specialist departments such as radiology, and the conventional hospital systems used to order such investigations and to receive imaging study reports. It is working closely with DICOM and HL7 in this area.

Its most recent specification, still in draft form, is for Cross-Document Sharing (XDS). It defines registry and repository services that can function as a centralised or distributed warehouse for clinical documents. Through specific collaborations between the parties involved, it will be capable of supporting HL7 CDA documents and EHRcom (13606) equivalent structures, but not a full EHR. It is a primarily a storage, indexing and distribution mechanism, and is a practical complement to these other standards.

8.6 Other Standards and Specifications

It is not possible in this chapter to summarise all of the potentially relevant standards, industry standards and specifications that might pertain to parts of an EHR, such as particular data sets or data types. Examples of these include the Object Management Group Health Domain Task Force (OMG-HDTF) and the American Society for the Testing of Materials (ASTM). For example, ASTM is developing a standard "Continuity of Care Record" which is a rich data set of clinical and administrative data items that ought to be considered for inclusion in a shared care clinical communication. This is not a replacement for a comprehensive EHR, but the work on generic EHR specifications reported above either has or is evolving links with these related standards bodies.

Figure 7-13 illustrates the roles within a distributed healthcare environment of several of the standards referred to in this section. Interoperability of specific clinical data sets is shown in purple and those supporting generic clinical information interoperability are shown in pink.

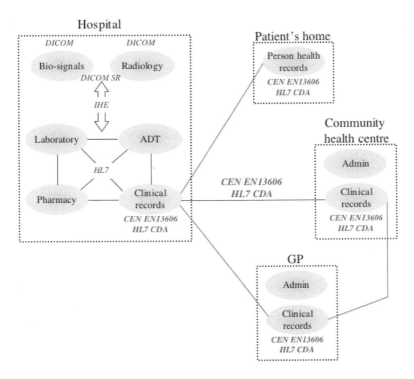

Figure 7-13 Domains of communication of health information covered by different industry and legislative standards.

9 Integrating Reminders, Alerts and Decision Support

Systems to compare patient-specific observation values with population norms or scientific evidence are now widely used. The use of the term *decision support* is variably applied to:

- simple logical algorithms such as an alert to a user that a patient's screening test is overdue; these are sometimes described as reminder systems,
- calculations derived from one or more clinical observation parameters such as a cardiovascular disease risk score,

- algorithms that compare new entries with existing record entries and with reference databases, such as drug prescribing systems; these sometimes function as alerting systems,
- rule-based systems incorporating probabilistic algorithms to determine the most likely clinical decision or pathway from a set of predetermined options, based on informal description logic or formal languages such as Arden Syntax, GLIF, *pro*Forma or Prodigy.

The enactment of an electronic guideline and decision support function is of greatest clinical value when it is linked to the circumstances and needs of an individual patient. Guidelines therefore need to be linked to the EHR. An appropriately linked guideline system would, for example, enable a clinical system to:

- accept a random blood glucose of 4.2 mmol/l and pass it directly to the EHR,
- warn the clinician when entering a blood glucose of 7.4 mmol/l, invoking a textual message or initiating a protocol depending upon whether the patient is diabetic,
- reject a blood glucose of 74 mmol/l as a typing error.

If decision support and EHR systems are to interoperate safely the metadata defining clinical data elements needs to be held in common, including the permitted data value ranges and the units or terminology systems to be used. The clinical use of a decision support system needs itself to be documented within the EHR, including the origin, name, version and step of the guideline influencing or generating a particular entry, and a copy of any message or recommendation provided to the user. Decision support systems also need to be much more interoperable than at present, so that a tailored guideline can "follow the patient" as well as their EHR might soon do.

10 The *open*EHR Foundation

The *open*EHR Foundation is an independent, not-for-profit organisation and community, facilitating the creation and sharing of health records by consumers and clinicians via open-source, standards-based implementations [59]. Its mission statement is:

> "To improve the clinical care process by fostering the development and implementation of open source, interoperable EHR components. These components should be based on internationally agreed requirements and address the need for privacy and security,

while supporting the development of interoperable and evolving clinical applications."

The goal of *open*EHR is to exemplify good designs for interoperable EHR systems through open source components, and to validate and refine these through practical clinical demonstrators. The *open*EHR Foundation was formalised as a not-for-profit company in 2003. *open*EHR aims to:

- promote and publish the formal specification of requirements for representing and communicating EHR information, based on implementation experience, and evolving over time as healthcare and medical knowledge develop,
- promote and publish EHR information architectures, models and data dictionaries, tested in implementations, which meet these requirements,
- manage the sequential validation of the EHR architectures through comprehensive implementation and clinical evaluation,
- maintain open source "reference" implementations, available under licence, to enhance the pool of available tools to support clinical systems, and
- collaborate with other groups working towards high-quality, requirements-based and interoperable health information systems, in related fields of health informatics.

Technically, *open*EHR brings together many of the strong threads of R&D in the field of electronic and federated health record systems described in this chapter, underpinned by published requirements, and with the goal of evolving best practice in the design of the EHR information architectures through collaboration and the evaluation of implementations in live clinical settings. *open*EHR seeks to foster this collaborative approach through openly available specifications, open source components and hosting e-mail discussion fora to debate the issues and challenges that arise in working towards its mission. The process and deliverables of its activities are managed by a formal change control process.

The *open*EHR technical specifications define design principles, reference and archetype models and will in the future include other middleware service specifications. This work is becoming regarded internationally as the most complete and best-validated EHR information architecture.

11 The Challenge of Access Control

The foundations of the relationship between a clinician and a patient are the delivery of clinical care to the highest possible standard and the respect for patient autonomy [27]. This inevitably means that the right to informed consent and the right to confidentiality are important moral principles for a good health record system. Patients should exercise as much choice over the content and movement of their health records as is consistent with good clinical care and the lack of serious harm to others. Records should be created, processed and managed in ways that optimally guarantee the confidentiality of their contents and legitimate control by patients in how they are used. The communication of health record information to third parties should take place only with patient consent unless emergency circumstances dictate that implied consent can safely be assumed. Around the globe these principles are progressively becoming enshrined in national data protection legislation.

In an ideal world, each fine-grained entry in a patient's record should be capable of being associated with an access control list of persons who have rights to view that information, which has been generated or at least approved by the patient and which reflects the dynamic nature of the set of persons with legitimate duty of care towards patients through their lifetime. The access control list will ideally include those persons who have rights to access the data for reasons other than a duty of care (such as health service management, epidemiology and public health, consented research) but exclude any information which they do not need to see or which the patient feels is too personal for them to access. On the opposite side, the labelling by patients or their representatives of information as personal or private should not hamper those who legitimately need to see the information in an emergency, nor give genuine healthcare providers such a filtered perspective that they are misled into managing the patient inappropriately. Patients' views on the inherent sensitivity of entries in their health record may evolve over time, as their personal health anxieties alter or as societal attitudes to health problems change. Patients might wish to offer some heterogeneous levels of access to family, friends, carers and members of their community as well as to those in healthcare professions. Families may wish to provide a means by which they are able to access parts of each other's records (but not necessarily to equal extents) in order to monitor the progress of inherited conditions within a family tree.

Such a set of requirements is arguably more extensive than that required of the data controllers in most other industry sectors. It is in practice made extremely complex by:

- the numbers of health record entries made on a patient during the course of modern healthcare,
- the numbers of healthcare personnel, often rotating through posts, who might potentially come into contact with a patient at any one time,
- the numbers of enterprises with which a patient might come into contact during his lifetime,

- the difficulty (for a patient or for anyone else) of classifying in a standardised way how sensitive a record entry might be,
- the difficulty of determining how important a single health record entry might be to the future care of a patient, and to which classes of user,
- the logically indelible nature of the EHR and the need for revisions to access control to be rigorously managed in the same way as revisions to the EHR entries themselves,
- the need to determine appropriate access very rapidly, potentially in less than one second,
- the low level of concern the majority of patients have about these requirements,
- the high level of concern expressed by a growing minority of patients to have their consent for disclosure recorded and respected.

In order to support interoperable EHRs, and seamless communication of EHR data between providers of healthcare, the negotiation that is required to determine if a given requestor of EHR data should be permitted to receive the data needs to be capable of automation. If this were not possible, the delays and workload of managing human decisions for every or most record communications would obviate any value in striving for data interoperability: paper would probably be just as quick!

In practice, efforts are in progress to develop international standards for defining access control and privilege management systems that would be capable of computer-to-computer negotiation. However, this kind of work is predicated upon health services agreeing on a mutually consistent framework for defining the privileges they wish to assign to staff, and the spectrum of sensitivity they offer for patients to define within their EHRs.

The main principles of the approach to standards development in the area of EHR communications access control are to match the characteristics and parameters of a request to the EHR provider's policies, and with any access control or consent declarations within the specified EHR, to maintain appropriate evidence of the disclosure, and to make this capable of automated processing.

This requires consistency in the way the relevant information is expressed, to make this sensibly scalable at definition-time (when new EHR entries are being added), at run-time (when a whole EHR is being retrieved or queried), and durable over a patient's lifetime. It is also important to recognise that much diversity will exist across Europe on the specific approaches to securing EHR communications — including differing legislation — and that a highly prescriptive approach to standardisation is not presently possible.

The view taken by the authors, and reflected in work currently in progress within CEN (towards EN13606) is that a coarse-grained categorisation is needed for staff privilege, for record sensitivity and for their interrelationship. Such a framework needs to be underpinned by a sound set of defaults, in which the public have a high degree of confidence, since the vast majority of record accesses will occur in situations where patients do have trust in their clinical carers, and will wish to exercise few if any specific constraints, if those defaults are seen to be adequate.

This is a rapidly progressing aspect of health informatics standardisation, and the reader is encouraged to review the latest versions of publications from ISO TC/215 in this field.

12 Summary

Joining up diverse and sometimes discipline-specific and culturally specific kinds of clinical information to compose a whole-person EHR that can safely, legally and useably replace paper records is a complex challenge. There is currently considerable activity on the EHR front: specifying, standardising and implementing components to demonstrate comprehensiveness and interoperability. In practice, these different efforts are each tackling slightly different aspects of the interoperability challenge, and where overlap exists there is a good working relationship between the groups, including cross-membership, and harmonisation is actively sought. It is the hope of the authors that, for example, future standards arising from CEN and from HL7 can have a good degree of fit and be mutually compatible.

The delivery of high-quality clinical care depends upon a well-recognised triad of information services: health records, medical knowledge and protocols of care (Figure 7-14).

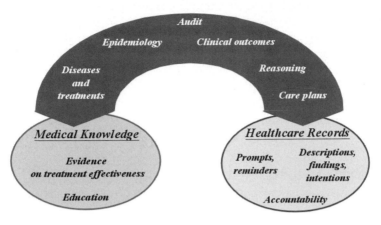

Figure 7-14 Clinical information services supporting patient care.

It is likely that the next generation of healthcare systems will be designed as a set of collaborating middleware components in which this triad of clinical middleware itself interoperates with a range of other middleware services as illustrated in Figure 7-15.

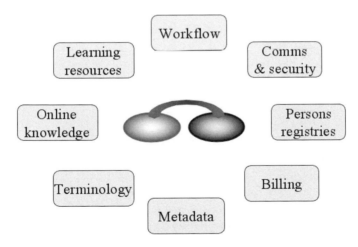

Figure 7-15 Other components and services supporting the clinical middleware.

This kind of interoperability, particularly between vendor products, has yet to be embraced by industry. It is the view of many in the health informatics community that this interoperability between the core clinical middleware components will best be stimulated by the availability of good-quality Open Source reference examples, such as those presently being developed by *open*EHR.

It should be remembered that human and organisational factors play a significant role in the rate of acceptance of health informatics innovations. A key component of the EHR challenge will be to nurture the necessary skills within the clinical workforce to adopt the EHR as part of a modern and integrated health service. This will require an investment in training and, most importantly, the recognition that major change is often best implemented incrementally. Concerns about protecting the confidentiality of sensitive personal information must also be recognised and addressed if consumer confidence is to be maintained when EHRs are widely accessible.

13 Bibliography

[1] Allaert F.A. and Dusserre L. *Telemedicine: responsibilities and contractual framework.* Medinfo 9. 1998; 1:261-4

[2] Alvares R. *Integrating Telehealth – Infoway perspective.* In: Proceedings of the 7th Annual Meeting of the Canadian Society for Telehealth; 2004 Oct 3-5; Quebec City, Canada. Available from: URL: http://www.infoway-inforoute.ca/pdf/CST_TelehealthV8_E.pdf

[3] Anderson J.G. *Evaluating clinical information systems: a step towards reducing medical errors.* MD Computing. May 2000-Jun 2000; 17(3):21-3

[4] Australian Department of Health and Ageing. *HealthConnect – an overview;* 2004. Available from: URL: http://www7.health.gov.au/healthconnect/pdf/HealthConnect_overview_May2004.pdf

[5] Ball M.J. and Lillis J. *E-health: transforming the physician/patient relationship.* International Journal of Medical Informatics. 2001; 61:1-10

[6] Barnett G.O. and Shortliffe E.H. *Medical Informatics: Computer Applications in Health Care.* Addison Wesley. 1990

[7] Bates D.W., Cohen M., Leape L.L., Overhage J.M., Shabot M.M., and Sheridan T. *Reducing the frequency of errors in medicine using information technology.* J Am Med Inform Assoc. Jul 2001-Aug 2001; 8(4):299-308

[8] Beale T. *The GEHR software architecture for a reliable EHR.* Toward an Electronic Health Record Europe '99. Nov 1999; 328-39

[9] Berg M. *Medical work and the computer-based patient record: a sociological perspective.* Methods of Information in Medicine. Sep 1998; 37(3):294-301

[10] Brennan P.F. *Health informatics and community health: support for patients as collaborators in care.* Methods of Information in Medicine. Dec 1999; 38(4-5):274-8

[11] Burns F. NHS Executive. *Information For Health - An Information Strategy For The Modern NHS 1998-2005.* HMSO Ltd, London; Sep 1998; ISBN: 0 95327190 2

[12]Carl F. and Gribble T.J. *HealthDesk for Haemophilia: an interactice computer and communications system for chronic illness self-management.* Medinfo 8. 1995; 829-33

[13]cited by Douglas J.V. *Health Data Online.* MD Computing. Jan 2001-Feb 2001; 18(1):9

[14]Clinton W. *State of the Union Address;* Feb 1997

[15]Department of Health (UK). *Delivering 21st Century IT Support for the NHS - National Strategic Programme.* The Stationery Office; 2002

[16]Department of Health (UK). *The NHS Improvement Plan - Putting people at the heart of public services.* The Stationery Office; 2004

[17]Dick R.S., Steen E.B., and Detmer D.E. *The Computer-Based Patient Record, an Essential Technology for Healthcare.* National Academy Press, Washington DC; 1991

[18]Dixon R., Grubb P.A., Lloyd D., and Kalra D. *Consolidated List of Requirements. EHCR Support Action Deliverable 1.4.* European Commission DGXIII, Brussels; May 2001. 59pp. Available from http://www.chime.ucl.ac.uk/HealthI/EHCR-SupA/del1-4v1_3.PDF

[19]Dolin R.H. *Outcome analysis: considerations for an electronic health record.* MD Computing. Jan 1997-Feb 1997; 14(1):50-6

[20]Dolin R.H., Alschuler L., Beebe C., Biron P.V., Boyer S.L., Essin D., Kimber E., Lincoln T., and Mattison J.E. *The HL7 Clinical Document Architecture.* J Am Med Inform Assoc. Nov 2001-Dec 2001; 8(6):552-69

[21]*EHR fanfare masks complicated IM&T spending plan.* Br J Healthcare Comput Inf Manage. 2001; 18(2):4

[22]*Good Medical Practice. Third edition.* General Medical Council (UK), London; May 2001. http://www.gmc-uk.org/standards

[23]Grimson J., Grimson W., Berry D., Stephens G., Felton E., Kalra D., Toussaint P., and Weier O.W. *A CORBA-based integration of distributed electronic healthcare records using the synapses approach.* IEEE Trans Inf Technol Biomed. Sep 1998; 2(3):124-38

[24]*Harnessing information technology to improve health care.* United States Department of Health and Human Services. 6 May 2004. Available from http://www.hhs.gov/news/press/2004pres/20040427a.html Last accessed 4 November 2004

[25]Haughton J. *A paradigm shift in healthcare. From disease management to patient-centered systems.* MD Computing. Jul 2000-Aug 2000; 17(4):34-8

[26]*Health Online: a health information action plan for Australia.* The National Health Information Management Advisory Council, Commonwealth of Australia; 1999

[27]Heard S., Doyle L., Southgate L., and others. *The GEHR Requirements for Ethical and Legal Acceptability.* European Commission, Brussels; 1993; The Good European Health Record Project: Deliverable 8. 9 chapters, 68 pages

[28]Heard S., Grivel A., Schloeffel P., and Doust J. *The benefits and difficulties of introducing a national approach to electronic health records in Australia* in: National Electronic Health Records Taskforce. A Health Information Network for Australia. Department of Health and Aged Care, Commonwealth of Australia; Jul 2000

[29]Hopkins R. and others, Editors, Project Team 1-028. ENV 13606: *EHCR Communications: Part 3 Distribution Rules.* CEN TC/251, Stockholm; 1999

[30]Hurlen P., Editor, Project Team 1-011. ENV 12265: *Electronic Healthcare Record Architecture.* CEN TC/251, Brussels; 1995

[31]Iakovidis I. *From electronic medical record to personal health records: present situation and trends in European Union in the area of electronic healthcare records.* Medinfo 9. 1998; 1 Suppl:18-22

[32]Iakovidis I. *Towards personal health record: current situation, obstacles and trends in implementation of electronic healthcare record in Europe.* International Journal of Medical Informatics. 1998; 52(1-3):105-15

[33]Ingram D., Hap B., Lloyd D., Grubb P., and others. *The GEHR Requirements for Portability.* European Commission, Brussels; 1992; The Good European Health Record Project: Deliverable 5

[34]Ingram D., Lloyd D., Baille O., Grubb P., and others. *The GEHR Requirements for Communication Capacity.* European Commission, Brussels; 1992; The Good European Health Record Project: Deliverable 6

[35]Ingram D., Murphy J., Griffith S., Machado H., and others. *GEHR Educational Requirements.* European Commission, Brussels; 1993; The Good European Health Record Project: Deliverable 9

[36]Ingram D., Southgate L., Kalra D., Griffith S., Heard S., and others. *The GEHR Requirements for Clinical Comprehensiveness.* European Commission, Brussels; 1992; The Good European Health Record Project: Deliverable 4. (19 chapters, 144 pages)

[37]Institute of Medicine (US). *To Err is Human.* Washington: The Institute; 2000

[38]Jones R., Pearson J., McGregor S., Cawsey A.J., Barrett A., Craig N., Atkinson J.M., Gilmour W.H., and McEwen J. *Randomised trial of personalised computer based information for cancer patients.* BMJ. Nov 1999; 319(7219):1241-7.

[39]Kalra D., Ingram D., Austin A., Griffith V., Lloyd D., Patterson D., Kirstein P., Conversin P., and Fritsche W. *Demonstrating wireless IPv6 access to a Federated Health Record Server.* In Bubak, M.; van Albada, G. D.; Sloot, P. M. A.; Dongarra, J. J. (eds) Computational Science - ICCS 2004 4th International Conference Krakow, Poland, June 6-9, 2004 Proceedings, Part IV. pp1165-1171. Lecture Notes in Computer Science. ISSN: 0302-9743

[40] Kalra D., Singleton P., Ingram D., Milan J., MacKay J., Detmer D., and Rector A. *Security and confidentiality approach for the Clinical E-Science Framework (CLEF).* Proc Health Grid 2004, Clermont-Feraud. European Commission. Available from http://clermont2004.healthgrid.org/ Last accessed 6 September 2004

[41] Kalra D. and Spence M. *Seeking a consensus on discharge communications with City and Hackney GPs.* City and East London Medical Audit Advisory Group, London; 1998

[42] Kalra D. *Clinical Foundations and Information Architecture for the Implementation of a Federated Health Record Service.* PhD Thesis. University of London, 2003 [Available from http://www.ehr.chime.ucl.ac.uk/docs/Kalra,%20Dipak%20(PhD%202002).pdf]

[43] Kay S. and Marley T., Editors, Project Team 1-026. ENV 13606: *EHCR Communications: Part 1 Electronic Healthcare Record Architecture.* CEN TC/251, Stockholm; 1999

[44] Lloyd D., Kalra D., Beale T., Maskens A., Dixon R., Ellis J., Camplin D., Grubb P., and Ingram D., Editors., *The GEHR Final Architecture Description.* European Commission, Brussels; 1995; The Good European Health Record Project: Deliverable 19. 11 chapters; 250 pages. Available from http://www.chime.ucl.ac.uk/HealthI/GEHR/EUCEN/del19.pdf

[45] Markwell D. and others, Editors, Project Team 1-029. ENV 13606: *EHCR Communications: Part 4 Messages for Exchange of Information.* CEN TC/251, Stockholm; 1999

[46] McKay H.G., Feil E.G., Glasgow R.E., and Brown J.E. *Feasibility and use of an Internet support service for diabetes self-management.* Diabetes Educator. 1998; 24:174-9

[47] Papagounos G. and Spyropoulos B. *The multifarious function of medical records: ethical issues.* Methods of Information in Medicine. Dec 1999; 38(4-5):317-20

[48] Patterson D., Ingram D., Kalra D. *Information for Clinical Governance, In Clinical Governance: Making it Happen.* The Royal Society of Medicine Press Ltd.; 1999. ISBN 1-85315-383-4

[49] Pringle and Purves, Editors. *ScopeEPR Project Report.* Royal College of General Practitioners, London; 1997

[50] Pringle M. *Ensuring patient safety.* Br J Gen Pract. Nov 2001; 51(472):876-7

[51] Ramsaroop P. and Ball M.J. *The "bank of health". A model for more useful patient health records.* MD Computing. Jul 2000-Aug 2000; 17(4):45-8

[52] Rector A.L., Nowlan W.A., Kay S., Goble C.A., and Howkins T.J. *A framework for modelling the electronic medical record.* Methods of Information in Medicine. Apr 1993; 32(2):109-19

[53] Richards T. *Patients' priorities.* BMJ. Jan 1999; 318(7179):277-8

[54]Rogers R. *Overcoming the barriers: national to European to G7.* International Journal of Medical Informatics. Feb 1998; 48(1-3):33-8

[55]Rossi Mori A., Kalra D., Rodrigues J.M. and others, Editors, Project Team 1-027. ENV 13606: *EHCR Communications: Part 2 Domain Termlist.* CEN TC/251, Stockholm; 1999

[56]Sackett D.L. and Straus S.E. *Finding and applying evidence during clinical rounds: the "evidence cart".* JAMA. Oct 1998; 280(15):1336-8

[57]Schloeffel P., Editor. *Requirements for an Electronic Health Record Reference Architecture.* ISO/TS 18308: 2002

[58]Schloeffel P., Heard S., Beale T., and Rowed D. *The Good Electronic Health Record (GEHR) in Australian General Practice.* Toward an Electronic Health Record Europe '99. Nov 1999; 340-6

[59]Schloeffel P., Lloyd D., Beale T., Ingram D., Heard S., and Kalra D. *The openEHR Foundation [Web Page].* Accessed Nov 2004. Available at: http://www.openehr.org

[60]Shortliffe E.H. *The evolution of health-care records in the era of the Internet.* Medinfo 9. 1998; 1 Suppl:8-14

[61]Slack W.V. *Cybermedicine: how computing empowers patients for better health care.* Medinfo 9. 1998; 1:3-5

[62]Smith R. *The future of healthcare systems.* BMJ. May 1997; 314(7093):1495-6

[63]Sottile P.A., Ferrara F.M., Grimson W., Kalra D., and Scherrer J.R. *The holistic healthcare information system.* Toward an Electronic Health Record Europe '99. Nov 1999; 259-66

[64]Southgate L. *Professional competence in medicine.* Hosp Med. Mar 1999; 60(3):203-5

[65]Southgate L., Berkson L., Fabb W., and others. *Towards Better Definitions of Competence:* a Paper From the Cambridge Conference. Office of the Regius Professor of Medicine, Cambridge University, Cambridge; 1989

[66]Summerton N. *Trends in negative defensive medicine within general practice.* Br J Gen Pract. Jul 2000; 50(456):565-6

[67]Tange H.J. *Consultation of medical narratives in the electronic medical record.* Methods of Information in Medicine. Dec 1999; 38(4-5):289-93

[68]Vincent C., Neale G., and Woloshynowych M. *Adverse events in British hospitals: preliminary retrospective record review.* BMJ. Mar 2001; 322(7285):517-9

[69]Waegemann C.P. *Medical Record Institute's survey of electronic health record trends and usage.* Toward an Electronic Health Record Europe '99. Nov 1999; 147-58

[70]Waegemann C.P. *The five levels of electronic health records.* MD Computing. May 1996-Jun 1996; 13(3):199-203

[71]Wagner M.M. and Hogan W.R. *The accuracy of medication data in an outpatient electronic medical record.* J Am Med Inform Assoc. May 1996-Jun 1996; 3(3):234-44

[72]Weed L.L. *Clinical judgment revisited.* Methods of Information in Medicine. Dec 1999; 38(4-5):279-86

[73]Williams J.G. and Morgan J. *The clinician-information interface.* Greenes R. A. and others, Editors. Medinfo 8. 1995; 801-5

8 Decision Support Systems in Medicine

Jana Zvárová[1, 2, 3]

[1]   European Center for Medical Informatics, Statistics and Epidemiology
[2]   Charles University and Academy of Sciences of the Czech Republic
[3]   Institute of Computer Science AS CR, Pod Vodarenskou vezi 2, 182 07 Prague, Czech Republic

One of the greatest appeals of a career in medicine is the challenge to one's intellect to solve an endless variety of problems. Medical care is often said to be the art of making decisions without adequate information. Physicians must frequently choose treatment long before they know which disease is present. Even when the illness is known, one must usually select from among several treatment options, and the consequences of each cannot be foretold with certainty.

In medical decision-making it also means to collect data on patients in the framework of a diagnostic and therapeutic cycle (Figure 8-1). For each patient a diagnostic and therapeutic cycle can occur once (e.g. during the examination of a patient) or it may be repeated (e.g. in monitoring of a patient on the intensive care unit).

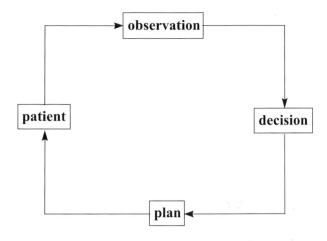

Figure 8-1 Diagnostic and therapeutic cycle.

Information gathered in the diagnostic and therapeutic cycle about a patient from medical interviews, physical examinations and diagnostic tests usually does not reveal the patient's true state. Patient's signs, symptoms and diagnostic tests are usually representative of more than one disease, and there is no certain way to distinguish among these possibilities. Considering the basic features that are used in diagnostic processes (e.g. anatomic defects, specific etiological factors, genetic deviations, physiological and biochemical abnormalities, clinical signs), we can divide diseases into five classes according to the degree of certainty of diagnostic conclusions [8]. However, in diagnostic decision-making, diagnoses are often considered as convention symbols that only mark clinical states that are very similar.

To the first class of diseases, diagnosed with the *highest degree of certainty* (sometimes with total certainty), belong diseases that are, under current medical knowledge, well defined, with known etiology and clear clinical manifestation that is not changed by the type of individual or external conditions. This class includes major anatomic deviations, some inherited diseases and injuries. The second class involves diseases with known and well-defined etiology, but with different clinical presentation in individuals and influenced by external conditions. This class includes malnutrition, microbiological infections, and allergic reactions to given substances and poisonings. In the third class are diseases of the descriptive type, where something is known about etiology or the general type of a pathologic reaction of the organism. The name of the diagnosis is derived from a description of the principal symptoms and signs, e.g. liver cirrhosis, essential hypertension. The fourth class includes diseases where the physical effects of the disease are apparent but the cause is unknown and the picture of the disease shows great individual differences. Here degenerative diseases like osteoarthritis or whole groups of benign and malignant tumors are placed. The fifth class of diseases covers diseases with nearly unknown etiology, where many signs and symptoms show great variability influenced by external conditions and individuals. Inflammatory rheumatic diseases are examples of diseases in this class.

Therefore diagnostic conclusions based on examinations of a patient are the basis for further therapeutic decisions made by a physician. In a medical decision-making task a physician can be supported by information and communication technologies using an appropriate decision support system.

1   Decision Support Systems

Medical decision-making diagnostic processes are based on collected data and knowledge, their analysis, and different ways of reasoning. In expert systems different methodologies are used to formalize the reasoning processes using gathered data and knowledge. Considering the support of diagnostic and therapeutic decision-making, attention is restricted to systems which would come into play when or after the patient data is collected. Electronic information sources such as hypertext systems and medical databases can be used to assist in decision-making, but they are not specifically designed to do so. It must be noted that technology itself cannot (yet) generate the knowledge base and identify what are the significant features required for the confirmation of a diagnostic situation. Specification of rules for identification can be achieved in other ways. Mostly clinical experts can express the factors and the interactions that they feel are clinically significant to identify a particular clinical condition. As clinical resources become more and more scarce, and the necessary competencies become even more in short supply, the expert system will act as a tool for practice guidance and also "insurance" when more junior staff, or those who do procedures less frequently, have to undertake diagnostic procedures that they are not fluent in. So for specific training, the reference and ongoing supervision expert systems, which reflect clinical "good practice" and leading edge-knowledge, will be increasingly useful. Resources, which need to be input into the current mechanisms for expert systems and artificial intelligence, will ultimately migrate from being research exercise to being cost-effective operational support both diagnostic support and clinical intervention activities.

Decision support systems in medicine should help physicians support their medical decision-making in an interactive way. They can be used in many fields, e.g. in diagnostic and prognostic decision-making, interpretation of laboratory tests, therapy planning, monitoring of treatment and diseases as well as in clinical management. However, if we are trying to design an "intelligent" system we are facing the problem how to model the intelligent behavior of human decision-making. The broad field that is now referred to as *artificial intelligence* deals with the problems that have until recently only been able to be tackled by humans because their formulation and solutions require some abilities that only exist in humans (such as the ability to memorize, think, observe, learn, see and similar senses). To these belong problems such as speech and pattern recognition, chess playing and diagnostic, therapeutic and prognostic medical decision-making. Turing [20] proposed an interesting test to find out if a computer exhibits intelligent behavior. His proposal was: "A computer could be considered to be thinking only when a human interviewer, conversing with both an unseen human being and unseen computer, could not determine which is which." This definition of artificial intelligence was focused on the comparison between the abilities of humans and the abilities of computers. Other definitions of artificial intelligence focus on decision-making and problem solving. In summary, the goal of artificial intelligence is to develop systems that behave intelligently. It aims to create computer hardware and software capable of emulating human reasoning.

The costs of hardware and software are declining whereas the capabilities of computer systems are continuously increasing. However, despite all the technological and methodological developments, many physicians or health managers are not using computers at all, or are using them primarily to support simple decisions. *Decision support systems*, especially *knowledge-based systems* and *expert systems*, are designed to change this situation. The classical definition of decision support system, provided by Keen and Scott-Morton[11], is: "A decision support system couples the intellectual resources of individuals with the capabilities of the computer to improve the quality of decisions. It is a computer-based support system for management decision makers who deal with semi-structured problems". As a special case of decision support systems we can consider *knowledge-based* or *expert systems*. We will work with the following definitions: "A knowledge-based system is a computer system that embodies knowledge, including inexact, heuristic, and subjective knowledge the results of knowledge engineering" [19]. An expert system is defined as "a computer system that simulates a human expert in a given area of specialization" [5]. Therefore an expert system can be seen as a knowledge-based system used for simulation of human expertise in a given area of specialization.

Medicine is the area where expert systems can rely on two basic types of medical knowledge [3]: *scientific knowledge* (based on results of biomedical research) and *empirical knowledge* (based on experience gathered from diagnostic and treatment processes). Both types of knowledge are described in textbooks and other publications and especially scientific knowledge is taught at medical faculties. Scientific "know how" knowledge is of a cognitive type, i.e. it helps in recognizing the basis of biological processes, relationships among pathophysiological conditions and symptoms of diseases. Clinical experience is concentrated in medical documentation and it can be stored in medical databases. This empirical "know why" knowledge helps a physician to recognize a disease from observed features of a patient. In practice physicians consider both types of knowledge. Mostly physicians have sufficient scientific and empirical knowledge and no decision support systems are needed. However, there are situations when decision support systems are desirable. In expert systems different methodologies are used to formalize the reasoning processes using gathered data and knowledge.

Formalization and structuring of medical data and knowledge is not easy. Even in the case where we admit that all scientific and empirical knowledge is stored in computer we only can propose expert systems based on our currentmethodological achievements on how to make decision proposals. Till recently we have not known how the human brain process collects data and knowledge. In contrast to the human brain, decision-making using an expert system has been well described. Thus, the dream of the computer that performs at a high level of competence over a wide variety of tasks that people perform well seems to rest upon knowledge in the task areas.

In the paper by Feigenbaum [9] the knowledge principle was formulated as: "a system exhibits intelligent understanding and action at a high level of competence primarily because of the specific knowledge that it contains about its domain of endeavor". The knowledge principle simply says that reasoning processes of intelligent systems are generally weak and are not the source of power that leads to high levels of competence in behavior. Therefore one of the basic requirements to solve decision-making problems is to collect sufficient knowledge about it. The significance of research oriented to intelligent systems development for management and decision support in medicine and healthcare, including knowledge-based system, is increasing for the needs of the information society in healthcare.

2   Knowledge-Based and Expert Systems

Problems that decision support systems (in special cases knowledge-based systems and expert systems) in medicine and healthcare deal with can be both deterministic and cope with uncertainty. Classical expert systems have two famous origins: MYCIN and PROSPECTOR. MYCIN [17] is one of the first examples of the work in the field of medical decision support. MYCIN is a consulting system which provides advice on diagnosis and therapy of infectious diseases. PROSPECTOR [7] is a geological system; but both were soon transformed into domain independent inference machines (empty expert systems) accepting knowledge bases as data. Origins of many diagnostic strategies and medical expert systems can be found in papers published in the last century, e.g. van Bemmel, Gremy and Zvarova[2]. Expert systems can be classified into two main types according to the nature of problems they are designed to solve: *deterministic* and *stochastic expert systems*.

Deterministic expert systems work under certainty. Stochastic expert systems deal with uncertain situations. In stochastic expert systems it is necessary to introduce some method of dealing with uncertainty. One of the intuitive measures of uncertainty is *probability*. Other uncertainty measures are based on *certainty factors* used in expert systems such as MYCIN, *fuzzy logic* [21] or Dempster and Shafer's *theory of evidence* [16]. Expert systems that use probability as a measure of uncertainty are known as *probabilistic expert systems*. Expert systems that are deterministic or use measures of uncertainty based on fuzzy logic, theory of evidence or certainty factors are called *logical expert systems*.

Another classification of expert systems can based on a generic categorization by problem areas addressed by expert systems. A brief description of some categories follows. *Interpretation systems* infer situation descriptions from observations. These include systems for speech recognition, image analysis or signal interpretation.

Prediction systems provide predictions and prognoses including demographic predictions or health economic forecasting. *Diagnostic systems* typically relate observed behavioral irregularities to underlying causes. To this category belong also medical diagnostic systems. *Design systems* develop configuration of objects that satisfy the constraints of the design problem, for example reconstruction of body outlines from mummies found in ancient tombs. *Planning systems* specialize in problems of planning, for example planning antibiotic therapy. *Monitoring systems* compare observations of systems behavior with standards that seems crucial for successful goal attainment. These systems can be used for monitoring of ECG on cardiology intensive care unit. *Instruction systems* help diagnose weaknesses in the medical student's knowledge and identify appropriate remedies to overcome the deficiencies. *Control systems* adaptively govern the overall behavior of a process examined. These can be used in medical treatment processes.

We will first look at general structure and then knowledge representation.

2.1 General Structure of Expert System

The basic components of an expert system are displayed in Figure 8-2 which is a slight modification of the version published in Castillo, Gutiérrez and Hadi [5]. The main components of the structure are: Knowledge base, Knowledge acquisition subsystem, Information acquisition subsystem, User interface subsystem, Explanation subsystem, Coherence control subsystem, Learning subsystem, Action execution subsystem and Inference engine.

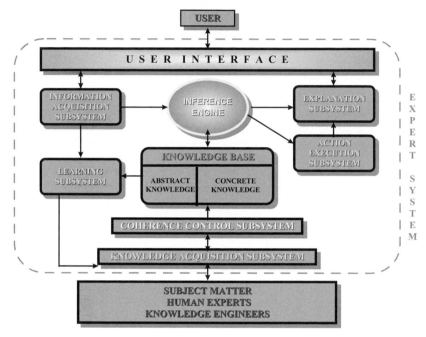

Figure 8-2 General scheme of expert system.

2.1.1   Knowledge Base

The nucleus of the expert system is the knowledge base. A knowledge base is everything necessary for understanding, formulating and solving the problem. It includes two basic elements: *concrete knowledge base*, i.e. a database of facts such as the problem situation (e.g. facts on actual cases to be solved) and the theory of the problem area (e.g. facts on previously observed cases) and *abstract knowledge*, i.e. special heuristics or rules that direct the use of knowledge to solve problems in a particular domain. For example, in medical diagnosis, the symptoms, diseases and the relationship among them form the abstract knowledge, whereas particular symptoms of given patients form the concrete knowledge.

2.1.2   Knowledge Acquisition Subsystem

A knowledge acquisition subsystem accumulates, transfers and transforms problem-solving expertise from various knowledge sources to a computer system in order to construct or expand the knowledge base. Potential knowledge sources in the subject matter include textbooks, databases, special research reports, human experts and the users' own experience. The reason why not all expertise is documented is that most human experts are unaware of the exact mental process by which they diagnose or solve a problem; therefore knowledge engineers help the human experts structure the problem area. Sometimes a number of human experts collaborate and difficult situations can occur if the experts disagree.

2.1.3   Information Acquisition Subsystem

An information acquisition subsystem provides information that is utilized by an inference engine to make conclusions and for a learning subsystem and knowledge acquisition subsystem. This procedure assures that any information provided by the user is checked for consistency before it is entered into the knowledge base.

2.1.4   User Interface Subsystem

A user interface subsystem is the interface between the expert system and the user. Thus, in order for an expert system to be an effective tool, it must incorporate efficient mechanisms to display and retrieve information in an easy way. A language processor for friendly, problem-oriented communications between the user and the expert system must be included. Another important aspect of the user interface subsystem is that users commonly evaluate expert systems based on the quality of the user interface rather than on that of the expert system itself.

2.1.5   Explanation Subsystem

An explanation subsystem provides an explanation of the conclusions drawn or of the actions taken by the expert system. This makes it possible to trace responsibility for conclusions to their sources, both in the transfer of expertise and in problem solving.

2.1.6   Coherence Control Subsystem

A coherence control subsystem controls the consistency of the knowledge base and prevents any incoherent knowledge from entering the knowledge base. In complex situations, even an expert can give inconsistent statements. A coherence control subsystem therefore checks the knowledge and informs human experts about inconsistencies.

2.1.7   Learning Subsystem

A learning subsystem enables expert systems to learn from available data. These data can be collected by both experts and non-experts and can also be used by the knowledge acquisition subsystem. Learning which improves estimation of frequencies or probabilities associated with the symptoms and diseases belongs to *parametric learning* whereas some aspects related to the structure of the knowledge base (e.g. new rule, type of probability distribution) belong to *structural learning*.

2.1.8   Action Execution Subsystem

An action execution subsystem enables the expert system to take actions. For example to trigger an alarm to signal a critical health situation of a monitored patient can be a solution.

2.1.9   Inference Engine

An inference engine is the heart of the expert system. This component is essentially a computer program that provides a methodology for reasoning based on information already gathered in the knowledge base and acquired information from the user. The conclusions drawn by the inference engine may be based either on *deterministic knowledge* or *uncertain knowledge*. Uncertain knowledge can occur in a concrete knowledge base (e.g. patient is not sure about his symptoms) or in an abstract knowledge base (e.g. a given combination of symptoms occurs in a given disease very frequently but not always). The inference engine must also be able to handle uncertain knowledge.

2.2   Knowledge Representation

Knowledge acquisition is the accumulation, transfer and transformation of problem-solving expertise from a knowledge source to a computer system to construct or expand the knowledge base. The information in the knowledge base includes everything necessary for understanding, formulating and solving the problem. Knowledge, not mere facts, is the primary material of expert systems. For example a knowledge base of rule-based expert systems consists of a set of objects and a set of rules. Rule-based systems belong among *logical expert systems*. However, to construct the knowledge base of a *probabilistic expert system,* we need to specify the joint probability distribution of variables. The most general model is based on a direct specification of the joint probability distribution. Unfortunately, the direct specification often involves a huge number of parameters. Simplifications of the most general model can be obtained by exploiting independence of variables or other additional assumptions about the joint probability distribution.

3 Probabilistic Decision Support Systems

Processing uncertain, incomplete and vague data has been stressed as one of the typical features of probabilistic decision support systems, especially probabilistic expert systems. At the early stages of probabilistic expert systems several obstacles, due to the difficulties encountered in defining the joint probability distributions, slowed down their development. With the introduction of *probabilistic network models* these obstacles have been largely overcome. More detailed information about probabilistic network models can be found in [5]. We all have an intuitive feel for *probability* but often we can see that the terms *relative frequency, odds, odds ratio* or *likelihood ratio* are used synonymously. Mathematicians do not use them that way. In practice the *relative frequency* can be considered as an estimate of the probability of a random event **A**. In the number (*n*) of independent trials we observe the number (*m*) of outcomes of the random event **A**. It can be seen that for a large *n* of the trials the relative frequency (*m/n*) is nearly the same as the probability **P(A)**.

Therefore the relative frequency of **A** is

$$\hat{P}(A) = \frac{m}{n}.$$

The main purpose of allotting numerical values to probabilities is to allow calculations to be performed on these numbers. The odds of the random event **A** is calculated as

$$O(\mathbf{A}) = \frac{P(A)}{1 - P(A)}.$$

In medicine we often use odds for calculating an odds ratio (OR) that is given by the ratio of the odds of **A** given that the condition **B** is satisfied (**B**) to the odds of **A** given that the condition **B is** not satisfied (**nonB**). Therefore the odds ratio is calculated as

$$OR = \frac{O(A \mid B)}{O(A \mid nonB)}$$

and the likelihood ratio (LR) is calculated similarly using the probabilities $P(A \mid B)$ and $P(A \mid nonB)$ as

$$LR= \frac{P(A \mid B)}{P(A \mid nonB)} .$$

More details about probabilistic and statistical concepts can be found for example in Armitage and Colton[1].

3.1 Bayesian Decision Support Systems

We can demonstrate the Bayesian approach to decision support in the process of screening. An implicit assumption underlying the concept of screening is that early detection of disease will lead to a more favorable prognosis because of earlier treatment. Some diseases are not suitable candidates for application of a screening program. To be appropriate for screening, a disease should be serious and treatment given before symptoms develop but should also be more beneficial in terms of reducing morbidity or mortality than that given after they develop. Moreover, the prevalence of pre-clinical disease should be high among the population screened.

We intend to evaluate the quality of screening test used for detection of the disease D. The observed data concerning the screening test T and the disease D are presented in the following way (Table 8-1)

Table 8-1 Results of screening test

Screening test T	Disease D +	Disease D -	Total
+	a	b	$a + b$
-	c	d	$c + d$
Total	$a + c$	$b + d$	n

Sensitivity and specificity are two measures of the validity of a screening test. *Sensitivity (SE)* is defined by the probability $P(T+|D+)$ of testing positive, if the disease is truly present. From given data it is estimated by

$$SE = a/(a+c).$$

Specificity (SD) is defined as the probability $P(T-|D-)$ of testing negative, if the disease is truly absent. It is estimated by

$$SP = d/(b+d)$$

Obviously, it would be desirable to have a screening test that would be both highly sensitive and highly specific. Usually that is not possible, and there is generally a trade-off between the sensitivity and specificity of a given screening test. However, the costs of a screening test include not only those related to the procedure itself, but also those arising from subsequent evaluation of individuals with a positive test result.

Predictive values of screening test measure whether an individual actually has the disease, given the results of the screening test. *Predictive value positive* ($PV+$) is the probability $P(D+|T+)$ that a person actually has the disease in case of a positive test. It is estimated by $PV+=a/(a+b)$. Similarly, *predictive value negative* ($PV-$) is the probability $P(D-|T-)$ that a person actually does not have the disease in case of a negative test. It is estimated by $PV-=c/(c+d)$. *Prevalence* of the disease ($P(D+)$) is the probability of the occurrence of the disease ($D+$) in the population.

The interrelationship of sensitivity, specificity and prevalence $P(D+)$ with predictive values can be expressed using *Bayes' formula* as

$$PV+ = \frac{SE \cdot P(D+)}{SE \cdot P(D+) + (1-SP)(1-P(D+))}$$

and

$$PV- = \frac{SP \cdot (1-P(D+))}{SP \cdot (1-P(D+)) + (1-SE)P(D+)} \,.$$

Some methods for decision support in medicine and healthcare are derived from the following model, which can (in a simplified form) be described as follows. Let us consider that the patient can suffer from one of k diseases $\mathbf{D}^{(1)}$, $\mathbf{D}^{(2)},\dots, \mathbf{D}^{(k)}$ only. We let π_{I} denote the prevalence (*prior probability*) of the disease $\mathbf{D}^{(i)}$, $\sum_{i=1}^{k}\pi_i=1$.

We can observe m different features (variables) $X_1, X_2,\dots,X_m$ on a patient. $\mathbf{X}$ denotes the vector or all features ($X_1, X_2,\dots,X_m$). The relationship of features $\mathbf{X}$ to the disease $\mathbf{D}^{(i)}$, is described by probabilities $P(\mathbf{x}\,|\,\mathbf{D}^{(i)})$ for discrete features $\mathbf{X}$ (e.g. sex, marital status, presence of fever) and by probability distribution $f_i(\mathbf{x})$ (for continuous features $\mathbf{X}$ (e.g. weight, height, body temperature)).

Let $L(\mathbf{D}^{(i)}, \mathbf{D}^{(j)})$ denote the *loss* that occurs by making the decision $\mathbf{D}^{(i)}$ when the correct decision is actually $\mathbf{D}^{(j)}$. Then $\delta(\mathbf{X})$ denotes a *decision function* that gives the decision $\delta(\mathbf{x})=\mathbf{D}^{(i)}$ for examined features $\mathbf{x}$. The quality of the decision function $\delta(\mathbf{X})$ is expressed by the *average risk*, written as

$$r(\delta) = \sum_{i=1}^{k} \sum_{x} (L(\mathbf{D}^{(i)}, \delta(x))\pi_i P(x | \mathbf{D}^{(i)})$$

for discrete features X and similarly for continuous features X.

The *optimal (Bayesian) decision function* δ^* (if such exists) is that for which $r(\delta^*)$ is the minimum of $r(\delta)$ from all considered decision functions δ. We often choose the *loss function* $L(\mathbf{D}^{(i)}, \mathbf{D}^{(j)})$ in such a way that

$$L(\mathbf{D}^{(i)}, \mathbf{D}^{(j)})=1 \text{ for } \mathbf{D}^{(i)} \neq \mathbf{D}^{(j)} \text{ and } L(\mathbf{D}^{(i)}, \mathbf{D}^{(j)})= 0 \text{ for } \mathbf{D}^{(i)} = \mathbf{D}^{(j)}.$$

Then the average risk $r(\delta)$ of a decision function δ equals $e(\delta)$, the *total probability of misclassification* (TPM), and therefore the optimal (Bayesian) decision function δ^* (if such exists) yields the *minimal total probability of misclassification $e(\delta^*)$*.

Using the above-mentioned Bayesian decision-making approach we face many different problems in practice. Often we do not know either the prior probabilities of diseases π_i, i=1,2,...k or conditional probabilities $P(\mathbf{x} | \mathbf{D}^{(i)})$ (or probability densities $f_i(\mathbf{x})$). We therefore have to replace them by sample estimates from population studies or subjective estimates of experienced physicians. In practice we can often receive good estimates of conditional probabilities $P(\mathbf{x} | \mathbf{D}^{(i)})$ (or probability densities $f_i(\mathbf{x})$) from population studies. However, we would like to know other conditional probabilities $P(\mathbf{D}^{(i)} | \mathbf{x})$ which are known as *posterior probabilities* of diseases for measured $\mathbf{x}$.

In addition, merely having knowledge of the prior probabilities of diseases $\mathbf{D}^{(i)}$ can help physicians to make diagnostic estimates before examining the patient. This occurs only when a prior probability of one of the considered diseases is close to one. However, if the prior probabilities of all considered diseases are nearly the same, prior diagnostic estimates are impossible.

Let us judge how the knowledge of one feature $X_l = x_l$ might influence the ability of a physician to decide better on diagnosis $\mathbf{D}^{(i)}$. Using Bayes formula we can calculate posterior probabilities $P(\mathbf{D}^{(i)} | x_l)$ as

$$P(D^{(i)}|x_1) = \frac{\pi_i P(x_1|D^{(i)})}{\sum\limits_{j=1}^{k} \pi_j P(x_1|D^{(j)})}$$

for i=1,2,...,k.

We can continue in this way for measured values of two features (x_1 and x_2) and calculate posterior probabilities $P(\mathbf{D}^{(i)}|x_1,x_2)$ as

$$P(D^{(i)}|x_1,x_2) = \frac{\pi_i P(x_1,x_2|D^{(i)})}{\sum\limits_{j=1}^{k} \pi_j P(x_1,x_2|D^{(j)})}$$

It is much more difficult to estimate the conditional probabilities for combinations of features from population studies. Under the assumption that the features are independent for considered diagnoses, then the conditional probability

$$P(x_1,x_2|D^{(i)}) = P(x_1|D^{(i)}) \, P(x_2|D^{(i)})$$

and Bayes' formula can be simplified. In the same way, we can proceed for more than two measured features.

It follows that all combinations of values of features $\mathbf{X}=(X_1, X_2,....,X_m)$ can be divided into k disjoint sets $\mathbf{X}^{(1)}, \mathbf{X}^{(2)},..., \mathbf{X}^{(k)}$. For the measured values $(x_1, x_2,....,x_m)$ belonging to the set $\mathbf{X}^{(i)}$ we accept the decision $\mathbf{D}^{(i)}$.

Let us consider that the optimal TPM decision-making, i.e. the total probability of misclassification, $e(\delta)$ is minimal. Decision-making is based on searching for decisions with the maximal posterior probability. Therefore, for the measured values of features $(x_1, x_2,...,x_m)$ we will decide for $\mathbf{D}^{(i)}$ if

$$P(D^{(i)}|x_1,x_2,....,x_m) = \max_{j \in 1,2,...,m} P(D^{(j)}|x_1,x_2,....,x_m).$$

TPM optimal decision-making is based on maximal posterior probabilities. For measured values of features $\mathbf{x}=(x_1,x_2,..,x_m)$, we determine the conditional probabilities $P(\mathbf{x}|\mathbf{D}^{(i)})$ (or conditional densities $f_i(\mathbf{x})$ for continuous features), which we multiply by prior probabilities $P(\mathbf{D}^{(i)})$. Posterior probabilities of all decisions $\mathbf{D}^{(i)}$, according to Bayes' formula, are expressed as the ratio of the product $P(\mathbf{D}^{(i)}) \, P(\mathbf{x}|\mathbf{D}^{(i)})$ divided by the same constant. Therefore, the optimal

TPM decision-making is equivalent to searching for the decision $\mathbf{D}^{(i)}$ where the product $P(\mathbf{D}^{(i)}) \, P(\mathbf{x} \,|\mathbf{D}^{(i)})$ is maximal. This decision-making is the ideal one when we know all the probabilities and/or probability distributions or we can estimate them well. Using Bayes' model of decision-making, very good results were achieved in diagnostics of acute abdominal pain [6]. Let us consider the results reached in computer-supported diagnostics of acute abdominal pain. For this purpose the system called MEDICL (Medical Diagnosis and Computer-aided Learning) was created. Using the MEDICL system, physicians collect data about examined patients using standardized questionnaires and forms. After entering the collected data into the MEDICL computer system, the data are compared with a large database of patients who have already been examined for acute abdominal pain. Using Bayes' formula, posterior probabilities for considered diagnoses are computed. However, these probabilities are made available to the physician only after his own diagnostic conclusion is made. When the physician's diagnostic conclusion differs from the conclusion made by the computer, the MEDICL system provides further information, which shows reasons for the computer's conclusion.

3.2   Discriminant Analysis

As already mentioned, the application of Bayesian decision-making in practice is sometimes uneasy due to difficult estimation of conditional probabilities. However, sometimes we can restrict ourselves to situations where further assumptions are justified. Often the assumptions concern the independence of features, normality of conditional probability distributions or types of decision function (such as linear, quadratic). It can be proved that for features with conditional distributions described by the multivariate normal distribution, optimal decision-making (Bayesian decision-making) can be done by quadratic discriminant (decision) functions. Moreover, if the covariance matrices of these multivariate normal distributions are the same, optimal decision-making is based on linear discriminant (decision) functions.

In medical decision-making the principal problem is to assign a patient with an unknown disease to one of two (or more) diagnostic and/or treatment groups on the basis of the values of observed features (clinical signs, laboratory tests, history and so forth). This is also the task of *discriminant analysis*. First we can consider that the patient population consists of two diagnostic groups $\mathbf{D}^{(1)}$ and $\mathbf{D}^{(2)}$. Physicians observe features $\mathbf{X} = (X_1, X_2, ..., X_m)$ on patients. Based on this information, each patient is assigned to one of diagnoses $\mathbf{D}^{(1)}$ or $\mathbf{D}^{(2)}$. This means that the observed features $\mathbf{X}$ in medical decision space are divided into two subsets $\mathbf{X}^{(1)}$ and $\mathbf{X}^{(2)}$. It is the ideal case of the diagnostic situation, when the correct classification using $\mathbf{X}$ is always possible.

Fisher in the 1930s developed a method for choosing the coefficient of a linear combination of features so as to maximize the ratio of the difference of means of the linear combinations in two diagnostic groups to its variance. *Fisher's criterion of goodness of classification* can be written as follows. Suppose we look for a linear function

$$z = b_1 x_1 + b_2 x_2 + \ldots + b_m x_m.$$

If this is going to discriminate well between the groups we should expect the mean values of z in the two groups to be reasonably far apart in comparison with the variation of z within groups. We could therefore try to find values of the b's in such a way that the ratio expressed by

$$\Delta^2 = \frac{(\bar{z}_{D^{(1)}} - \bar{z}_{D^{(2)}})^2}{\text{variance of } z \text{ within groups}}$$

is as large as possible. The estimated variance of z will in general be different in the two groups, but a pooled estimate could be calculated.

The square root of Δ^2 is the so-called *Mahalanobis distance* Δ. If Δ is greater than about 4 the situation is like two univariate distributions whose means differ by more than 4 standard deviations: the overlap is quite small, and the probabilities of misclassification are correspondingly small.

To use z for allocating future patients to one of two diagnoses we need to find a cut point z_0.

The allocation rule based on the Fisher criterion for $\bar{z}_{D^{(1)}} > \bar{z}_{D^{(2)}}$ that is intended to come close to minimizing the total probability of misclassification (TPM) is as follows:

Allocate a patient to $D^{(1)}$ if $z > z_0$, otherwise allocate a patient to $D^{(2)}$, where z_0 is

$$z_0 = \frac{\bar{z}_{D^{(1)}} + \bar{z}_{D^{(2)}}}{2} + \ln \frac{\pi_2}{\pi_1},$$

and π_1, π_2 are prior probabilities.

Many computer programs calculate the value of z for each patient in the two original samples. It is thus possible to count how many patients in the two groups would have been wrongly classified by the allocation rule. This unfortunately gives an overoptimistic picture, because the allocation rule has been determined to be the best (in above-specified sense) for these two particular samples, and it is likely to perform rather less well on the average with subsequent observations from the two groups.

Where the prior probabilities are equal, i.e. $\pi_1 = \pi_2 = 0.5$, then $\ln\dfrac{\pi_2}{\pi_1} = 0$.

One particular form of distribution is called the *multivariate normal distribution*. It implies, among other things, that all regressions of one feature follow a normal distribution and that all regressions of one feature on any set of other features are linear. If the $\mathbf{X}$ followed multivariate normal distributions $f_i(\mathbf{x})$, $i=1,2$ with the same variances and correlations in both diagnostic groups $\mathbf{D}^{(1)}$ and $\mathbf{D}^{(2)}$, but with different means, the Fisher and TPM minimization criteria lead to the same results. As has been shown, the discrimination by TPM criterion is as follows.

Allocate a patient to $\mathbf{D}^{(1)}$ if $\pi_1 f_1(\mathbf{x}) > \pi_2 f_2(\mathbf{x})$, otherwise to $\mathbf{D}^{(2)}$.

This allocation yields the minimization of the TPM criterion.

The discriminant analysis can be generalized to more than two groups. One approach is that we allocate the patient to the diagnostic group with the maximal posterior probability. In cases in which simultaneous distributions of features in diagnostic groups are normal ones, the discrimination will coincide with minimization of the total probability of misclassification. Other ways of generalization lead to methods of *canonical analysis*.

4 Logical Decision Support Systems

Logical decision support systems, especially logical knowledge-based and expert systems, are often deterministic. In order to cope with uncertainty, they are based on concepts different from probability. We will describe some logical decision systems and ways of representing knowledge in rule-based expert systems, frame-based expert systems, semantic nets and other systems.

4.1 Rule-Based Expert Systems

Rules are the most widely used way to represent heuristic knowledge in expert systems. Rules are, abstractly formulated, as follows:

IF <condition> THEN <conclusion/action>.

Rules were already used before the era of artificial intelligence in research on formal logic and on transformational grammars. Rules state that whenever the condition part of the rule is true, the conclusions are true (*declarative rule*) or the specified actions should be taken (*procedural rules*). It is the task of the inference engine to check whether the conditions are indeed true for the problem at hand. Most medical expert systems use rules in one form or another. Weaknesses of the rule formalism include the fact that they do not represent the basic or deep knowledge of a domain, but merely compiled, shallow knowledge. This limits the amount of explanation the system can give. The rules in knowledge base can be displayed in the form of AND/OR graphs. In this case the nodes of graphs are statements and the edges are rules.

However, it is often difficult to specify when a certain rule is valid. Although a rule may state a generally valid association between the condition and conclusion part, there might be many exceptional situations in which the rule is not valid. Therefore a knowledge base often consists of rules of the form

IF <condition> THEN <conclusion/action> with the weight w,

where w is a degree of certainty (degree of belief) of the rule validity.

A typical knowledge base has hundreds to thousands of rules formed from tens to hundreds of propositions. The rules are obtained from experts with their subjective beliefs. Therefore, for condition satisfied with certainty the expert believes in conclusion/action with the degree of certainty w. The activity of the rule-based expert system is the following. The system asks the user some questions concerning his/her degree of belief into some propositions and propagates his/her answers through the system of rules, finally obtaining degrees of belief (or degrees of certainty) for some other propositions including some diagnoses. The example of a declarative rule with the degree of certainty is a rule of the expert system MYCIN:

IF
> The site of the culture is blood, and
> The identity of the organism is not known with certainty, and
> The stain of the organism is gramneg, and
> The morphology of the organism is rod, and
> The patient has been seriously burned

THEN
> There is weakly suggestive evidence (.4) that the identity of the organism is pseudomonas

4.2 Frame-Based Expert Systems

The weakness of frame-based representation is that reasoning is not defined. Frames are only formalism for data recording. Frames were originally proposed by Marvin Minsky [15] as the tool for representation of knowledge. Originally frames had to represent stereotype situations. The main idea behind the concept of frames came from the imagination of how a human being perceives the world that surrounds him. The frame is a structure, a list, which consists of some items, attributes and their values. Some values can be fixed, some could be predefined and some values can be left empty and they will be filled in when an actual object will be examined. Frames are assumed to represent *static knowledge* well; meaning the concepts hierarchy or decomposition. Association among frames can be shown by a graph. Nowadays frames penetrated into programming languages, where they are named *objects* and the corresponding way of programming using objects is called *object-oriented programming*. Although frames are basically used for the representation of static knowledge, they also allow for some sort of inference. One of the strong points of frame formalism is that it includes the generation of instances. The mechanism which accompanies this generation of instances and that allows us to draw inferences is often called *inheritance*. It implies that the attributes of a frame are inherited by its instance. It is even possible to inherit attributes from multiple "parents". Hence the properties of different generic classes are combined in one specific instance. Not only can attributes be inherited, but attribute values may also be passed from the parents to the children. It is obvious that rules have to be defined to determine how attribute values from different parents are to be combined when they have the same attribute names. The inheritance is often defined to be dynamic. This means that when the value of an attribute of a frame is changed during the reasoning, the attribute values for all instances are changed as long as no constraints are violated. This can be considered as a strong point as well as a weakness of inheritance. However, it is also difficult to represent uncertain inheritance.

4.3 Semantic Nets

Semantic nets were designed in the 1960s to model the storage of knowledge in the human brain. They tried to represent every fact separately and to connect all facts that are in some sense connected. The model of associative memory was designed using an oriented graph, called *semantic network*. The nodes of this graph represented words in natural language and the edges represented associations and meanings between two terms in a language. It can be generally stated that a semantic network simply offers a graphical notation for logical formulas restricted to unary and binary predicates and the two types of quantification: *is member of* some set, which represents the relationship between the object and some notation (set of objects), and *is part of*, which represents the relationship between the notion and some more general notion. Semantic nets are useful for descriptive purposes, because they give a simple structure of the body of facts. The major idea is that the meaning of a concept comes from its relationship to other concepts, and that the information is stored by interconnecting nodes with labeled arcs. A weakness of a semantic net is that heuristics are difficult to express, while a reasoning strategy for dealing with the knowledge in the network is also not obvious.

4.4   Other Decision Support Systems

4.4.1   Hypothesize-and-Test (H&T)

Knowledge that is encoded in rules relates facts to conclusions or diagnoses. In medicine, this diagnostic knowledge is seldom directly available. In most textbooks, knowledge is presented in the reverse order: The symptoms are described which occur in a certain disease. Diagnosis can be defined as a searching problem in which one has to match the patient's pattern of symptoms with all possible descriptions to come to a list of possible diagnoses. By querying the patient and by doing diagnostic tests, one tries to reduce the list of possible diagnoses to the one or two that explain the symptoms of the patient best. Disease descriptions can relatively easily be stored in frames. The inference engine has to match the symptoms of the patient against the various disease descriptions to find possible diagnoses. In the case more than one diagnosis is likely, the system should be able to provide information on which test or symptoms might give additional information to decide between the competing diagnoses. INTERNIST-1 [13] as well as QMR [14] are based on this type of inference. However, this knowledge representation is limited in the sense that correlations between observed symptoms are not taken into account.

4.4.2   Event-Driven Reasoning

Event-driven reasoning is an interesting approach to problem solving. It is particularly suitable for simulation and monitoring. The basic idea is that when the value of an attribute changes or exceeds a threshold, some procedure is activated. This procedure is often called a "demon". The "demon" might be some computational algorithm or another inference procedure that might be based on the previously described methods.

4.4.3 Predicate Calculus

Predicate calculus is one form of knowledge representation. Predicate calculus was originally proposed to study relation of logical consequence, but it became mainly the prototype of schemes for knowledge representation.

The knowledge is represented by logical sentences in which predicates occur to define relations or properties.

It is clear that the formal description of knowledge is not easy for non-logicians to read and understand. On the other hand, formal theories are available for chaining expressions to arrive at inferences. A basic disadvantage is the difficulty of modelling uncertainty in predicate calculus.

4.4.4 Neural Networks

Neural networks are a special kind of decision support method. They consist of networks of elements, each element or node computes a weighted sum of its input and applies a function of some kind to generate an output, hence the analogy with neurons. Nodes are arranged in layers. The input layer receives input, which may be raw image data, processed image data or information about the features of an interpreted image. The output layer provides the response of the system. Most neural networks used in object recognition systems include a single "hidden" layer between the input and output. To use the systems for object recognition, they must first be trained. Training consists of providing the system with examples of the possible input and allowing a control loop to adjust the weights of the system's nodes to produce the required output. The system is considered a success if it is able to generalize what it has learned and classify new examples correctly.

5 Summary

Decision support systems may improve patient care through a number of different decision-making strategies. Although the need seems obvious, there are only a few medical decision support systems running in practice. The evaluation of decision technology is often neglected, education is not appropriate [10] and there are still remaining problems to solve mainly in processing uncertain, incomplete and vague information. However, it seems to be promising that various approaches are not developed in isolation, but under mutual influence. The effectiveness of appropriate decision support systems (especially knowledge based systems) in medicine and healthcare must reach the healthcare goals of the information society.

6   Bibliography

[1] Armitage P, Colton T (eds): *Encyclopedia of Biostatistics*, John Wiley & Sons, New York 1998

[2] Bemmel van JH, Gremy F, Zvarova J: *Diagnostic Strategies and Expert Systems*. Elsevier, Amsterdam 1986

[3] Bemmel van JH, Musen A: *Handbook of Medical Informatics*. Springer, Berlin 1997

[4] Blois MS: *Clinical Judgment and Computers*. New Engl. J. Med. 303, 1980, 192-197.

[5] Castillo E, Gutiérrez JM, Hadi AS: *Expert Systems and Probabilistic Network Models*. Springer, New York 1997

[6] Dombal de FT, Leaper DJ., et al: *Computer-aided Diagnosis of Acute Abdominal Pain*. British Medical Journal 2, 1972, 9-13

[7] Duda RO, Hart P, Nilsson NJ: *Subjective Bayesian Methods for Rule-Based Inference Systems*. In: Proceedings of AI FPS Conference, SRI International, Stanford, 1976, 1075-1082

[8] Engle RL, Davis BK: *Medical Diagnosis: Present, Past and Future*. Arch. Intern. Med. 112, 1963

[9] Feigenbaum EA: *Autoknowledge: From the File Servers to Knowledge Servers*. In R Salamon, B Blum and M Jorgensen (eds), MEDINFO´86, Amsterdam, North-Holland 1986

[10] IT-EDUCTRA, CD, Commission of European Communities, 1998

[11] Keen PGW, Scott-Morton MS: *Decision Support Systems: An Organizational Perspective*. Addison-Wesley, Reading, MA 1978

[12] Ledley RS, Lusteed LB: *Reasoning Foundations of Medical Diagnosis*. Science 130, 1959, 9-12

[13] Miller RA, Pople HE, Myers JD: *Internist-1: An Experimental Computer-based Diagnostic Consultant for General Internal Medicine*. New England Journal of Medicine 307, 1982, 468-476

[14] Miller RA, Masarie FE, Myers JD: *Quick Medical Reference (QMR) for diagnostic assistance*. M.D. Computing 3, 5, 1986, 34-35

[15] Minsky ML: *A Framework for Representation Knowledge*. In: Winston (ed.): The Psychology of Computer Vision. McGraw-Hill, 1975, 975-982

[16] Shafer G: *A Mathematical Theory of Evidence*. Princeton University Press, Princeton, NY 1976

[17] Shortliffe EH: *Computer-based Medical Consultations: MYCIN*. American Elsevier, New York 1976

[18] Sox CS, Blatt MA, Huggubs MC, Marton KI: *Medical Decision Making*. Butterworth-Heinemann, Boston 1988

[19] Turban E: *Decision Support and Expert Systems*. Macmillan, New York 1988

[20] Turing AM: *Computing Machinery and Intelligence*. Mind 59, 1950

[21]Zadeh LA: *The Role of Fuzzy Logic in the Management of Uncertainty in Expert Systems.* Fuzzy Sets and Systems 11, 1983

9 Health Telematics Networks

Piotr Nawrocki[1], Dominik Radziszowski[1]

[1]   Department of Computer Science, AGH University of Science and Technology, Krakow, Poland

The healthcare sector [7] is characterized by increasing specialization among the parties: hospitals, either public or private, practitioners, pharmacies, social insurance etc. which generate an intensive structured communication flow. A major driving force behind the development of telematics for health is to more efficiently manage the healthcare delivery process, while providing more user-oriented applications and integrated solutions in such areas as continuity of care, patient records, regional healthcare telematics networks and health information to the citizen.

This chapter presents the problems of the health telematics network. Some technical aspects of the network communication are presented in Chapter 5 – ("Wireless Systems in e-Health"). Information about security in the e-health systems is found in Chapter 4 – ("Security and Safety of Telemedical Systems").

1   Transport Layer in Telematics Networks

One of the most important issues when designing telematics networks is assuring reliable and suitable communication [10] between computer nodes. Due to the specific conditions in medical networks (among others, data protection), telematics networks should have a very high level of security. The transport layer describes all communication aspects of telematics computer networks.

1.1   Packet-Based Communication

Along with the evolution of the Internet, a wide range of services and capabilities of computer networks has been developed. Existing network protocols such as TCP/IP[1] and UDP/IP are based on packet transmission and predominate in backbone of telematics networks. This conception of transmission is suitable for multimedia of audio/video streams, and hence is of great importance for telematics networks. Modern telematics applications make use of picture, video and sound for sending information. Multimedia transmission requires specific network conditions and parameters. The possibility of losing packets, lack of retransmission of packets, and unauthorized access are problems which programmers of telematics (and particularly teleconsultation) applications must tackle. DSL and ADSL solutions are recently becoming increasingly popular. This technology is not expensive and remains suitable for most users, but it is not satisfactory for streaming A/V data. These solutions exhibit transmission asymmetry and only one direction has good bandwidth, while the opposite direction transmission bandwidth is comparable to dial-up technology (and it is not adequate for multimedia transmission).

1.1.1   Edge Access Technologies

The base backbone technology for communication in telematics networks is based on packet transmission in wire media. Additionally, for communication between nodes (for example between doctors and patients at home or hospitals and ambulances), modem communication or wireless technology can be used. In scenarios where patients exchange medical information with doctors the cheapest way of communication is a modem (and new DSL and ADSL technology). This solution is sufficient for exchanging textual data (for example blood pressure) but the bandwidth is too low for examination results presented as audio/video. New wireless technologies are sufficient for audio/video streams and also provide communication with mobile nodes (for example ambulances). There are some wireless technologies (see Chapter 5) for communication in networks. Among the diverse wireless technologies available, users can choose the networks most suitable for telematics.

1.1.2   Quality of Service

Modern computer networks enable connecting independent (until now) topologies for data, video and voice transmission into one infrastructure that uses IP technology. Bringing together so many applications with diverse requirements for parameter values in the network layer forces one to consider

---

[1] The IP standard version 4 is being used currently but technological developments and a rapid increase in numbers of people using IP addresses (as a result of an increase in the number of network devices) have spurred the development of a new standard - IP version 6. The new standard also solves the problem relating to a large number of network addresses.

Quality of Service (QoS) mechanisms. These mechanisms make it possible to unify all available computer networks' usage with assurances of an appropriate service level. QoS mechanisms are indispensable where traffic overloads may potentially appear, to assure that traffic sensitive to packet losses and delays (e.g. real-time audio and video) is prioritized with respect to computer data where such faults are better tolerated. Usage of QoS solutions is critical at the point of contact of local networks with bandwidths of hundreds of megabits per second, and slow WAN links, where aggregation of hundreds of kilobits of available bandwidth is performed.

2 Health Digital Data Standards

Thus far, we have discussed generic network communication standards; there is also a set of standards specific to the healthcare industry. Some of these concern equipment, and some concern patient records. Problems arise when there is a need for integration of different hospital systems in one functionally-coherent system, e.g. the creation of HIS (Hospital Information System) based on RIS (Radiological Information System), LIS (Laboratory Information System) and PACS (Picture-Archiving and Communication System). In such situations, dedicated programmer interfaces and data conversion dictionaries have to be created. A better solution is to set up standards for medical data interchange, standards sufficiently open and universal that they would allow for effective integration of systems working on different system and hardware platforms and using different data representations.

The current situation is that there exists a large number of inconsistent standards. Major health informatics standards applicable to medical data representation, interchange and secure communication, originate from CEN (Comité Européen de Normalisation - Technical Committee 251) [9], [1].

2.1 ENV 13606: EHCR Communication (1999)

This four-part European pre-standard (ENV) [9] governs the representation of EHR information as it might be communicated between two repositories or between a client and a server. In its four parts it defines:

- the object model that must be used to represent the EHR,
- a set of term lists that must be used to populate key attributes defining the classes of information being communicated,
- a set of rules and an information model governing how access control requirements should be specified,
- a set of message specifications to support message-based exchange e.g. using XML.

In December 2001 CEN TC/251 confirmed a new Task Force, known as "EHRcom", to review and revise the 1999 four-part pre-standard ENV 13606 relating to Electronic Healthcare Record Communications. The intention of this work is to propose a revision that could be adopted by CEN as a formal standard during 2004. The overall mission statement of the EHR communications standard proposed by the Task Force is to produce a rigorous and durable information architecture for representing the EHR, in order to support the interoperability of systems and components that need to interact with EHR services:

- as discrete systems or as middleware components,
- to access, transfer, add or modify health record entries,
- via electronic messages or distributed objects,
- preserving the original clinical meaning intended by the author,
- reflecting the confidentiality of that data as intended by the author and patient.

A combination of good working relationships between CEN, openEHR [13] and HL7 [12] has led to an intention to harmonise the proposed new standard both with openEHR (reference model and archetype approach) and with HL7 [1].

2.2   Health Information Systems Architecture (HISA)

ENV12967 defines an open systems architecture facilitating the development of products and services by different vendors. It defines the structure for how healthcare information systems should be built, implemented and used. It specifies the interactions between hospital information systems, organisations and users, and the control, storage and manipulation of the different types of data in the various components of the system.

HISA services are divided into:

- *Generic Common Services* which would be found in the core information systems in any business domain,
- *Healthcare Common Services* which are more specific to healthcare but common to most applications within healthcare: subject of care, activities, resources, authorisation, patient health characteristics.

A new HISA Task Force was established in early 2002 to revise this standard, and this work is expected to be completed during 2003-4 [1].

2.3   Health Level 7

This US-based international organisation, generally known as HL7 [12], is responsible for the most widely adopted standard for message-based communication in healthcare. HL7, whose message specifications were first published in 1988 as an industry standard, was awarded Standards Development Organisation (SDO) status in 1993 so that newer versions of the specification are official ANSI legislative standards. The messages primarily support the interoperability of components of a hospital information system and purchaser-provider contractual communications.

HL7 Version 2 messages have been developed to reflect standardised reporting data sets for several aspects of a patient's care in hospital:
- patient admission, transfer or discharge (ADT),
- orders for drugs, procedures or tests and their results,
- messages relating to finance and billing information,
- clinical observations focussing primarily on measurements.

Despite its wide international usage, the problems of inconsistent implementations of Version 2 and the unsystematic growth of message segment definitions have limited the realisation of interoperability, leading to the drafting of a new v3 standard. A key feature of Version 3 is the Reference Information Model (RIM): a means of specifying the information content of messages through an information model that clarifies the definitions and ensures that they are used consistently. The RIM is a formal object model, expressed using UML, representing the superset of core classes and attributes that will be required (in various combinations) by the different HL7 Version 3 messages.

The HL7 Clinical Document Architecture (CDA) is a proposal for the generic structure of clinical documents, and is sometimes regarded as the HL7 equivalent of a record architecture. Only "Level One" of the CDA has at present been ratified: this XML-based specification includes a header with document authorship information, organisational origin and patient identifiers, and a body whose basic structure is loosely defined at this stage.

HL7 version 2 is presently being used in the United States, Australia, Canada, Germany, the Netherlands, Israel, Japan and New Zealand. Additional countries are joining each year [1].

2.4 Standards for Images - DICOM

The Digital Imaging and Communications in Medicine (DICOM) [11] standard arose out of a precursor standard for images (ACR-NEMA) that was first published in 1985 by the American College of Radiology (ACR) and the National Electrical Manufacturers Association (NEMA). The DICOM standard is the most widely used common data representation internationally for the various medical images acquired and communicated. It has addressed many of the issues of vendor-independent data formats and data transfers for digital medical images. CEN and ANSI have adopted DICOM by reference in their imaging standards.

DICOM is a result of efforts to create a standard method for the transmission of medical images and their associated information which started in the 1980s. Having an open architecture, DICOM enabled equipment from different manufacturers covering a range of examination types (so-called modalities) to be interconnected. This is why it soon has become the industry standard.

Distinct from various general-purpose graphical formats, DICOM files offer very good, diagnostic quality of the images, although, where worse quality is clinically acceptable, lossy compression can be applied. DICOM files contain many so-called tags (name-value pairs) precisely describing not only the image and how to properly display it but also information with patient demographic data and examination annotations. The operations which are the most characteristic of DICOM format are the following: adjusting Hounsfield window value, animating dynamic images (e.g. from coronarography examinations), displaying contained tags and marking annotations. Hounsfield window scale adjusting is necessary to notice the subtle differences between some tissues, and two parameters are used here: the value, expressed in Hounsfield Units (HU), and the window's width; the values outside the window border are non-distinguishable.

DICOM is not only the specialised file format but also a client-server protocol. It introduces different services (e.g. storage, printing, displaying) called the Service Class and their providers (SCP) and users (SCU). For example, a laser printer is the SCP providing printing service for a workstation (being Print SCU). Infrastructure of hospital PACS systems consists of many such devices.

The security issues pertaining to medical information have come under more serious consideration in recent years. This manifests not only in installing firewalls in hospitals but also in DICOM protocol changes. DICOM standard authors, in consecutive annexes, address, among others, secure transport connection, data integrity and authentication of users and media security (e.g.

encryption of the file while storing DICOM data on media). Altogether, this allows efficient transfer of medical data over insecure networks [3].

Integrating the Health Environment (IHE) is a recently-formed industry-sponsored organization seeking to promote interoperability between systems within specialist departments such as radiology, and the conventional hospital systems used to order such investigations and to receive imaging study reports. It works closely with DICOM and HL7 in this area [1].

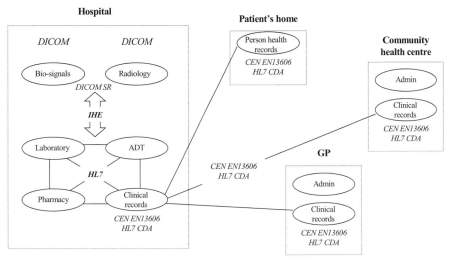

Figure 9-1 Domains of communication of health information covered by various industry and legislative standards.

2.5 Data Security Standards

There are several CEN standards relating to the secure handling of EHR information. The key ones are listed below; in practice many of the general security requirements are similar to those adopted by other industry sectors. They are therefore not discussed further.

- Algorithm for Digital Signature Services in Health Care, ENV 12388:1996,
- Security Categorisation and Protection for Healthcare Information Systems, ENV 12924:1997,
- Secure User Authentication for Health Care: Management and Security of Authentication by Passwords, ENV12251:2000,
- Security for Healthcare Communication, ENV13608:1999,
- Secure User Identification for Healthcare — Strong Authentication using Microprocessor Cards, ENV 13729:1999.

Use of electronic certificates for signature and encrypted communication between healthcare professionals has to be regulated by national law e.g. Belgium is currently introducing identification cards (2004) with selected attributes (certification, PKI, TTP). The processing of personal health data must also comply with the 1995 EU Directive [8] and the 1997 Council of Europe Recommendations [4] regarding its acquisition, storage, communication and analysis. Each member state has passed national legislation to reinforce these instruments, such as the 1998 Data Protection Act in the UK [1].

3 Telematics Network Organizational Model

There are two main models of organization in telematics networks, from the information flow point of view:
- Centralised,
- Dispersed.

The centralised model [5] hinges on a central point of the system – a reference centre (hospital, clinic) where medical experts are located. Some of the local points of care connect with the referential centre for the purposes of (tele)consultation.

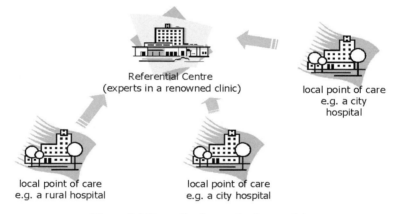

Referential Centre
(experts in a renowned clinic)

local point of care
e.g. a city
hospital

local point of care
e.g. a rural hospital

local point of care
e.g. a city hospital

Figure 9-2 Centralised organisation model.

In the dispersed model, local points of care can consult with the referential centre, but there is also a possibility of consultation between respective local points. Potential experts are situated at some of the hospitals and clinics. This model can be more complicated to organize (equipment, coordination, etc.). On the other hand, the dispersed model extends the possibility of exchanging information (experience) between doctors and increases the quality of healthcare.

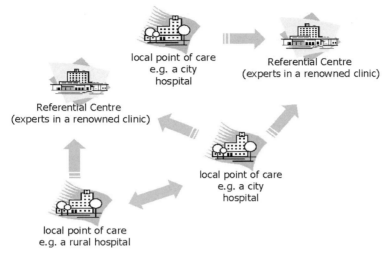

local point of care
e.g. a city
hospital

Referential Centre
(experts in a renowned clinic)

Referential Centre
(experts in a renowned clinic)

local point of care
e.g. a city
hospital

local point of care
e.g. a rural hospital

Figure 9-3 Dispersed organisation model.

3.1 Models for Team-Oriented Healthcare Practice

"Integrative healthcare" is a common term for describing teams of healthcare providers working together to provide patient care. There are several models [2] for describing, comparing and evaluating different forms of team-oriented healthcare practices that have evolved in modern healthcare systems throughout Europe.

Seven different models of team-oriented healthcare practice are described below:

- Parallel
  - characterized by independent healthcare practitioners working in a common setting,
  - each individual performs his/her job within his/her formally-defined scope of practice.
- **Consultative**
  - expert advice is given from one professional to another; this may be via direct personal communication, but is often via a formal letter or referral note.
- **Collaborative**

- practitioners, who normally practice independently from each other, share information concerning a particular patient who has been (is being) treated by each of them,
- these collaborations are ad hoc in nature and usually occur informally on a case-by-case basis.
- **Coordinated**
  - a formalised administrative structure requires communication and the sharing of patient records among professionals who are members of a team intentionally gathered to provide treatment for a particular disease or to deliver a specific therapy,
  - a case coordinator (or case manager) is responsible for ensuring that information is transferred to and from relevant practitioners and the patient.
- **Multidisciplinary**
  - is characterized by teams and managed by a leader (usually not a physician) who plans patient care,
  - one or two individuals usually direct the services of a range of ancillary members who may or may not meet face-to-face,
  - each individual team member continues to make their own decisions and recommendations which may be integrated by the team leader,
  - is a highly articulated and formalised outgrowth of coordinated practice.
- **Interdisciplinary**
  - emerges from multidisciplinary practice when the practitioners who make up the team begin to make group (usually based on a consensus model) decisions about patient care facilitated by regular, face-to-face meetings.
- **Integrative**
  - consists of an interdisciplinary, non-hierarchical blending of both conventional medicine and complementary and alternative healthcare that provides a seamless continuum of decisionmaking and patient-centric care and support,
  - is based on a specific set of core values which include the goals of treating the whole person, assisting the innate healing properties of each person, and promoting health and wellness as well as the prevention of disease,
  - employs an interdisciplinary team approach guided by consensus building, mutual respect, and a shared vision of healthcare that allows each practitioner and the patient to contribute their particular knowledge and skills within the context of a shared, synergistically charged plan of care.

There are many trends in healthcare practices. These models help patients and healthcare practitioners to determine what styles of practice meet their needs, and they are also helpful to healthcare managers and researchers, who document the evolution of team practices over time.

3.2   Telematics Networks Overview

In this section some interesting examples of health telematics networks in Europe and Canada are presented.

3.2.1   HYGEIAnet

HYGEIAnet (http://www.hygeianet.gr/), the regional health information network of Crete that interconnects the public healthcare facilities of the island, provides an information infrastructure for the evolution of the lifelong integrated electronic health record, and promotes telemedicine as an accountable reimbursable medical act. HYGEIAnet empowers individuals and communities to make informed choices about their own health, the health of others and Crete's health system. In an environment of strengthened privacy protection, it builds on a regional healthcare information infrastructure to improve the quality and accessibility of healthcare and to enable the delivery of integrated healthcare services. It provides information and services that are the foundation for accountability, continuous improvement to healthcare and better understanding of the determinants of the health of the population.

3.2.2   Health Telematic Network (HTN)

Health Telematic Network (HTN) (http://www.e-htn.it/), based in Italy, provides telemonitoring services for the following services: teleconsultation, triage, second opinion, telematic instrumental services reporting. HTN — Telemedicine Services started in December 1998 based on the scientific research project called Boario Home Care.

The HTN Service centre is a call centre, which is open 24 hours a day, all year round. With its technologically advanced platform and specialised staff, it can satisfy sanitary demands presenting real-time telematic solutions:
- monitoring the state of health in any circumstances, 24 hours a day,
- taking an active part in one's health management,
- activating protected discharges (public or private hospitals, rehabilitation centres).

HTN services assure telematic medical assistance and personal monitoring for:

- users who want to check their health conditions,
- users with previous specific diseases.

3.2.3   MBTelehealth

MBTelehealth (http://www.mbtelehealth.ca/) is one of 27 federally-funded telehealth projects established in the spring of 2001. The goal of MBTelehealth is to provide quality information and knowledge at the point of care, for all Manitobans (Canada), wherever they reside. MBTelehealth utilizes the latest in information technology to achieve that goal.

Telehealth is the use of information technology to link people to healthcare expertise at a distance. A satellite or ground link is used to connect a specialist or other healthcare provider to a patient. The centrally-administered MBTelehealth Network uses broadband information and telecommunications technology, such as Internet-based (IP) video-conferencing, to bring and improve health services closer to home for rural Manitobans.

3.2.4   HealthNet Luxembourg

HealthNet Luxembourg (http://www.healthnet.lu/) is a secure telematic network for healthcare professionals in the Grand Duchy of Luxembourg. The main goals of HealthNet are:
- to develop a technical infrastructure allowing healthcare professionals to communicate safely,
- to offer basic services such as professional electronic mail, medical databases, secure access to the Internet, etc.,
- to help healthcare professionals integrate or develop specialised applications in the areas of tele-radiology, laboratory results exchange, telepathology, etc.

The network utilises leased lines, ISDN or DSL connections (via VPN), according to the required bandwidth and the needs of the participants. All hospitals of the Grand Duchy, some laboratories and around 200 physicians are connected to HealthNet, as are health insurance providers and the Entente des Hopitaux (the organisation that represents all hospitals).

4   E-health Network Services

The activities going by the term "eHealth network services" should cover the concept of eHealth as defined in the context of eEurope [6] – the application of information and communications technologies (ICT) across a whole range of functions and services which, one way or another, affect the health of citizens and patients, specifically:

- health-related information,
- delivery of care to patients by healthcare professionals,
- electronic trading of healthcare goods.

Internet-based electronic trading of healthcare goods is already developed very widely. A huge variety of Internet services offers an uncountable number of different applications supposed to improve our health and lifestyle. Yet, the quality and reliability of the information available is typically very low, mostly because these services operate just like other electronic trade markets. Hence, by eHealth network services we mean specialist, dedicated information centres oriented towards serving competent information to patients and physicians.

4.1 General Information Oriented Services

Facilitating patient involvement in the process of getting better access to high-quality information is a key point in the speed-up of the recovery process. The first source of trustworthy, independent, competent and complete information is usually the patient's GP but it has become increasingly difficult for one person to provide all this information during the limited time of consultations. This situation has led to the creation of many health-related Internet services, authored by medicals, whose intention is to improve access to quality information for their patients. Several of them, selected from the thousands available on the net, are described below.

Table 9-1 Selection and descriptions based on Dr Steven S. Overman, http://www.dr-overman.com/

Site	Description
http://www.medmatrix.org	Highly suggested site as it has a *ratings system* to help you determine the value of a listed Web site, very useful. **The Medical Matrix Project** is devoted to posting, annotating, and continuously updating "full content, unrestricted access, Internet clinical medicine resources." Medical Matrix assigns ranks to Internet resources based on their utility for point-of-care clinical application. Quality, peer review, full content, multimedia features, and unrestricted access are emphasized in the rankings. To ensure that the ranks are applied systematically, and as objectively as possible, they are reviewed by

	editorial board and assigned 1–5 stars according to the guidelines.
http://www.mayoclinic.com	This site is produced by a team of writers, editors, multimedia and graphics producers, health educators, nurses, doctors, and scientists. The presence on the Web is a natural extension of Mayo's longstanding commitment to provide health education to their patients and the general public. MayoClinic.com is the only Web site that gives an access to the experience and knowledge of the more than 2,000 physicians and scientists of the Mayo Clinic.
http://www.netwellness.com	NetWellness is a non-profit consumer health Web site that provides high-quality information created and evaluated by medical and health professional faculty at the University of Cincinnati, Case Western Reserve University and The Ohio State University. NetWellness is dedicated to improving the health of Ohioans and people worldwide through information that is scientifically sound, high quality, and unbiased. One of their more popular features, Ask an Expert has nearly 200 health professionals, including physicians, nurses, pharmacists, dieticians, dentists, genetics counsellors, optometrists, athletic trainers, and social workers who answer all legitimate questions, usually within 2 to 3 days.
http://www-hsl.mcmaster.ca/ /tomflem/ill.html	**An interesting collection of links. HealthCare Information Resources** is compiled and maintained by Tom Flemming: "I have been developing this page since Canada Day (1 July) 1995 as a collection of links to sources of healthcare information of interest to a broad spectrum of potential users, both in Canada and beyond. Among the users I have in mind in the development of this resource are: patients, their families and friends, and their healthcare workers. The resources presented here are not intended exclusively for those who are

	ill. Anyone with an interest in health (maintaining it, protecting it and improving it, especially), and everyone interested in the quality of healthcare will find electronic information sites of interest in the various sections of this page".
http://www.medscape.com	**CBS Healthwatch, a health consumer development by Medscape:** Over 2.8 million healthcare professionals and consumers have become members of Medscape's network since 1995 to get trusted health information on the Web. Founded by Medscape, Inc., as a site primarily for healthcare professionals, www.medscape.com has earned a strong following among consumers who seek cutting-edge, authoritative content that they cannot find on traditional consumer health sites. Now Medscape takes consumer health information to a new level with CBSHealthWatch, which offers an array of high-quality information and interactive tools to help consumers and their families manage their daily personal health.
http://www.healthfinder.gov	**Healthfinder®** is a free gateway to reliable consumer health and human services information developed by the U.S. Department of Health and Human Services. Healthfinder can lead you to selected online publications, clearinghouses, databases, Web sites, and support and self-help groups, as well as the government agencies and not-for-profit organizations that produce reliable information for the public. Launched in April 1997, served Internet users over 1.7 million times in its first year online; in 1999, the site received 94 million hits and 4,549,810 visits!

Many of these services are built on the potential for citizen empowerment through widespread availability of high-quality appropriate health information on the Internet. However, most still do not correspond with the average citizen's needs (i.e. they are more oriented towards the business and commercial needs of the authors) located at the centre of attention in the development of high-quality health-related information services.

Implementation and sharing best practices related to e-health result in creating more and more personalised services, where patients look for more and more detailed information suitable for their problems. The next natural step in the development of such services is reorientation-shifting emphasis from information to the patient himself.

4.2   Patient-Oriented Services

Most existing medical systems expose their interfaces to hospital staff, but usually not to the general public. Therefore, detailed information about the services (availability, preconditions, waiting time) is not widespread and assistance of specialised medical staff is often mandatory.

The problem of making some information available to outside hospital users is very complex. Security of legacy systems, unauthorised access control in particular, is mainly based on total access blockade to the systems from the outside world (firewalls, non-routable IP addresses, etc.) Attempts to allow access to a part of the data for a wide group of external users within the confines of existing systems cause a huge security risk for data which ought to remain confidential. Hence we can safely say that common medical systems cannot be accessed by the public.

4.2.1   Public Transparent Access to Medical Services

Expectations concerning public transparent access to medical services are very wide. Public access means not only access for patients at a point of care; it should also cover potential patients and external physicians (i.e. GP doctors). Such circumstances carry strong ambiguity and decrease the level of confidence in medical services. Public transparent access means access to information about medical services, equipment, hospital personnel and examination results, first and foremost as a method for booking a medical service selected from all those supported by a hospital, or a consultation with preferred medical specialists chosen from all hospital staff. Additionally, it requires setting clear rules for access to short-supply services (e.g. transplants). Creation of various standards of services access makes the procedures complex and unclear. This leads to patients' confusion and the necessity of clarifying rules. In this context, transparent and public access to medical services begins to play a more and more important role.

4.2.2   Home Care

Home care treatment is especially important for chronic or fatally ill persons. Home care requires that computer systems be extended beyond simple information servers; they need to be able to monitor all parameters that are important from the medical treatment point of view. Currently-available systems are usually installed and configured at patient homes in an experimental fashion, not as part of normal treatment practices. They are usually able to monitor only a limited number of very basic critical parameters. Communication between equipment at the patient's home and a hospital is based on dial-up lines or SMS.

Parameters sent from the patient's home are stored in hospital systems and later used for tracing changes in patient health state. There is a lack of advanced automated reaction mechanisms to possible patient's condition deterioration, mostly because of the small set of parameters subject to monitoring.

There is also a notable lack of return communication, which would enable interaction with the patient and quick reaction in urgent situations. Existing services should therefore be extended with patient interaction – bilateral audio and video communication, modules for sending and storing more detailed medical data and the possibility of remote control over medical devices installed at the patient's home.

5   Case Study — CAS

In order to validate medical data integration and security in a heterogeneous access environment and J2EE architecture [16], [15], [14] the Clinical Appointment System (CAS), a set of Web-based systems that transparently expose their functionality to the wide public, has been developed. The work has been carried out by the Dept. of Computer Science, AGH University of Science and Technology as part of the 6WINIT grant.

CAS is an application that gives patients the possibility to make an appointment with a doctor for a specified examination at a selected clinic using a Web browser. The system works as follows: patients issue requests specifying the type of examination, the doctor, the clinic and the time when they want the examination to occur. Requests are served by appointment clerks who validate patients' requirements and approve the requests, modify or refuse them in accordance with the doctors' timetables. If a clerk modifies appointment prerequisites, the patient is able to accept or rearrange them to suit his needs. This dialog lasts until both sides of the conversation are satisfied.

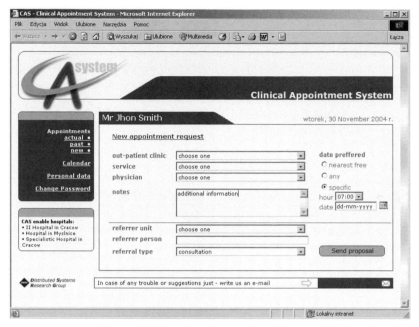

Figure 9-4 Creation of a new appointment.

The application distinguishes three separate groups of users who access its functionality. Besides patients and appointment clerks described previously, there are administrators who handle all system management tasks e.g. adding clinics, doctors, appointment clerks, etc.

The mentioned basic functionality is accompanied by several extensions:

- patients can review the schedule of their visits,
- patients can review the information about completed visits,
- patients can review their personal data,
- appointment clerks are able to create new visits on behalf of the patient,
- appointment clerks validate and correct patients' personal data.

One important characteristic of the system is that appointment clerks have the possibility to act on behalf of the patient. In this way, the system can be used in a traditional way when a patient calls clerks or makes an appointment at an appointment desk. This feature enables seamless progress towards Web-based functionality.

The CAS user interface has been designed to enable use of the system from PCs and PDAs. Other client devices can access the system as well, but the overall page layout wouldn't look as good as it does on displays of these two types of end machines.

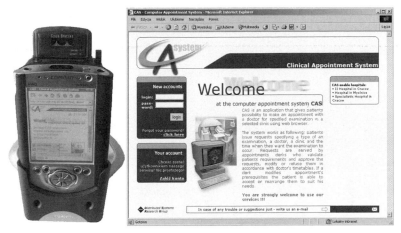

Figure 9-5 CAS on PDA and PC displays.

CAS functionality is accessible only for authenticated users. Every system client is equipped with a login and password and must use them to access the system. Authorisation mechanisms allow every patient to use only the part of the sensitive information gathered by the system that concerns him/her. Appointment clerks can read all the information connected with appointments and personal data. To prevent data exchange between browser and server from being vulnerable to malicious users' attacks, the secure HTTP protocol is used.

CAS was deployed at the John Paul II hospital in Krakow in order to validate its usefulness and performance.

The CAS system has proven that there are no significant technical obstacles to creating transparent public access to medical services. Pilot deployment has revealed significant demand from both patient and medical staff for this kind of system. Unfortunately, current legal regulations effectively prevent us from progressing towards systems fulfilling the goals pointed out by the authors.

6 Summary

The functionality of health telematics networks presented in the chapter requires dedicated, reliable computer networks with huge throughput and guaranteed QoS. Detailed technical requirements are also described in other chapters in this book, but it is not the case that they are the main reason for the very slow development and sparse dissemination of such services.

Many sociological, ethical, technical and legal issues have to be overcome to bring such services to a proper level. In the authors' opinion, existing solutions present an opportunity to surmount technical problems, while other issues still remain unsolved. Another very sensitive problem is appropriate selection of information and its presentation to the right access groups – general public, hospital staff, individual doctors etc. Hence, organisational and legal problems appear more troublesome than technical ones.

7 Bibliography

[1] 6WINIT project IST-2000-25153, *deliverable D15.*
[2] Boon H., Verhoef M., O'Hara D., Findlay B.: *From parallel practice to integrative healthcare: a conceptual framework.*
http://www.biomedcentral.com/1472-6963/4/15
[3] Cala J., Czekierda Ł.: *TeleDICOM - environment for Collaborative medical consultations.* International Conference on e-Health in Common Europe, Kraków - Poland, June 5 - 6, 2003
[4] Council of Europe Recommendation, R(97)5: *On the Protection of Medical Data.* Council of Europe, Strasbourg, 12 February 1997
[5] Duplaga M., Radziszowski D., Dul M., Nawrocki P., Zielinski K.: *Technical and non-technical factors influencing the process of teleconsultation services development carried out in Krakow Centre of Telemedicine.* Tromso Telemedicine Conference, Tromso - Norway, September 15 - 17, 2003
[6] eEurope2005: *An Information Society for all.*
http://www.europa.eu.int/information_society/eeurope/2005/index_en.htm
[7] eTEN – Work Programme, http://europa.eu.int/information_society/
[8] European Community Directive 95/46/EC: *On the Protection of Individuals with Regard to the Processing of Personal Data and on the Free Movement of such Data.* OJ L281/31 - 50, 24 October 1995
[9] *European Standardization of Health Information.* http://www.centc251.org
[10] Kosiński J., Nawrocki P.: *Technical aspects of teleconsultation organization.* International conference on E-health in Common Europe, Kraków - Poland, June 5 - 6, 2003.
[11] *Main DICOM standard web.* http://www.dicom.org
[12] *Main HL7 organization web.* http://www.hl7.org
[13] *Main Open Health Record Community web.* http://www.openehr.org
[14] Radziszowski D., Rzepa P.: *Enterprise Java Beans.* TelenetForum, April 2002
[15] Roman E.: *Mastering Enterprise JavaBeans and the Java 2 Enterprise Edition.* Wrox Press Ltd, 2001
[16] *Specification of Java 2 Enterprise Edition Platform.* http://java.sun.com/j2ee

10 IT Applications for the Remote Testing of Hearing

Andrzej Czyżewski[1], B. Kostek[1,2], H. Skarżyński[2]

[1]   Gdańsk University of Technology, Faculty of Electronics, Telecommunications and Informatics, Multimedia Systems Department

[2]   Institute of Physiology and Pathology of Hearing

Telemedicine can play an important role in diagnosing and treating hearing losses. This fact is associated, among others, with the methodology of audiometric measurements and with supporting hearing through hearing aids and cochlear implants. Current problems related to treating hearing impairments and total deafness pose a distinct challenge for science, which must provide ever more effective methods for application in diagnostics and audiology as well as otolaryngology practice. Scientific experiments in these fields also indicate ways of supplementing methods of acoustic signal analysis and processing used in hearing diagnostics and prosthetics with modern technological advances, so that patients can benefit from methods whose history is so short that they may be classified as experimental.

Similar needs for wider introduction of electronics and computer science technologies can be recognised in phoniatry and speech therapy, where the diagnostic process, devoid of advanced signal analysis tools, remains very difficult and therapy is often arduous and laborious.

Choosing hearing aids according to patients' needs and hearing characteristics is yet another problem which has not been solved yet. Experience shows that even the preliminary step, i.e. adjusting the aid's acoustic path to the patient's hearing track, is very important, especially in the case of major hearing losses. The process of regulating parameters of signal track for electronic hearing aids should utilise, insofar as possible, the knowledge on the patient's hearing characteristics, with the aim of allowing him to understand speech. The multimedia hearing aid fitting system presented in this paper is based on research concerning the degree of understanding speech in the presence of noise and on determining (on that basis) the optimum characteristics of the multi-band dynamic compressor, which is an important part of advanced hearing aids. This process utilises so-called fuzzy reasoning, which marks our application as one of the first in audiology to employ soft computing methods.

Advances in teleinformatics as well as its wide employment in recent years have opened new possibilities for conducting mass screening of hearing, tinnitus (ear noises), speech and vision. Diagnostic and recovery systems associated with the interactive medical portal *Telezdrowie (www.telewelfare.com)* designed by the institutions mentioned in the header of this paper serve as an example of how simple diagnostic methods employed in screening tests can be mass-deployed thanks to teleinformatics, thus defining a new quality for widespread diagnostic tests of communication senses. In addition, one cannot neglect the influence of advances in the field of network database systems on epidemiology tests and associated studies on hearing deficiency and vision deficiency.

The aspects mentioned above will be briefly illustrated by sample applications deployed under the supervision of the head of the present project. For practical reasons, the presentation is limited to selected applications associated with hearing. Information on other applications can be found in [4], [6], [8], [2].

1 Methodology of Hearing Screening

Screening methods employed thus far can be divided into three groups: The first one includes methods which only use questionnaires for the person being diagnosed or for people from his/her vicinity (e.g. parents). The second group employs physiological and audiometric measurements. The third group of methods is comprised of tests employing both questionnaires and measurements. Several measurement methods can be distinguished among screening tests. Screening can utilise audiometric tests. According to the standard proposed by ASHA (American Speech-Language-Hearing Association) in 1985, an audiometric screening test should determine whether a child can hear in both ears three 20-dB HL tones of frequencies of 1000 Hz, 2000 Hz and 4000 Hz, respectively. The above procedure may be extended by supplying an additional 500-Hz tone of the same level of 20 dB HL. If the child cannot hear at least one of the tones presented, he or she must undergo detailed audiometric tests. In the case of adults, the test signal levels are increased, usually by 5 dB.

Screening tests associated with the project show that speech audiometry can also be employed for screening tests. The main advantage of speech audiometry is that, unlike tonal audiometry, it allows not only for measuring receptive or conductive hearing, but also for assessment of the whole complex hearing-perception mechanism. That is why speech audiometry is proposed for use in screening children and teenagers. Two main types of thresholds are associated with speech audiometry. The first one is *speech detection threshold* (SDT). It is defined as the lowest signal level for which speech is heard 50% of the time. The second threshold type is *speech reception threshold* (SRT), defined as the lowest signal level for which speech is understood 50% of the time. These thresholds are presented in Figure 10-1.

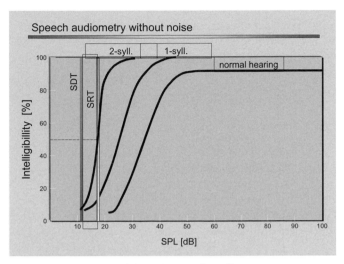

Figure 10-1 Sample speech audiograms.

Sound material presented during audiometric tests may vary in type. For example, it may involve logatoms, monosyllabic words, disyllabic words or whole sentences. The degree of understanding is directly influenced by the type of verbal material and, more importantly, acoustic pressure level. This effect is presented in Figure 10-2, where curves marked "1-syll." and "2-syll." correspond to monosyllabic and bisyllabic (spondey) tests, respectively. In the case of regular hearing the speech audiograms are rising curves, which describe an increase in the understanding of speech, coupled with increasing sound exposure. However, for certain hearing impairments increasing the speech signal level causes the degree of understanding to decrease. Analysis of this phenomenon may be facilitated by the so-called audiogram curvature index defined by the following formula:

$$RI = \frac{(Y_{max} - Y_{min})}{Y_{max}} \tag{10-1}$$

where: *RI* is the audiogram curvature index,

Y_{max} is the maximum understanding value,

Y_{min} is the minimum understanding value for the sound levels presented at the uncomfortable hearing level.

A value of the audiogram curvature index exceeding 0.45 may indicate hearing damage.

When designing tests for speech audiometry, one must take into account the number of words in the test, since it influences test reliability. For example, Figure 10-2 presents a graph of standard deviation as a function of the number of words in the test and of speech understanding. This graph was constructed on the basis of the following relation:

$$\sigma = 100\sqrt{\frac{p(1-p)}{n}} \qquad (10\text{--}2)$$

where: σ is the standard deviation,

p is the speech understanding ratio,

n is the number of words in the test.

As can be seen from the graph, test reliability decreases (i.e. standard deviation grows) with a decrease of the number of words used in the test. Tests using 10 or even fewer words are particularly unreliable.

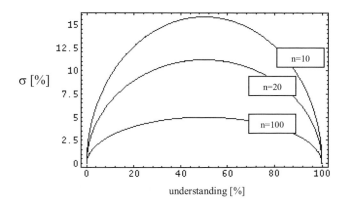

Figure 10-2 Standard deviation σ as a function of the number of words in the test and of speech understanding.

When speech audiometry tests are performed using noise masking the investigated ear, we speak about so-called speech-in-noise audiometry. The masking noise makes speech understanding harder, although in this case it is done on purpose. This effect can be seen on audiograms as classic noiseless speech audiograms "shifted" to the right by a value equal to the masking noise level (Figure 10-3).

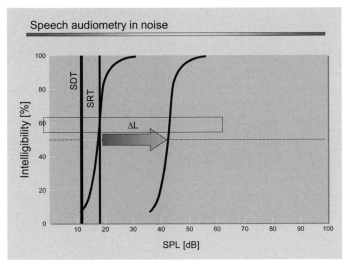

Figure 10-3 Example of audiogram being "shifted" due to influence of masking noise of level ΔL.

Widely-used measurement methods are based only on three-tone tonal audiometry. Within the presented project a new method, based on additional use of speech-in-noise audiometry, was proposed. Besides simple tones this method utilizes a speech signal mixed with noise in appropriate proportions. This method, in conjunction with the three-tone test and with a system of electronic questionnaires, forms the basis for a mass hearing screening system, which has so far been used to test above 150,000 school pupils. The patronage of MENiS (Polish Ministry of Education and Sport) over this system allows us to expect that the tests will become ever more widespread, covering schools in the whole country, similar to screening ear noises, speech [4] and sight [7]. Figure 10-4 illustrates typical results obtained from tests performed in schools. A criterion of min. 70% correct answers in the speech-in-noise test causes up to 20% of children to require clinical diagnosis in order to exclude hearing difficulties. Performing the full set of tests, i.e. analysing the electronic questionnaires and the results of the three-tone test, often reveals that over 15% of children have difficulties with attaining satisfactory results of the screening test. A standard audiometric test allows us to detect hearing problems in up to 20% of the population being tested. This result confirms the frightening extent of hearing impairment, even in young people.

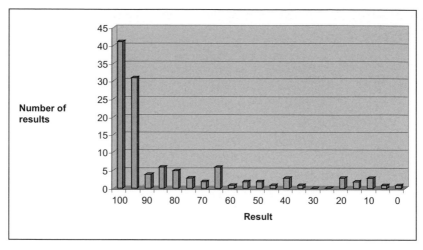

Figure 10-4 Summary of results of the picture test (utilizing speech in noise).
The x-axis represents the percentage of correct answers.

2   Method of Computer-Aided Adjustment of Hearing Aids

Widely-used systems for adjusting hearing aids allow for setting optimum parameters of a hearing aid, which usually does not mean that the optimum characteristics of hearing loss correction are obtained. The idea of a multimedia system for adjusting hearing aids (developed within the scope of a Ph.D. thesis by Piotr Suchomski [12]) was to create a computer utility allowing for unrestrained shaping of the characteristics of the prospective hearing aid which would optimally compensate for the given hearing damage. Since in a general case the problem of adjusting a hearing aid can be boiled down to the problem of adjusting the wide dynamics of speech to the narrowed dynamics of impaired hearing, the presented system focusses mainly on determining the characteristics of impaired hearing and then on deriving the dynamics of the sought-after hearing aid that would compensate for the damage. This is, however, a simplification, because in a real hearing aid the quality of hearing loss correction is also influenced by other factors, such as noise reduction algorithms, equalising of the processed signal and acoustic elements of the hearing aid itself [3], [12].

This paper presents the general principles of operation of the designed system as well as the results of experiments utilising implementations of this system. Several important stages of operation can be distinguished in the designed system (Figure 10-5). First, dynamics characteristics of the diagnosed hearing impairment are determined. These are then used to determine dynamics characteristics of the desired hearing aid. On the basis of the derived dynamics characteristics of the desired hearing aid, hearing training is conducted, utilising an extensive base of speech signals (100 logatoms, 200 words, 630 sentences).

The properties of hearing dynamics can be determined on the basis of results of a loudness scaling test. The designed system includes an implementation of the loudness scaling test based on an algorithm for evaluating the sensation of Loudness Growth in half-Octave Bands (LGOB) [1]. The test utilises signals in the form of white noise samples filtered in half-octave bands, with central frequencies of 0.5 kHz, 1 kHz, 2 kHz and 4 kHz respectively. During the test the person being diagnosed is exposed to randomly-presented test signals of various sound levels. The person being diagnosed evaluates the loudness sensation using a seven-degree scale of categories of loudness sensation (Figure 10-6).

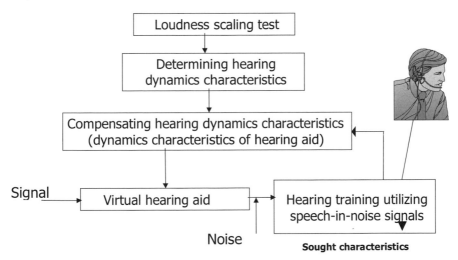

Figure 10-5 Scheme of adjusting hearing aid parameters.

The presented system utilizes a special module for converting results of loudness scaling into hearing dynamics. It uses fuzzy processing to map the results of scaling derived from the categories of the loudness sensation evaluation onto an objective scale of input sound levels, expressed in decibels. The category scale is represented by 7 fuzzy sets described by membership functions. These membership functions have been derived on the basis of statistical analysis of loudness scaling for 20 persons with no hearing impairments. The output of the fuzzy logic system is described by 13 membership functions which represent the differences between any given result of scaling and analogous results for unimpaired hearing [9], [11], [10].

As there are four frequency bands, with central frequencies of 500 Hz, 1000 Hz, 2000 Hz and 4000 Hz, which are tested in the LGOB test, four sets of membership functions are required. In order to derive these membership functions one has to perform the LGOB test on several dozens of regular-hearing persons. During the method design phase we prepared the required membership functions on the basis of generally-accepted approximation of LGOB test results for normal hearing (Figure 10-7). In order to obtain a much more reliable and realistic set of membership functions, one had to test loudness scaling using the LGOB test on several dozens of healthy individuals.

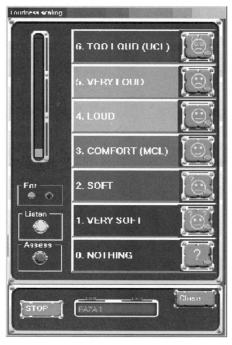

Figure 10-6 Scale of loudness sensation evaluation (graphical interface of a developed computer program).

One of the basic methods of approximation that come to mind when analyzing typical fuzzy logic systems and the sets of theoretical membership functions (as in Figure 10-7) is the approximation of the result-containing set boundary with triangle-shaped functions. It can be performed e.g. through mean-square approximation. In order to perform this task, one should determine the equations of two straight lines approximating triangle sides in the mean-square sense. The algorithm used by the authors to determine the triangular membership functions involves the following steps:

- finding the value of the first element belonging to the given fuzzy set (value of the first argument, for which the factual membership function assumes a non-zero value);
- to determine the position of the first arm of the triangle, one considers all the elements of the factual membership function MF satisfying equation (10–3):

$$x : \left\langle \forall_{x_i} \left(MF(x_i) - MF(x_{i-1}) \right) > 0 \right\rangle \qquad (10\text{–}3)$$

where: i - consecutive indices of arguments of membership functions MF satisfying condition (10–3)

- calculating coefficients a_1 and b_1 of the straight line equation $y=a_1x+b_1$;
- to determine the position of the second arm of the triangle, one considers all the elements of the factual membership function MF satisfying equation (10–3):

$$x : \left\langle \forall_{x_i} \left(MF(x_i) - MF(x_{i-1}) \right) <= 0 \right\rangle \qquad (10\text{–}4)$$

where: i - consecutive indices of arguments of membership functions MF satisfying condition (10–3).

- calculating coefficients a_2 and b_2 of the straight line equation $y=a_2x+b_2$;
- calculating the point of intersection of the straight lines $y=a_1x+b_1$ and $y=a_2x+b_2$;
- calculating zeros of both lines.

An example of a set of membership functions for the frequency band of 500 Hz obtained by approximating actual values is illustrated in Figure 10-8.

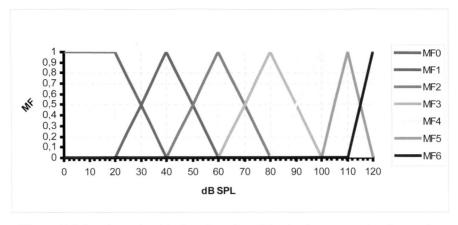

Figure 10-7 Set of membership functions describing loudness sensation for regular hearing, derived from theoretical data.

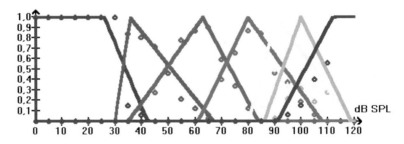

Figure 10-8 Approximation of values of membership functions with triangles performed on actual data.

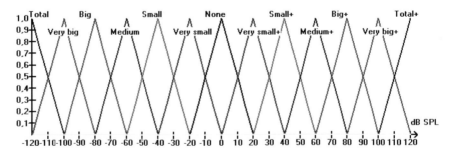

Figure 10-9 Initial membership functions describing the difference between regular and abnormal loudness scaling.

The next step of the described method involves defining the system output. As the aim of the designed method is determining the dynamics of impaired hearing, the designed system should "calculate" the difference between the given loudness sensation evaluation and the correct loudness sensation evaluation corresponding to the given test signal. This difference should be expressed in decibels.

Analysis of a typical plot of LGOB test results reveals that in between the seven categories of loudness sensation evaluations, one can define six differences which point to hearing loss (area below the LGOB curve for regular hearing) and six differences which point to hypersensitivity (area above the LGOB curve for regular hearing). No difference is a treated as a special case of difference. The above analysis leads to the conclusion that the output of the described fuzzy system can be expressed by a set of thirteen membership functions (Figure 10-9) representing the difference between the factual loudness sensation evaluation and the evaluation for regular hearing. Fuzzy sets obtained in this fashion can be described with the following labels (indicating the size of the difference): *none, very small, very small+, small, small+, medium, medium+, big, big+, very big, very big+, total, total+*. Labels marked with "+" sign denote positive difference (hypersensivity).

Fuzzy processing depends on a properly defined rule basis. Fuzzy logic rules take on the following form:

If <premise1> **AND** <premise2>**AND**...<premise_n> **THEN** decision

In the discussed case there are two premises. The first one is associated with information on regular loudness scaling. The other premise is associated with the investigated results of the LGOB test. Since both premises apply to the results of the LGOB test, they both use the same categories describing loudness sensations. In order to differentiate between the fuzzy sets associated with individual premises, labels of fuzzy sets for the first premise use lowercase letters while those of fuzzy sets for the second premise utilize capital letters.

Generally speaking, the rule base is designed on the basis of expertise. In our case, such expertise can be derived from the analysis of the LGOB test. The analysis of LGOB test results for healthy persons shows that the loudness scaling is linear in character, albeit the factor of proportionality increases from 1:1 to 2:1 (the loudness sensation rises twice as fast) for test signals exceeding 100 dB SPL. Based on this information, a rule base was prepared. It is presented in Table 10-1. Categories associated with regular hearing are marked in lowercase (e.g. "loud"), while categories written in capitals (e.g. "LOUD") represent hearing impairment.

The last stage of the system's operation is defuzzyfication, i.e. conversion of the obtained categories to a numerical value. After performing this process (using the centre of gravity method) we obtain the relations between sound levels expressed in decibels and the expected subjective assessment of loudness sensation for a given patient. This relation is the sought-after characteristic of hearing dynamics).

In order to determine the entire scope of dynamics characteristics for a given patient we had to create an algorithm which would calculate the desired characteristics on the basis of LGOB test results using the designed method of determining the difference between regular and impaired loudness scaling. The general scheme of the procedure is shown in Figure 10-10.

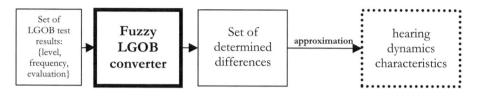

Figure 10-10 Diagram of fuzzy processing-based algorithm for determining characteristics of hearing dynamics.

Table 10-1 Rule base for the fuzzy system (the decision attribute is the difference between regular perception and perception associated with hearing impairment)

	I DON'T HEAR	VERY SOFT	SOFT	MCL	LOUD	VERY LOUD	TOO LOUD
I don't hear	None	V.small+	Small+	Medium+	Big+	V.big+	Total+
very soft	V.small	None	V.small+	Small+	Medium+	Big+	V.big+
soft	Small	V.small	None	V.small+	Small+	Medium+	Big+
mcl	Medium	Small	V.small	None	V.small+	Small+	Medium+
loud	Big	Medium	Small	V.small	None	V.small+	Small+
very loud	V.big	Big	Medium	Small	V.small	None	V.small+
too loud	Total	V.big	Big	Medium	Small	V.small	None

The system is fed a stream of results of the given LGOB test and produces a stream of consecutive differences for each result of the test. An LGOB test result consists of three parameters (level, frequency, evaluation), where "level" is the level of the given test signal (expressed in decibels), "frequency" is the frequency band encompassing the given test signal (expressed in hertz) and "evaluation" is the loudness sensation category used to evaluate the loudness sensation caused by the given test signal.

A fundamental advantage of the presented method is the mechanism of automated mapping from the category scale to the scale of sound levels expressed in dB. Moreover, the designed method of determining hearing dynamics utilizes all the available information on regular loudness scaling in the LGOB test, while standard methods of adjusting hearing aids rely on averaged data only. In the course of the standard determination of loudness scaling (LGOB test) the diagnosed person is presented with multiple filtered noise samples and the obtained results are subsequently processed in a statistical manner, while the proposed method only requires presenting the diagnosed person with filtered noise samples corresponding to seven loudness levels in four frequency ranges. The resulting difference in test-related effort and duration is of fundamental importance for audiologic practice.

Figure 10-11 presents a sample plot of loudness scaling results with the LGOB test, obtained for test signals from the frequency band centred around 500 Hz.

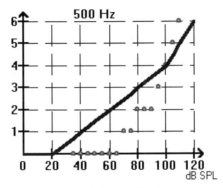

Figure 10-11 Sample results of LGOB test (Y axis represents category scale).

The derived dynamics characteristics of impaired hearing can be additionally used by the presented system for approximate simulation of hearing loss. In order to derive the dynamics characteristics of any hearing aid, the system compensates for the characteristics of impaired hearing. This compensation is based on flipping the hearing dynamics characteristics around the $y = x$ straight line (Figure 10-12).

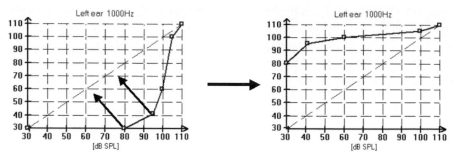

Figure 10-12 Compensating for the dynamics characteristics of impaired hearing.

The obtained hearing dynamics characteristics have been verified on the basis of training with speech-in-noise signals, processed according to the virtual hearing aid module algorithm (Figure 10-13). The speech signal is first filtered into 4 octave-wide bands with central frequencies identical to those used in the loudness scaling test. For each band, the signal dynamics are processed in a way adequate for the dynamics characteristics of the hearing aid, for the given band. When the dynamics have been processed, signals from individual bands are added to form a common channel. The module also allows for adding arbitrary noise, at both input and output. Moreover, we can equalize the level of the processed signal in individual bands, critical for speech.

The obtained degrees of speech understanding for individual listening tests are presented in Table 10-2. The degree of speech understanding is expressed as percentage values. The first value denotes the degree of speech understanding without dynamics processing, while the second value (to the right) denotes the degree of speech understanding following dynamics processing, based on the obtained dynamics characteristics of the hearing aid.

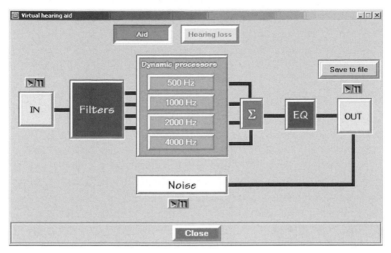

Figure 10-13 Algorithm for signal processing in a virtual hearing aid.

Table 10-2 Averaged degrees of speech understanding for patients suffering from severe hearing deficiency (without compression)-> with compression adjusted on the basis of investigation of loudness discrimination)

Patient	Logatom test	Word test + CCITT noise	Sentence test + cocktail-party noise
Patients 1-10	55% › 66%	11% › 33%	55% › 77%

3 Digital Technology in Diagnosing and Treating Tinnitus

Tinnitus (ear noises) often appears in cases of elevated hearing threshold associated with hearing loss due to inner-ear diseases. Such a condition may be caused by degeneration of external hair cells, causing neurons to be activated by stronger-than-normal signals. In such cases, an elevated activation threshold is present. However, before such elevated threshold appeared for the given patient e.g. due to a disease or development of otosclerosis, signals had been received and interpreted as hearing stimuli at higher levels of the hearing track. This fact results in the introduction of an additional mechanism of threshold quantisation of weak acoustic stimuli, which in turn relates to the elevated activation threshold of nerve cells. Existing audiology theories attempting to explain this phenomenon do not directly take into account the mechanisms of signal quantisation occurring due to the presence of threshold characteristics in the transmission system. Such interpretation becomes possible only with the knowledge of electric signal processing developed in other fields of science, e.g.

in digital signal processing. Using this approach, we have proposed a new interpretation of the phenomenon of tinnitus generation on the basis of the audio signal quantisation theory [4]. Moreover, using digital signal processing concepts we have proposed a theoretical explanation of a method to eliminate threshold quantisation-related tinnitus, basing on the dithering technique. Generally speaking, this technique involves supplementing low-level useful signals with certain levels of noise, which has the effect of stopping the process of spontaneous noise generation in the hearing track (resulting from threshold characteristics). One can easily notice that a similar approach is used to reduce tinnitus in audiology, where masking noise generated by a special masker device is utilised. The widely known effectiveness of such techniques for reducing both ear noises and quantisation noises generated spontaneously in electronic circuits indicates that ear noises can indeed be interpreted as a direct consequence of quantisation of weak signals in threshold systems. At this point it may be useful to present several aspects of analysis of quantisation phenomena. They will be further used to show how the interpretation of the phenomenon of noise generation in quantising systems and its elimination with additional "masking" dither noise may be useful for explaining the phenomena observed in the case of ear noises [5].

As is widely known, typical transition functions of a quantizer are described by the following formulae:

$$Q(x) = \Delta \left[\frac{x}{\Delta} + \frac{1}{2} \right]$$

(10–5)

or:

$$f(x) = \Delta \left[\frac{x}{\Delta} \right] + \frac{\Delta}{2}$$

(10–6)

where: x – value of the sample before quantization (at input)
Δ – height of quantization step
[ ] – operator returning the integer nearest to the given real number.

In the case of complex input signals of high amplitudes, successive errors are uncorrelated and therefore the power density spectrum is similar in character to that of white noise. Error signal is also uncorrelated with the input signal. The distribution of error probability density for a quantiser of the transition function described by formula (10–6) is a rectangular window function:

$$p_\delta(x) = \begin{cases} \dfrac{1}{\Delta} & dla \,|x| \le \dfrac{\Delta}{2} \\ 0 & dla \,|x| > \dfrac{\Delta}{2} \end{cases} \tag{10--7}$$

For complex input signals the maximum error is equal to the least significant byte (LSB) and, given a good approximation, samples of quantisation error δ_n can be considered independent of the input signal. For input signal of such type, uniform quantisation can be easily modelled by adding white noise to the input signal. However, for low-level input signals the model of additive white noise is no longer valid. In such a case the error becomes significantly dependent on the input signal. Signals from the range $[-\Delta/2, \Delta/2]$ are ascribed zero value by the converter and therefore are not conducted along the track; this effect is known as "digital deafness". In such case there is no signal at the output and the error is equal to the input signal, but has the opposite sign. This type of error is noticeable by ear and therefore constitutes a disadvantageous phenomenon associated with quantisation.

The dither technique is aimed at modifying statistical values of the total error. In quantising systems which do not use the dither technique the instantaneous error is a defined function of the input signal. If the input signal is simple and comparable in amplitude to the quantisation step, the error depends strongly on the input signal and it introduces audible distortion and modulation noise. Use of a dither signal with appropriately-shaped statistical properties may cause the audible distortions to become similar in character to stationary white noise.

Modern digital audio tracks use the dither technique, with noise described by a triangular function of probability density and peak-to-peak values of 2 LSB. The dither noise is therefore additive in nature, and it is usually introduced into the signal before the quantisation step. The averaged response obtained at the conversion system output is the following function of the input signal:

$$\overline{y}(x) = \int_{-\infty}^{\infty} y(x+\upsilon)p_\upsilon(\upsilon)d\upsilon \tag{10--8}$$

where: $p_\upsilon(\upsilon)$ is the probability distribution density of noise, in the case of noise with a rectangular distribution, defined as:

$$p_\upsilon(\upsilon) = \begin{cases} 1/\xi, dla \,|\upsilon| \le \xi/2 \\ 0 \end{cases} \tag{10--9}$$

where: ξ is the peak-to-peak amplitude of the dither noise.

Figure 10-14 illustrates the fundamental phenomena taking place when a signal of amplitude comparable to the quantization threshold is fed to the A/C converter input.

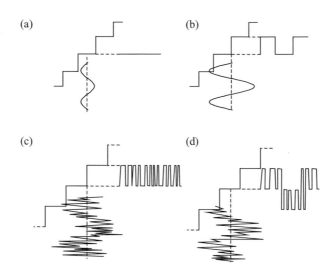

Figure 10-14 Effects associated with quantisation of small amplitudes and the influence of the dither noise: (a) "digital deafness"; (b) "binary quantisation"; (c) dither removes the insensitiveness range of the converter; (d) "response blurring" in the case of binary quantization.

Analysis of the influence of the dither noise on quantisation within the first part of the quantiser's characteristics (see Figure 10-15) shows that if the continuously-present dither noise is related to the quantiser's characteristics in a certain fashion, for properly adjusted noise level its steps become blurred and it approximates linear characteristics, therefore reducing the quantisation error and the related noise decrease.

FIGURE 10-16 a shows the result of quantization of a sinusoidal signal obtained without introducing dither noise, while FIGURE 10-16 b shows the result of quantisation of the same signal in the presence of the dither signal. The same figure (FIGURE 10-16 c and d) proves that averaging the representation (b) can lead to almost perfect reproduction of the original waveform that was subject to quantisation. We can also note that, as the sense of hearing possesses noticeable integrating properties, similar processes can certainly take place in the hearing track.

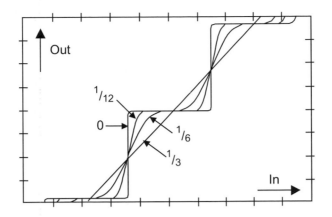

Figure 10-15 Effect of linearisation of conversion characteristics under the influence of dither noise at various levels corresponding to fractions of the quantisation step.

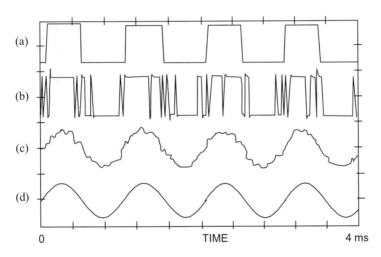

FIGURE 10-16 Effects of quantisation of waveform of amplitude corresponding to quantisation step:
(a) harmonic signal directly after quantisation; (b) quantisation using dither noise; (c) signal from the previous plot averaged over 32 periods; (d) result of averaging over 960 periods.

FIGURE 10-17 shows how adding dither noise affects the reduction of harmonic distortions.

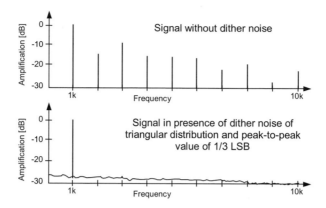

FIGURE 10-17 Spectrum of a quantised harmonic signal with an amplitude corresponding to the quantisation threshold (a) and a spectrum of the same signal in the presence of dither noise added at input of the A/C converter (b)

Noise power at output for the static input signal can be defined as:

$$P_n^{\,2}(x) = \int\limits_{-\infty}^{\infty} [y(x+v) - \overline{y}(x)]^2 \, p_v(v) dv \qquad (10\text{--}10)$$

In the case of dither noise with a Gaussian distribution defined as:

$$p_v(v) = \frac{1}{\sqrt{2\pi}\sigma_v} \exp(\frac{-v^2}{2\sigma_v^{\,2}}) \qquad (10\text{--}11)$$

$$\overline{v} = \sum_k v_k p_v[v_k] \qquad (10\text{--}12)$$

$$\sigma_v^2 = \sum_k (v_k - \overline{v})^2 p_v[v_k] \qquad (10\text{--}13)$$

modulation with noise is practically absent. Adding Gaussian noise allows for reducing quantisation errors, while being relatively simple to implement.

Introducing the "masking" dither noise lets us obtain the desired results of eliminating the quantiser's insensitiveness range and minimising distortions occurring for very low amplitudes of the signal being quantised. Audibility of the introduced noise can be decreased by preliminary shaping of its spectrum so that noise energy rises towards higher frequencies. The same principles remain valid for masking tinnitus, which suggests direct similarities between the phenomena occurring in electronic and biological signal-transmission systems.

The possibilities resulting from the above statements have been employed practically in the process of creating a Web-based application for people suffering from ear noises, which is accessible at www.telezdrowie.pl (or www.telewelfare.com). This application includes a system of electronic questionnaires and a database of signals useful for masking ear noises. It allows the patient to diagnose his/her own ear noises using a computer. Subsequently, after consulting a doctor, the patient can download a masking noise appropriate for him/her and store it in a portable mp3 player, which allows for effective treatment by masking tinnitus.

4 Summary

Results of over 200,000 tests performed so far show that multimedia computers running appropriate software are effective tools for performing hearing screening tests. In this approach, it is important to use tests adapted for individual age groups and use noised speech as test material.

Choosing hearing aids according to patients' needs and hearing characteristics is yet another problem, which has so far remained unsolved. Experience shows that the process of regulating the signal track parameters of electronic hearing aids should utilise knowledge on the patients' hearing characteristics in the maximum degree possible, with the aim of allowing them to understand speech. In order to face this challenge, we had to design new methods of adjusting hearing aids that would involve computers to a greater extent than before. An example of such a method is the multimedia hearing aid selection system presented in the paper, which is based on research regarding the degree of understanding speech in the presence of noise and on determining the optimum characteristics of the multi-band dynamics compressor, which is an important part of advanced hearing aids. This process utilises fuzzy reasoning, which marks the final application as one of the first in audiology to employ soft computing techniques.

Besides hearing deficiency, the problem of ear noise remains one of the principal hindrances for patients seeking audiological aid. The reasons behind this problem are not always understood by the patients, which hinders diagnostic and therapeutic interactions. Nevertheless, modern sound engineering and computer science can significantly improve the situation in both fields. Computers can be used effectively in tinnitus diagnosing and miniaturised recording and playback devices are successfully utilised in the therapy process. Moreover, the biocybernetics-inspired approach to scientific problems aimed at exploiting the analogies between nature and technology lets us search for ear noise origins and formulate hypotheses concerning the process of their generation.

As mentioned in the introduction, projects described in the present paper do not exhaust the scope of the application of sound and vision engineering in biomedicine. In fact, many other systems can be mentioned as well: e.g. a system for vision screening designed by the authors, a diagnostic system and therapeutic devices for correcting speech, and numerous other research projects that either have been or are being conducted at many research facilities around the world. Interdisciplinary applications of sound and vision engineering and multimedia techniques underlying telemedical applications result in increased effectiveness of diagnostic and therapeutic methods and therefore in increasing the effectiveness of detecting diseases and impairments, as well as of their prevention and therapy.

5 Acknowledgements

The research described in the paper has been partially subsidised by the Institute of Physiology and Pathology of Hearing and by the Polish Science Foundation.

6 Bibliography

[1] Allen B. J. B., Hall J. L., Jeng P. S., *Loudness growth in ½ octave bands (LGOB) – A procedure for the assessment of loudness*, J. Acoust. Soc. Am., vol. 88, No. 2, August 1990, pp. 745-753.

[2] Czyzewski A., Kaczmarek A., Kostek B., *Intelligent processing of stuttered speech,* J. of Intell. Inf. Syst., vol. 21, No. 2, Sept. 2003, pp. 143-171.

[3] Czyżewski A., Kostek B., *Expert Media Approach to Hearing Aids Fitting*, Int. J. Intell. Syst., 2002, pp. 277 – 294.

[4] Czyżewski A., Kostek B., Skarżyński H.: *Technika komputerowa w audiologii, foniatrii i logopedii (Computer technology in audiology, phoniatry and logopaedics)*, Akademicka Oficyna Wydawnicza EXIT, 2002: 441 pages (in Polish).

[5] Czyżewski A., *New Trends in Hearing Prostheses*, ICEBI'04 - XII International Conference on Electrical Bio-Impedance joint with EIT - V Electrical Impedance Tomography, Gdańsk University of Technology, Poland 20-24 June 2004.

[6] Czyżewski A., Skarżyński H.: *Interaktywne badania słuchu, wzroku i mowy (Interactive diagnosing of hearing, sight and speech)*, Elektronizacja, No. 10/2002, SIGMA-NOT 2002, pp. 27 – 30 (in Polish).

[7] Czyżewski A., Skarzyński H.: *Telemedycyna – czy może być interaktywna? (Telemedicine – Can It Be Interactive?)*, Expert Medyczny Nr 4 (6), 2002, pp. 39-41 (in Polish).

[8] Lorens A., Czyżewski A., *Model słuchu elektrycznego (Model of electric hearing)*, Presentation at the V Symposium "Modelling and Measurements in Medicine", Krynica 12-15.05.2003 (in Polish).

[9] McNally G. W., *Dynamic range control of digital audio signals,* J. Audio Eng. Soc., vol. 32, 1984 May, pp. 316-327.

[10] Skinner M.W., *Hearing Aid Evaluation*, Prentice Hall, New Jersey 1988.

[11] Stikvoort E. V., *Digital dynamic range compressor for audio*, J. Audio Eng. Soc., vol. 34, Jan/Feb 1986, pp. 3-9.

[12] Suchomski P., Kostek B., *Komputerowy symulator i korektor ubytku słuchu (Computer-based Simulator and Corrector of Hearing Loss)*, IX Symposium of Sound Directing and Engineering ISSET 2001, Warsaw 2001, pp. 293 – 300 (in Polish).

11 Model of Chronic Care Enabled with Information Technology

Mariusz Duplaga[1], Ole Martin Winnem[2]

[1]   Jagiellonian University Medical College, Krakow, Poland
[2]   SINTEF, Trondheim, Norway

The number of patients suffering from chronic diseases increased rapidly over the last few decades. As this group of patients consumes a considerable part of healthcare budgets in most countries, the need for consistent policies on chronic care is urgent nowadays. Chronic diseases do not resolve spontaneously and usually cannot be cured completely. As a result, patients with chronic diseases require care delivery over a prolonged period of time. Chronic conditions comprise several broad categories of diseases: noncommunicable diseases like cardiovascular disease, cancer or diabetes; persistent communicable diseases (AIDS); mental disorders like depression or schizophrenia; and impairments of structure (blindness, musculoskeletal disorders). Chronic diseases are the major health burden in developed countries; however, similar trends may also be seen in developing countries. The epidemiological data show that in the year 2000, noncommunicable conditions and mental disorders were responsible for 59% of total mortality in the world. In 46%, the general burden related to diseases was caused by these two categories of illnesses. The estimations indicate that in 2020, the disease burden resulting from noncommunicable diseases and mental disorders will increase to 60%. It should also be underlined that 70% of healthcare expenditures in Europe and in the USA is spent for management of chronic diseases. The number of patients suffering from chronic conditions is growing, but simultaneously many of them want to lead active professional and social lives.

All these circumstances result in growing pressure for improved efficiency of healthcare systems. For a long time, healthcare systems were usually designed for provision of care to patients with acute illnesses. The conclusions from the WHO 2002 Report "Innovative Care for Chronic Conditions" point to the fact that the patient's role in therapy and symptoms control, the importance of close patient follow-up, community services and prevention are not emphasized properly in healthcare systems[74]. However, nowadays healthcare systems are expected to maintain the continuity of care, shared care and the empowerment of patients in the management process[70]. E-health systems may add new quality to healthcare through shaping of an ambient care environment, enabling the automatic screening for trends indicating exacerbations of disease, improving the interactions between provider and patient and including the patient in the virtual supporting society. Improved model of chronic care incorporating the WHO recommendations and use of information technology tools is shown in Figure 11-1.

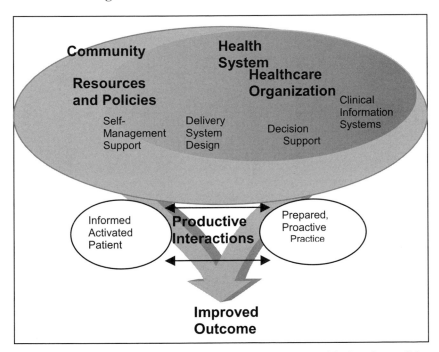

Figure 11-1 Enhanced model of healthcare delivery to patients with chronic conditions.

1   Systemic Approach to Chronic Conditions

Both in Europe and in the USA the systemic approaches to care delivered to patients with disorders having serious impact on their lives and status of the society were developed. The strategies implemented in the USA may be included in the term "disease management". The main elements of disease management programme according to the definition of the Disease Management Association of America are population identification process, evidence-based practice guidelines, collaborative practice model, patient self-management education including primary prevention, behaviour modification activities, compliance/surveillance process and outcomes measurement, evaluation and management, routine reporting and feedback loop as well as appropriate use of information technology[11]. The key factors critical for the success of disease management strategies include the support for the physician–patient relationship and plan of care, prevention of exacerbations and complications utilising cost-effective employment of evidence-based practice guidelines, development of patient empowerment strategies and evaluation of clinical, humanistic and economic outcomes with the goal of improving overall health. So, disease management programmes may be perceived as systematised activities undertaken in order to improve quality of care in relation to specific clinical problems. Disease management programmes, preserving high quality of care, strive for adherence to policies focused on cost-effectiveness. On the European ground, systemic approach to care was fulfilled comprehensively in the concept of integrated care covering also the features of continuity of care and patient empowerment[14][48].

As disease management or integrated care programmes may be quite complex, it is quite difficult to define these modes of care delivery on the basis of structure and functionality. There is a continuum of possible solutions developed for systemic care delivery in medical conditions, from those focused on the improvement of one aspect of care to those targeting the population of patients with multiple chronic conditions. Disease management programmes were generally criticized for the low cost-effectiveness ratio. The rapid development of e-health applications focused on the improvement of care and closer monitoring of patients' health status brought new opportunities for the employment of disease management or integrated care strategies[26][61]. The use of Web-based technologies for disease management programmes follows several scenarios. Such applications may be focused exclusively on patients, support primarily clinicians or enhance the collaboration between patients and clinicians[28][29][71].

The use of the emerging telematic technologies for care delivery to chronic patients resulted in the strategy described as Internet-enabled disease management. The use of Internet-based applications in chronic care is characterized by several advantages[38]. Relatively simple measures may bring considerable benefits, particularly if they are introduced on a large scale. Regular self-observations and self-measurements yield better symptoms control. Use of the Internet or computer modem for daily data transmission to monitoring centre results in improved patient's adherence to treatment regimens and recommended modes of behaviours. Automated data analysis may be the basis for tracing unfavourable trends in disease course and triggering the alerts forwarded to physicians and patients. The use of sophisticated algorithms of data analysis with implementation of data fusion techniques should exclude false alerts[12]. The important issue is the access to the patient's data for the health professional in every point of care at any time. Patients can also obtain access to specific health-related information remaining in the scope of their interest at any time. The decision process conducted by the physician during diagnostics and treatment of the patient may be further improved through the implementation of electronic guidelines into the e-health application[7][73].

2   Implementation of Information Technologies for Better Care

The use of electronic communication for delivery of care to patients is a real challenge, but technical barriers do not seem to be the main problem. Healthcare managers are well aware that the main obstacles are linked to political, legal and organisational aspects. It is obvious that the Internet brings not only opportunities but also threats which ought to be addressed efficiently if the e-health environment is to be shaped.

The benefits related to the use of such applications include improved data entry for patient's status monitoring, better communication between patient and physician, over-the-clock access to information for patients as well as increased access to information related to disease course and decision-supporting tools for physicians[3]. The communication between the patients and health professionals may be considerably enhanced as questions raised by the patients are answered without a visit to a physician's office. The doubts about disease course may appear quite often in patients anxious about their health status. Digital communication platform offers a more flexible solution for the provision of explanations by health professionals. Simultaneously, the change in the form of patient–physician communication brings new challenges to formal and legal regulations of standards of care[44][47].

Self-education is an important opportunity for chronic patients resulting from the widespread use of Web-based applications. Internet technologies enable individualised education and training processes[27]. More advanced solutions include the patient in an environment supporting self-management of his or her medical condition but also imposing the regularity of activities. Such environment supports the patient's feeling of safety as he or she may count on the transmission of appropriate information to a healthcare provider in the case of symptom deterioration.

The real advantage of the e-health applications may be fully explored in the populations having widespread access to the Internet. However, even in countries where Internet penetration reaches more than 50%, the phenomenon of "digital divide" considerably impairs the usability of e-health applications. Alternative forms of telemonitoring and data entry are searched for. In this context, cellular telephony seems to be the most promising option. Cellular phones are commonly used even in populations having limited access to the Internet. Health-related communication can also be accomplished with portable computers, handhelds or interactive TV.

Populations with low Internet penetration can be monitored with a computerized, telephone-linked communication system. This technology is quite inexpensive and may be an alternative to Internet-based applications in provision of long-term monitoring and education to patients with chronic diseases[22][23]. Fully automated telecommunications system plays the role of the monitor, the educator or the counsellor for chronic patients. Typical use of the system is based on regular automated telephone conversations conducted with the patients in periods between ambulatory visits in policlinics. Automated telecommunications systems are applied in management of patients with chronic diseases, in delivery of interventions aimed at the modification of health-related behaviours (promotion of smoking cessation, adherence to a medication regimen, sustaining regular physical activity and appropriate diet) and for provision of support to persons taking care of patients with severe disease[18][24][46].

Electronic systems supporting long-term monitoring and treatment of patients suffering from chronic conditions may follow several patterns of usage. They may differ according to the communication with health professionals as well as decision support options offered to patients and physicians. The functionality of such systems may be further extended by the use of devices measuring physiologic parameters essential for disease severity monitoring. Data transmission from these devices is performed through plain telephone line or personal computer with Internet access.

However, even if the benefits from the use of Internet-based solutions for care delivery are indisputable today, significant limitations for their use exist. Digital divide is a real problem; access to the Internet is not homogeneous and large parts of populations are excluded from the virtual community. Accessibility of the Internet solutions for physically or mentally handicapped people is not always assured. The reliability of health-related information on the Internet is frequently questioned. One should also remember that Internet-based applications designed to bring new quality into long-term care must respect legal issues[60].

Patients and their families are the driving force of the Internet use for access to health-related information and communication with health professionals. Surveys show that in highly Internet-literate societies like the USA, 90% of patients would like to contact their physicians by e-mail[56].

The attitudes towards Internet use in care delivery demonstrated by physicians are more complex. Their expectations are not so clear as they afraid of the additional burden put on them by electronic communication with patients[25]. It seems that nurses are the professional group developing quickly broad acceptance for home telecare and remote monitoring[66]. They play an important role in the process of moving the focus from hospital to home care. This is related to the fact that teleinformatic technologies may greatly support them in their routine activities including home visits and care for chronic patients.

The results of surveys performed among the users of Internet-based health-related applications indicate that the patients use them to obtain more information about specific diseases, their treatment strategies or physician-recommended medication, to diagnose medical conditions, to make the contact with physicians or other health professionals or to communicate with support groups. Some of them want to see how surgical or diagnostic procedures are performed. The benefits related to e-health solutions emphasized by potential users included time saving, convenience, improved knowledge about healthy lifestyles and behaviours. There were a considerable number of patients counting on enhanced communication with healthcare providers as well as support groups. Specific services which were appreciated to the greatest extent comprised appointment scheduling, e-prescribing, e-mail communication with physicians and possibility to see one's personal medical record. The patients searching the information on the Internet were focussed on types of treatment, the consequences of diseases and side effects of medication. They particularly appreciated the ability to ask specific questions. Internet-based applications play a role in education and training (symptom management, behaviour modification interventions). Those surveys were based on the expectation of the population of patients using specific Internet-based programmes in the USA and not all observations may be simply extrapolated to other societies. However, the survey results shed light on the perception of Internet-based solutions among the patients[52].

The use of e-health solutions is treated as the chance to assure the quality of care in the face of growing healthcare expenditures. The Institute of Medicine issued the report "Crossing the quality chasm: a new health care system for the 21st century" which addressed the problem of outdated models of care delivery and unsatisfactory management of chronic conditions. The Internet supplies patients with tools enabling efficient and safe self-management. The application of information technology was indicated as the possible remedy enabling the lowering of the number of medical errors, assuring appropriate quality of care and keeping the expenditures low[35].

3 Focus on Delivery of Care to Patient's Home

"Institutional" medicine developed fully in the 20th century, but in previous centuries almost all ailments were cared for at home. Now we face the shift to home care once again. This trend is driven by the pressure on medical cost reduction and availability of teleinformatic solutions improving home care quality. The patients usually prefer to stay at home than in a hospital ward. It is reasonable to let them remain in the environment they perceive as friendly and assuring. However, the quality of health services and safety of the patient must be impaired. Home telecare depends strongly on patient empowerment which is presently an obvious objective of successful long-term care. The majority of home visits of health professionals may be substituted by telecare. The estimations made in the USA indicate that the cost of a home telecare visit is one third of that of an on-site visit. On-site visits are related to considerable overhead costs dependent on transportation use and time of the health professional. Growing progress in electronic information and communications technologies has increased the clinical applicability of home telemonitoring systems. With every year these tools are more user-friendly for patients. This results in the situation that they may be used by patients without assistance from health professionals or caregivers.

Monitoring devices connected to computer modems allow for measuring and transmitting physiological parameters like blood pressure, heart rate, blood glucose level or oximetry. Data can be sent to the monitoring centre by a standard telephony line. This option is practical and even patients with limited education can successfully use such equipment, especially if Internet access is rare in the community. Home telecare offers cost-effective solutions — equivalent to home care visits[20].

One of the most successful initiatives in the area of home telecare was the Kaiser Permanente Tele-Home Health Research Project. The experience gained during the project is extremely instructive for developers of telecare applications. The main objective of the project was the evaluation of remote video technology in the home setting for healthcare services delivery. The evaluation undertaken by Johnston et al. within this project revealed that considerable reduction of total care costs could be achieved in the intervention group (access to a remote video system for real-time interaction between nurses and patients) due to lower hospitalization costs[41].

The change in the attitude towards home telecare may be best seen in the USA which seems to be currently the greatest market for the development of such services. In 2000 the Prospective Payment System was signed into law including the reimbursement by Medicare for home telecare. The new system of payments relies on the episode of care, so in-person home visits and remote visits are treated the same.

The attempts to develop home telecare solutions go even further and aim on the substitution of hospitalizations with extended home telecare. Researchers from the United Kingdom performed a study on the use of telemedicine approach in the treatment of patients with exacerbations of chronic obstructive pulmonary disease[72]. Apart from routine home care in such situation, eight patients were offered videophones installed in their home. The study was generally aimed on the evaluation of the feasibility of telemedical sessions with normal home visits in comparison to hospitalizations. The analysis was mainly based on questionnaires filled out by patients and nurses. Patients were more satisfied with the use of telemedical links than nurses; however, even nurses admitted that 80% of on-site visits in patients' homes could be replaced by home telecare.

4   Patient-Centred Role in Symptom Monitoring

Patient empowerment means his or her involvement in prolonged observations of disease course, conducting self-measurement of parameters essential for specific disease and, when appropriate, making decisions connected to further treatment. The main trace of self-management in chronic diseases is based on registration of self-observations and self-measurements in the longterm. Prolonged tracing of physiologic parameters enables the description of the course of disease and forecasting of exacerbations. Self-observations and self-measurements may be the basis for automatic triggering of alerts sent to health professionals and patients. The visualisation of data and ability to trace trends in the course of the disease brings valuable feedback for patient's activities. Trends observed in the disease course are also the basis for modification of medication by the patient (self-adjusted treatment).

Data transfer may be performed in two ways: directly — when measurements are conducted automatically, without patients' or caregivers' intervention and periodically downloaded from specialised equipment through appropriate telecommunication connection; or indirectly — when measurements are carried out manually by the patient or caregiver and transmitted online through Internet forms or by the use of telephone line and modem. Modern monitoring devices usually have enough memory for storing results of measurements from longer periods. These devices may be coupled with a modem for data transmission through telephone lines. Some of them feature special interfaces enabling the interaction[16]. Long-term monitoring of disease course requires specific outcomes measures. Asthma patients should proceed with regular measurements of the level of airway obturation with peak flow meters or portable spirometers. The airway obturation should also be assessed in patients with chronic obstructive pulmonary disease. Those of them who develop chronic respiratory failure may require pulse oximetry monitoring. The course of congestive heart failure is monitored with measurements of body weight, heart rate and blood pressure. Blood glucose level is the most essential parameter in diabetes but blood pressure should also be recorded. Daily measurements of blood pressure are essential for arterial hypertension control. There are other parameters which should be monitored in specific conditions, e.g. blood counts in AIDS/HIV infection or in patients receiving cancer chemotherapy.

New approach to monitoring includes the use of wireless systems[6][45]. Mobile phones are used commonly nowadays and it is natural they are perceived as a tool for healthcare communication. There is also great potential in the use of short message systems for transmission of data between patients and monitoring centres[1][55]. A study on feasibility of a wireless cardiorespiratory telemonitoring system was conducted by Johnson et al.[40]. The system was tested in a group of 14 elderly patients whose ECG, heart rate variability and breathing were recorded two times a day. The main focus of the study was demonstrating the ability of elderly patients staying at home to use such system.

Technological progress brings more sophisticated devices incorporated in textiles (wearables). These include different types of smart wearables like smart socks, shirts, and in future implantable chips[69]. The integrated telemonitoring environment may be embedded in the home environment in the form of "smart home". The system developed by Rialle et al. comprised networked sensors in an apartment operated by a communication system based on the Internet[62]. The sensors were connected wirelessly with a software module located in the home performing signal analysis and detection of critical situations (falls, sickness, sudden palsy, stroke, hypothermia). The in-home module communicated with the remote control station through mobile or Ethernet network. The system developed in the framework of this project was believed to be a powerful information and communication tool for medical and social professionals.

5 Management Plans Developed in e-Health Environment

The first-generation solutions for home-based treatment and care were based on old hospital-centred solutions with minimal integration giving minor support to the caregiver as well as medical professionals. Second-generation solutions are built on specific needs for specialist medical professionals with minimal focus on collaboration between levels and professions in the health chain (Figure 11-2). The second-generation systems are based on a point-to-point solution with telephone/broadband connection between patient home and a control center with medical professionals specialized on giving care to patients with many needs.

In order to support the WHO model[74] for care of chronic patients there is a need for the development of third-generation solutions focusing on collaboration between health levels and professions as well as supporting the local caregiver (e.g. patient relative). In Figure 11-3 a suggestion for an overall solution supporting this is described. Important issues regarding the new architecture are how roles and security are introduced at another level, but also how the architecture of the solution has changed into thinner clients with more central processing and storage. Only where sensors are presented, more powerful clients may be needed.

Empowering the patient by introducing a patient-centred role in symptoms and signs monitoring introduces a need for developing a common understanding between patients and the care providers of what and when to report. The patient has to know in which situations she should monitor and how different activities may impact the monitoring results. An example is the food eaten in relation to a measurement by a diabetes patient. The patient also needs to understand how the measurement should be carried out in order to create valid information.

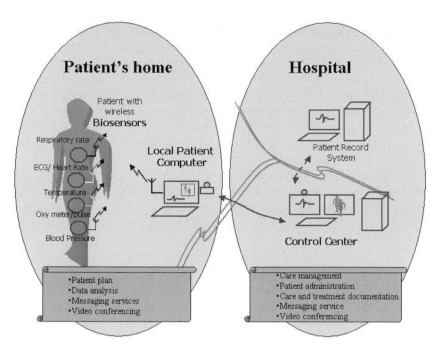

Figure 11-2 The second-generation technology for supporting advanced home care.

In order to support the patient at the point of care, health management plans are introduced. Plans support the patients in the day-to-day management of their problems and give specific support to carrying out the different tasks in the plan. The management plans are generated based on structured generic plans called patterns of care and contain two sequential steps. The first step is related to selection of pattern of care and the second is related to adapting the selected pattern of care to the available resources. The selection of pattern of care is the most knowledge intensive and difficult task. Diagnosis and available measurements give the input information which is mapped to available patterns of care in order to select the most promising pattern of care. Then a semiautomated process is used to adapt the management plan to available resources. Each activity in the pattern of care has a specific description in order to help the patient perform it. In this way the care in the patient homes is becoming more standardized which makes the measured data easier to study and take actions from.

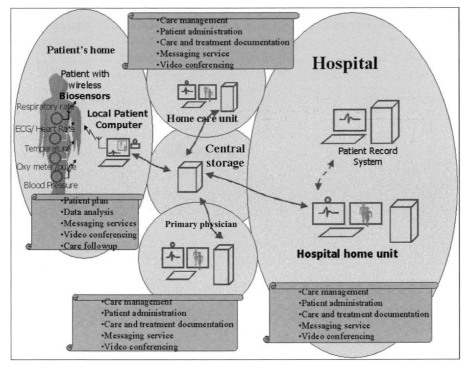

Figure 11-3 The third-generation technology for supporting advanced home care.

6 The Experience from Specific Areas of Chronic Care

Evidence from trials focused on e-health solutions application in chronic care reveals that their use may yield important outcomes: improved quality of patient life, diminished hospitalisation rate, lowered number of ambulatory visits, increased interactivity and satisfaction of patients and better continuity of care. The scope of possible applications of telemonitoring strategies in chronic care is extensive. The results of studies performed on patients with cardiological diseases (congestive heart failure, arterial hypertension), diabetes and respiratory conditions are summarized below.

6.1 Congestive Heart Failure

Integrated care encompassing the use of telemonitoring systems for patients with congestive heart failure was tested in several pilot projects[37][54][64]. The parameters monitored in these patients include body weight, blood pressure, heart rate as well as subjective assessment carried out by patients. Such options as electronic stethoscope and narrow bandwidth videoteleconferencing were implemented in some testbeds. The results obtained in long-term studies indicate that the use of telemonitoring systems may lead to diminished admission and readmission rate, shorter hospitalisation duration as well as decreased utilisation of emergency facilities by patients with congestive heart failure. The evaluation of patients' attitudes to telemonitoring systems reveals encouraging trends with average daily usage rate of the system equal to 94% in some studies. The use of telemonitoring systems also has an educational impact on the patients as their understanding of preventive measures increased considerably. An important finding from the assessment of patients with congestive heart failure using telemonitoring systems was improved quality of life. Satisfaction levels declared by patients were usually higher than revealed by physicians. The potential for improvement of care was evidenced in some studies on telemonitoring system use in this group of patients. Interestingly, the impact of telephone calls by nurses to patient homes on outcomes was similar to the impact of the telemonitoring system in one study.

6.2   Arterial Hypertension

The significance of regular blood pressure monitoring in successful antihypertensive therapy is well known and understood. Furthermore, it was evidenced that 20% of patients' self-reported blood pressure measurements may differ by more than 10 mm Hg[39]. These circumstances make patients with arterial hypertension a well-suited target group for telemonitoring applications. Telemonitoring systems designed for patients with arterial hypertension include systems using data transmission through standard telephone lines to those based on Internet technology and also offering educational and supportive information.

The results of the trials focussed on the use of telemonitoring systems for patients with arterial hypertension demonstrated high potential for better control of blood pressure and higher compliance with physicians' recommendations[2][5][21]. Nowadays, telemonitoring applications used by patients with arterial hypertension encompass such functions like automatic transmission of blood pressure measurement over telephone lines, computer conversion of data into report forms and periodic transmission of reports to health professionals and patients[63]. The feedback offered by telemonitoring systems strengthens the impact of established therapy and physicians' recommendation as well as increases the compliance of patients with arterial hypertension. The general conclusion from the use of telecommunication systems for monitoring of patients with hypertension is that greater reduction of the arterial pressure may be obtained with such approach. The cost of telemonitoring service can be lower than $30 per month per patient.

6.3 Other Solutions for Cardiology

ECG recording transmission through telecommunication links is one of the oldest examples of telemedical application. The first test of ECG recording transmission through telephone lines was made in the 1920s. ECG transmission systems are commonly available for patients with arrhythmias or implanted heart pacemakers. Tele-ECG service is also used in case of acute coronary symptoms. Transmission of the ECG signal can be an additional feature of more complex systems used for telemonitoring of cardiac and respiratory status of patients[76]. Furthermore, cellular telephony was quickly adapted for ECG transmission adding the feature of wireless communication to telemonitoring systems. There are medical centres which develop and implement advanced solutions for telesurveillance of high-risk cardiac patients, e.g. patients who underwent cardiac surgery or suffer from cardiomyopathy[33][58][75].

6.4 Diabetes

Successful diabetes management depends on strict patient adherence to the regimen of blood glucose monitoring, medication use, skin care, diet and exercise. Attempts to apply telemedicine for diabetic care were begun in the early 1990s. The solutions used in the early phase were based on communication through a standard telephony network. The first experience from the application of telemonitoring systems in patients with diabetes showed that they can be helpful in reduction of the incidence and severity of complications of type 1 diabetes and probably also in patients with type 2 diabetes[51][57][67].

The main objective of blood glucose measurements in diabetics is achieving optimum therapy. The monitoring process is based on sampling blood glucose levels carried out by the patient or the caregiver. Blood glucose measurements usually should be accompanied by blood pressure monitoring. The measurements are entered into a personal computer connected to the Internet and sent to the monitoring centre. In early solutions standard telephone lines were used for data transmission. In this scenario patient involvement in the measurements is necessary. Another option relies on the use of transcutaneous biosensors making automatic measurements of blood glucose levels and then transmitting the results to a personal computer linked to the Internet. Web-based systems with telemonitoring designed for use by patients and health professionals bring new advantages like long-term management options, access to electronic patient record and decision support[65].

The support received by patients with diabetes through e-health platforms may take various forms. Patients appreciate the educational and self-management applications, opportunity to stay in touch with support groups, intervention focused on specific activities included in diabetes management, e.g. physical training or enhanced communication with health professionals[15][49][59][78]. The results of trials on the use of telemonitoring systems in patients with diabetes showed favourable influence on monitored parameters (haemoglobin A1C level, body weight, blood glucose).

Within research and development programmes of the European Commission several projects focussed on telemonitoring of chronic patients were funded. The Multi-Access Services for the Management of Diabetes Mellitus (M2DM) Project was focussed on improvement of quality of diabetes management[4]. Its main objective was to provide patients and health professionals with around-the-clock support in order to improve quality of care. The service is accessible through the Web or interactive voice responder system. Data from the measuring devices may be sent due to use of smart modems. DIABtel Telemedicine Service described by Gomez et al. was based on the concept of "supervised autonomy"[30]. Such approach enables patients with chronic conditions to maintain an active professional and social life. The patient unit was developed as a handheld computer that can be used by the patient during daily activities. Telemedical systems addressing specific areas of diabetes care like pregnancy or foot care were also developed[43][50].

New York State financed one of the greatest projects in the field of home telemonitoring – the Informatics for Diabetes Education and Telemedicine Project (IDEATel)[34][68]. It is focused on patients with diabetes from urban and rural areas. The Project was initiated in 2000, and it is conducted as a randomized clinical trial. Its main objective is evaluation of how telemedical application can improve diabetes control. Patients were equipped with home telemedicine units with four functions: synchronous videoconferencing over standard telephone lines, electronic transmission of glucose and blood pressure readings, secure Web-based messaging and clinical data review as well as access to Web-based educational materials. The automatic alerts can be generated if the data entered by the patient exceed expected values. The concept of home telecare and remote monitoring is accompanied in this initiative with the notion of the patient's access to the electronic medical record. The home telemedicine unit gives patients numerous modes of interaction with their personal online charts.

6.5   Bronchial Asthma

The efficient treatment of asthma depends to a great extent on the empowerment of the patient, who is able to conduct regular self-observations and self-measurements. The monitoring of asthma course relies on regular measurements of airway obturation with a portable device. The appropriate preparation to self-management of asthma is based on education and training delivered by health professionals or specialised educators. This process may be considerably supplemented and enhanced with Internet-based applications. The advantage of such approach is continuous availability of the resources to the patient.

The results from feasibility studies indicate that airway obturation measurements performed by patients at home and sent via telecommunication links are reliable[17][18]. Patients with asthma usually show high acceptance for the use of telemonitoring systems and even patients without a computer background are able to use such systems properly. The systems used for remote telemonitoring by patients with asthma can be enhanced with the options supporting evidence-based medicine guidelines[36]. The appropriate modes of management incorporated in Internet applications bring opportunity for efficient guideline execution in relation to self-management as well as medical staff performance. The functionality of such system may be broadened with wireless solutions and portable devices. This is particularly important for patients who want to sustain an active professional life. The system structure may also be adjusted to the level of disease severity[13].

The range of parameters monitored in patients with asthma may exceed standard measures of pulmonary function tests. Some researchers tested the option to use continuous acoustic overnight monitoring of breath sounds as the means of evaluation of wheeze and cough in asthmatics[42]. They believe that breath sound monitoring would be more practical, cheaper and less time-consuming if performed in patients at home.

The use of telemonitoring option may be focused on a specific activity. One of the critical issues in asthma management is patients' adherence to medication regimens and systems monitoring compliance with the medication scheme were also developed[10].

General telemonitoring strategy implemented in asthma patients may be easily adapted to patients with chronic obturative pulmonary diseases. The feasibility of the telemonitoring systems (telephone-linked computer system and Internet-based systems) in long-term care delivered to these patients was tested with good results by the researchers[19][77].

6.6   Other Medical Conditions

The Comprehensive Health Enhancement Support System was developed as a computer-based tool for patients with several specific medical conditions including patients with AIDS or HIV in the USA[31]. The system enables access to information, referrals to health care providers, decision support as well as communication with experts or other people with the same health problems. The evaluation of the quality of life of patients using the CHESS revealed higher scores than in the group of patients who did not use the system. The users of the system also indicated the reduction of some healthcare expenditures related to hospitalizations. The feasibility and usability of the CHESS system were also evaluated in a population of elderly patients with breast cancer[32]. The conclusion was that age is not a barrier in using health-related Internet resources. The women included in the study use the system for obtaining basic information about the disease and treatment as well for communication with their peers.

Other areas of telemonitoring applications include the use of videophone technology for supervising therapy in patients with tuberculosis[8] or home monitoring of pulmonary function in patients after lung transplantation[53]. A computerized system for monitoring of dialysis remote sites and for follow-up of chronic patients was implemented with smart phones in G.Bosco Hospital in Torino, Italy[9]. The TELEDIAL system was designed for patients undergoing chronic ambulatory peritoneal dialysis at home. The data that may be transmitted by the patients include information about course of dialysis, symptom appearance, accidents or consumption of drugs unrelated to the main therapy scope. The physician taking care of the patients performing ambulatory peritoneal dialysis may change the mode of the therapy remotely.

7 Summary

The increase in prevalence of chronic disorders in modern societies has resulted in increasing organizational and financial pressure on healthcare systems. The challenge of adequate care delivered to patients with chronic conditions, who want to remain in their social context, promotes the search for effective models of care. Adequate use of information and communication technology may be an appropriate response to this challenge. Chronic patients require repetitive interactions with the healthcare system. High-quality care adhering to evidence-based medicine strategies must be delivered to a vast population of patients in a continuous manner. The experience from studies and pilot implementations of information technology tools in specific groups of patients suffering from chronic diseases indicates that considerable benefits may be gained related to improved cost-effectiveness and simultaneously maintained quality of care. It seems that e-health strategies may help to fulfill two contradictory requirements — provision of high-quality medical services and preservation of the cost-effective approach. Available evidence supports the use of e-health solutions for care delivery. The results of trials based on the use of integrated IT-enhanced model of care with focus on patient empowerment and better interdisciplinary team communication demonstrated improvement of such outcome measures like hospitalization rate, frequency of ambulatory visits and level of quality of life in populations of chronic patients. However, it must be emphasized that a new model of care based on the effective use of e-health solutions cannot be implemented without adherence to legal, ethical and psychosociological requirements existing in the healthcare environment.

8 Bibliography

[1] Anhoj J., Moldrup C.: Feasibility of Collecting Diary Data From Asthma Patients Through Mobile Phones and SMS (Short Message Service): Response Rate Analysis and Focus Group Evaluation From a Pilot Study. J Med Internet Res 2004; 6(4): e42 [http://www.jmir.org/2004/4/e42/]

[2] Artinian N.T., Washington O.G., Templin T.N.: Effects of home telemonitoring and community-based monitoring on blood pressure control in urban African Americans: a pilot study. Heart Lung 2001; 30(3): 191-199

[3] Baker D.B.: Patient-centered healthcare: The role of the Internet. Dis Manag Health Outcomes 2001; 9(8): 411-420

[4] Bellazzi R., Brugues E., Carson E., et al.: Multi-Access Services for the Management of Diabetes Mellitus: The M2DM Project. Diabetes 2002; 51 (Suppl. 2): A466

[5] Bondmass M.D., Bolger N.E., Castro G.M., Orgain J., Avitall B.: Rapid control of hypertension in African Americans achieved utilizing home monitoring. Circulation 1998; 98: I-517

[6] Boquete L., Bravo I., Barea R., Garcia M.A.: Telemetry and control system with GSM communications. Microprocessors Microsystems 2003; 27: 1-8

[7] Buchtela D., Anger Z., Peleska J., Vesely A., Zvarova J.: Presentation of Medical Guidelines on a Computer. In: Duplaga M., Zieliński K., Ingram D. (eds.): Transformation of Healthcare with Information Technologies. Amsterdam, IOS Press (2004) 166-171

[8] Chan D.S., Callahan C.W., Sheets S.J., Moreno C.N., Person D.A.: Store and forward technology: Telemonitoring of children using their asthma medication in their home (abstract). Telemed J e-Health 20002; 8(2): 244

[9] Contini E., Costantino G.P., Harti R., Quarello F., Sancipriano G., Selwood N.H.: Computerized monitoring of dialysis remote sites and follow-up of chronic patients using smart-phones. Medial Informatics Europe'96: Human Facets in Information Technologies. Amsterdam,: IOS Press (1996) 44-48

[10] DeMaio J., Schwartz L., Cooley P., Tice A.: The Application of Telemedicine Technology to a Directly Observed Therapy Program for Tuberculosis: A Pilot Project. Clin Infect Dis 2001; 33: 2082-2084

[11] Disease Management Association of America Webpag. Definition of Disease Management. [http://www.dmaa.org/definition.html]

[12] Dodd N.: Enhanced alarm detection for telemonitoring using the neural network alarm monitor. Br J Healthcare Comp Inf Manag 1997; 14(6): 20-22

[13] Duplaga M., Zielinski K., Szczeklik A.: Internet Telemonitoring Application for Improvement of the Quality of Severe Asthma Patient Care in Poland. 7th Int Conf on Medical Aspects of Telemedicine, Eur J Med Res 2002; 7(Suppl. 1): 21

[14] Ewers M.: The Advent of High-Tech Home Care in Germany. Public Health Nursing 2002; 19(4): 309-317

[15] Fail E.G., Glasgow R.E., Boles S., Mckay H.G.: Who participates in Internet-based self-management programs? A study among novice computer users in a primary care setting. Diabetes Educ 2000; 26(5): 806-811

[16] Field M.J., Grigsby J.: Telemedicine and Remote Patient Monitoring. JAMA 2002; 4: 423-425

[17] Finkelstein J., Cabrera M.R., Hripcsak G.: Internet-based home asthma telemonitoring: Can patients handle the technology? Chest 2000; 117(1): 148-155

[18] Finkelstein J., Hripcsak G., Cabrera M.R.: Patients' acceptance of Internet-based home asthma telemonitoring. Proc AMIA Symp 1998; 336-340

[19] Finkelstein J., O'Connor G., Galichina N.: Feasibility of Internet-based Home Automated Telemanagement in Patients with Chronic Obstructive Pulmonary Disease. Chest 2001; 120(4) Suppl.: 253S

[20] Forkner-Dunn J.: Internet-based Patient Self-care: The Next Generation of Health Care Delivery. J Med Internet Res 2003; 5(2): e8 [http://www.jmir.org/2003/2/e8]

[21] Friedman R.H., Kazis L.E., Jette A., Smith M.B., Stollerman J., Torgerson J., et al.: A telecommunications system for monitoring and counselling patients with hypertension. Impact on medical adherence and blood pressure control. Am J Hypertens 1996; 9: 285-292

[22] Friedman R.H., Stollerman J.E., Mahoney D.M., Rozenblyum L.: The virtual visit: using telecommunications technology to take care of patients. J Am Med Inf Assoc 1997; 4: 413-425

[23] Friedman R.H., Stollerman J.E., Rozenblyum L., Belfer D., Selim A., Mahoney D., Steinbach S.: A telecommunications system to manage patients with chronic disease. Medinfo 1998; 9 Pt 2: 1330-1334

[24] Friedman R.H.: Automated telephone conversations to assess health behaviour and deliver behavioural interventions. J Med Syst 1998; 22: 95-102

[25] Gerber B.S., Eiser A.R.: The Patient-Physician Relationship in the Internet Age: Future Prospects and the Research Agenda. J Med Internet Res 2001;3(2):e15

[26] Gillespie G.: Deploying an I.T. cure for chronic disease. Health Data Manag 2000; 8(7): 68-74

[27] Glick T.H., Moore G.T.: Time to learn: the outlook for renewal of patient-centred education in the digital age. Med Educ 2001; 35: 505-509

[28] Gomaa W.H., Morrow T., Muntendam P., Smith G.: Technology-based disease management: A low-cost, high-value solution for the management of chronic disease. Dis Manag Health Outcomes 2001; 9(10): 577-588

[29] Gomaa W.H.: High-Tech, Low-Cost, Huge Results. Health Manag Tech 2002; April: 32-33,38

[30] Gomez E.J., Del Pozo F., Hernando M.E.: Telemedicine for diabetes care: the DIABTel approach towards diabetes telecare. Med Inf 1996; 21(4): 283-295

[31] Gustafson D.H., Hawkins R.P., Boberg E.W., Bricker E., Pingree S., Chan C.L.: The Use and Impact of a Computer-based Support System for People Living with AIDS and HIV Infection. Proc Ann Symp Comp Appl Med Care 1994; 604-608

[32] Gustafson D.H., McTavish F., Hawkins R., Pingree S., Arora N., Mendenhall J., Simmons G.E.: Computer support for elderly women with breast cancer. JAMA 1999; 28(14): 1268-1269

[33] Hutten H.: Telesurveillance of Patients with Cardiac Risk. Eur Surg 2002; 34: 303-307

[34] Informatics for Diabetes Education and Telemedicine (IDEATel) Project Website [www.ideatel.com]

[35] Institute of Medicine, Committee on Quality of Care in America. A new health care system for the 21st century. Washington, DC: National Academy Press; 2001 Friedewald V.E., Pion R.J.: Returning home. Health Manag Technol 2001; 22(9): 22-26

[36] Jadad A.R.: Evidence-based decision making and asthma in the Internet age: the tools of the trade. Allergy 2002; 57 (Suppl. 74): 15-22

[37] Jerant A.F., Azari R., Nesbitt T.S.: Reducing the Cost of Frequent Hospital Admissions for Congestive Heart Failure. A Randomized Trial of a Home Telecare Intervention. Med Care 2001; 39(11): 1234-1245

[38] Joch A.: Can the Web Save Disease Management? Healthcare Informatics March 2000 [http://www.healthcare-informatics.com/issues/2000/03_00/cover.htm]

[39] Johnson A.L., Taylor D., Sackett D.L., Dunnett C.W., Shimizu A.G.: Self-recording of blood pressure in the management of hypertension. Can Med Assoc J 1978; 119: 1034-1039

[40] Johnson P., Andrews D.C., Wells S., de Lusignan S., Robinson J., Vandenburg M.: The use of a new continuous wireless cardiorespiratory telemonitoring system by elderly patients at home. J Telemed Telecare 2001; 7(Suppl 1): S1:76-77

[41] Johnston B., Wheeler L., Deuser J., Sousa K.H.: Outcomes of the Kaiser Permanente Tele-Home Health Research Project. Arch Fam Med 2000; 9: 40-45

[42] Kharitonow S.A., Kelly C., Meah S., Godfrey S., Pride N.B., Barnes P.J.: Home Overnight Monitoring of Breath Sounds in Normal and Asthmatic Subjects. ATS 98th Int Conf May 17-23, 2002, Atlanta, GA

[43] Ladyzyński P., Wójcicki J.M., Krzymień-Blachowicz J., Józwicka E., Czajkowski K., Janczewska E., Karnafel W.: Teletransmission system supporting intensive insulin treatment of out-clinic type 1 diabetic pregnant women. Technical assessment during 3 years' application. Int J Artif Organs 2001; 24(3): 157-163

[44] Leslie S.: Online consulting. The experience of a commercial service. J Telemed Telecare 2001; 7(Suppl. 2): S2:78-82

[45] Maglaveras N., Koutkias V., Meletiadis S., Chouvarda I., Balas E.A.: The role of wireless technology in home care delivery. Medinfo 2001; 10 (Pt 1): 835-839

[46] Mahoney D., Tennstedt S., Friedman R., Heeren T.: An automated telephone system for monitoring the functional status of community-residing elders. Gerontologist 1999; 39: 229-234

[47] Mandl K., Kohane I., Brandt A.: Electronic Patient-Physician Communication: Problems and Promise. Ann Intern Med 1998; 129(6): 495-500

[48] Mason A., Drummond M., Towse A.: Is disease management relevant in Europe: some evidence from the United Kingdom. Health Policy 1999; 48: 69-77

[49] Mc Kay H.G., King D., Eakin E.G., Seeley J.R., Glasgow R.E.: The diabetes network Internet-based physical activity intervention: a randomized pilot study. Diabetes Care 2001; 24(8): 1328-1334

[50] McGill M., Constantino M., Yue D.K.: Integrating telemedicine into a National Diabetes Footcare Network. Pract Diabetes Int 2000; 17(7): 235-238

[51] Mease A.: Telemedicine improved diabetic management. Milit Med 2000; 165(8): 579

[52] Molfenter T., Johnson P., Gustafson D.H., DeVries K., Veeramani D.: Patient Internet Services: Creating the Value-added Paradigm. J Healthcare Inf Manag 2002; 16(4): 73-79

[53]Morlion B., Knoop C., Paiva M., Estenne M.: Internet-based home monitoring of pulmonary function after lung transplantation. Am J Resp Crit Care Med 2002; 165(5): 694-697

[54]Nanevicz T., Piette J., Zipkin D., Serlin M., Ennis S., De Marco T., Modin G.: The feasibility of a telecommunications service in support of outpatient congestive heart failure care in a diverse patient population. Cong Heart Failure 2000; 6(3): 140-145

[55]Neville R., Greene A., McLeod J.: Mobile phone text messaging can help young people manage asthma. BMJ 2002; 325: 600

[56]NUA Internet Surveys. CyberAtlas: Americans want online access to doctors. 2002 April 12 [http://www.nua.com/surveys/index.cgi?f=VS&art_id=905357844&rel=true]

[57]O'Connor P., et al.: Continuous quality improvement can improve glycemic control for HMO patients with diabetes. Arch Fam Med 1996; 5: 502-506

[58]Palmer K., Parrott J., Scott R., Garnett D.: Hospital to home telemonitoring post cardiac surgery. Telemed J e-Health 2001; 7(2): 127-128

[59]Ploughmann S., Hejlesen O.K., Cavan D.A.: DiasNet – a diabetes advisory system for communication and education via the Internet. Int J Med Inf 2001; 64(2-3): 319-330

[60]Rabinowitz E.: Online MD programs must balance accessibility against legal risks. Managed Healthcare Executive 2001; 11(10): 35-37

[61]Regan M.: Utilizing an Intranet in Disease Management. Dis Manag Health Outcomes 2002; 10(3): 147-154

[62]Rialle V., Noury N., Herve T.: An experimental health smart home and its distributed Internet-based information and communication system: First steps of a research project. Medinfo 2001; 10(Pt 2): 1479-1483

[63]Rogers M.A.M., Small D., Buchan D.A., Butch C.A., Stewart C.M., Krenzer B.E., Husovsky H.L.: Home Monitoring Service Improves Mean Arterial Pressure in Patients with Essential Hypertension. A Randomized Controlled Trial. Ann Intern Med 2001; 134: 1024-1032

[64]Roglieri J.L, Futterman R., McDonough K.L., Malya G., Karwath K.R., Bowman D., Skelly J., Warburton S.W.: Disease management interventions to improve outcomes in congestive heart failure. Am J Manag Care 1997; 3(12): 1831-1839

[65]Roudsari A.V., Zhao S., Carson E.: Web-based decision support and telemonitoring system for the management of diabetes. Proc 22nd Ann Int Conf IEEE Engineering in Medicine and Biology 2000; 2: 1120

[66]Russo H.: Window of Opportunity for Home Care Nurses: Telehealth Technologies. Online J Issues Nursing 2001; 6(3) [http://www.nursingworld.org/ojin/topic16/ tpc16_4.htm]

[67] Selecky C.: Integrating technology and interventions in the management of diabetes. Dis Manag Health Outcomes 2001; 9(Suppl. 1): 39-52

[68] Shea S., Starren J., Weinstock R.S., Knudson P.E., Teresi J., Holmes D., Palmas W., Field L., Goland R., Tuck C., Hripcsak G., Capps L., Liss D.: Columbia University's Informatics for Diabetes Education and Telemedicine (IDEATel) Project. Technical Implementation. J Am Med Inf Assoc 2002; 9: 25-36

[69] Stammer L.: Future tech devices: Smart shirts. Healthcare Inf 2001; 18(9): 34

[70] Tattersall R.: The expert patient: a new approach to chronic disease management for the twenty-first century. Clin Med 2002; 2(3): 227-229

[71] Tsai C., Starren J.: Patient Participation in Electronic Medical Record. J Am Med Assoc 2001; 285(13): 1765

[72] Wilkinson M., Mair F., Bonnar S.A., Angus R.M.: Initial Experience with Telemedicine in the Home Care of Patients with Acute Exacerbations of COPD. Proc ATS 98th Int Conf 2002; May 17-23, Atlanta, GA

[73] Winnem O.M.: Integrating Electronic Guidelines into the Diagnostic Cycle. In: Duplaga M., Zieliński K., Ingram D. (eds.): Transformation of Healthcare with Information Technologies. Amsterdam, IOS Press (2004) 156-165

[74] World Health Organization "Innovative Care for Chronic Conditions: Building Blocks for Action. Global Report." 2002

[75] Yatim L.: Israeli telenursing call center: Home cardiac telemonitoring: revisiting Israel's Shahal. Telemedicine Today 1997; 5(6): 26-27,33

[76] Yonghong Z., Bai J., Lingfeng W.: Development of a home ECG and blood pressure telemonitoring center. Proc 22nd Ann Int Conf IEEE Eng Med Biol Soc 2000; 3: 2282-2285

[77] Young M., Sparrow D., Gottlieb D., Selim A., Friedman R.: A Telephone-Linked Computer System for COPD Care. Chest 2001; 119: 1565-1575

[78] Zrebiec J.F., Jacobson A.M.: What attracts patients with diabetes to an Internet support group? A 21-month longitudinal website study. Diabet Med 2001; 18(2): 154-158

12 Computer-Aided Interventions

Jon Harald Kaspersen[1], Thomas Langø[1], Frank Lindseth[1]

1   SINTEF Health Research, Medical Technology, 7465 Trondheim, Norway

Image-guided surgery (IGS) is an evolving technology used to carry out minimally invasive procedures. The majority of developed systems for IGS are designed for neurosurgery [7][14][18][19][27] although systems for other clinical applications are emerging, such as otologic procedures [32] and liver surgery [22][21][33]. In the most advanced systems available today, IGS may provide the surgeon with two- (2D) and three-dimensional (3D) visual "road maps" of a patient's anatomy corresponding to the position of the surgical instruments used. Minimally invasive surgery allows access to difficult-to-reach anatomy, minimizes trauma to the patient, and, hence, can result in a shorter convalescence and hospital stay and reduced pain for the patient after surgery. Prior to the development of IGS, surgeons performing e.g. minimally invasive laparoscopic surgery could only see the surface area visible from the laparoscope. This surface-view technology is limited because the surgeon must correlate the patient's medical images (MR/CT/ultrasound) mentally with the operative field to determine the location of vital anatomical structures that lie beyond the view of the monocular laparoscope. Stereoscopic laparoscopes add depth perception to the view, but this does not solve the problem of not knowing what it looks like beneath the surface. IGS overcomes this limitation and provides the surgeon with real-time enhanced visualization [9][10][11][12][22][21][33].

The use of intraoperative ultrasound has been found valuable due to its relatively low cost and the possibility to generate 3D anatomical visual information within seconds, especially in neurosurgery [9][10][11][12][54]. In other areas such as prostate brachytherapy, 3D ultrasound has been used for visual guidance when positioning seed implants [4][42].

An IGS system combines a high-speed computer system, specialized software and tracking technology. On this computerized system the actual movements of surgical instruments are correlated with the patient's preoperative medical images and are displayed on the system's monitor. The precision of computerized instrument localization and navigation is critical to maneuvering safely within concealed anatomy and for the surgeon to perform more precise and careful surgery. However, most IGS systems are based on preoperative images, sometimes acquired the day before surgery. This means that as surgery proceeds, the images are continuously becoming less representative of the true patient anatomy. Introducing intraoperative imaging modalities such as ultrasound can solve this problem [23].

In traditional laparoscopic surgery, only the endoscope camera is used for guidance of the procedure. However, by introducing other guidance methods, the outcome of laparoscopic procedures may be improved. In section 1, we present initial experience with 3D navigation technology based on preoperatively acquired MRI or CT data sets used in combination with a laparoscopic navigation pointer. This technology offers the surgeon a better overview of structures not readily visible with conventional endoscope technology, and, hence, improves the guidance of laparoscopic surgery.

Before we describe an in-house navigation system under development, we present a brief overview of image-guided minimally invasive surgery with reference to Figure 12-1. Patient treatment using IGS systems involves several important steps, of which some are more critical than others for obtaining the optimal therapy of the patient. These steps are shown in Figure 12-1, and involve: 1) preoperative image acquisition, data processing and preoperative image visualization for optimal diagnostics as well as satisfying preoperative therapy decision and planning, 2) accurate registration of preoperative image data and visualization in the operating room for accurate and optimal planning just prior to surgery, 3) intraoperative imaging for updating images for guidance as well as intraoperative visualization and navigation for safe, efficient and accurate IGS in the OR, and finally, 4) postoperative imaging and visualization for adequate evaluation of patient treatment.

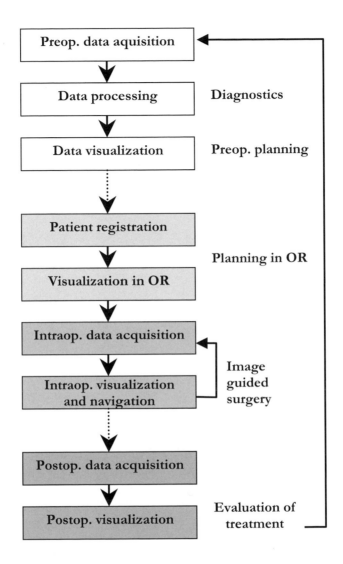

Figure 12-1 Important steps in image-guided surgery: 1) Preoperative data acquisition and planning, 2) patient registration and planning in the OR, 3) intraoperative data acquisition and navigation, 4) postoperative control of treatment.

1   Navigation in Laparoscopic Surgery

Our development navigation system, shown in Figure 12-2A, comprises a position tracker (Polaris®, NDI, Waterloo, Ontario, Canada), a desktop computer and the laparoscopic navigation pointer (LNP) with an attached tracking device on the shaft (Figure 12-2B). The pointer is approximately 40 cm long, i.e., approximately the same size as any other laparoscopic instrument. Furthermore, the pointer is normally used in combination with a Doppler device (SonoDoppler®, MISON, Trondheim, Norway) shown in Figure 12-2C. This Doppler device is a sheath with a 5 mm inner and 8 mm outer diameter and with an ultrasound transducer element at the tip for measuring Doppler shifts, i.e., blood flow. The Doppler device provides the surgeon with audio feedback on the blood flow as well as details on distance to the blood vessel in front of the instrument. The combined LNP and Doppler device (Figure 12-2D) comprise an advanced instrument for visualization control and blood vessel detection in laparoscopic surgery in the retroperitoneum.

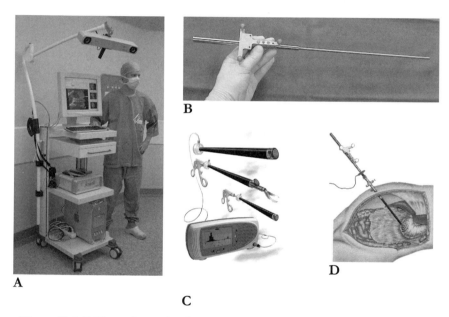

Figure 12-2 A) Photo shows development navigation system rack with optical tracking system cameras (Polaris®, NDI, Waterloo, Ontario, Canada) and a desktop computer. B) Laparoscopic navigation pointer (LNP) with a position-tracking device attached. C) Doppler device (SonoDoppler® MISON, Trondheim, Norway) in combination with a laparoscopic instrument. D) Intraoperative use of the LNP in combination with the Doppler device. The LNP controls visualization of 3D medical images on the navigation monitor based on position and orientation measurements of the attached tracking device, while the Doppler device provides detailed and real-time feedback on blood flow.

1.1 Preoperative Segmentation and Imaging

Prior to surgery, usually the day before, the MR/CT images (DICOM) are imported into the navigation software and reconstructed into a regular 3D volume. For laparoscopic surgery, the MR/CT images are acquired with the patient in the same position as what will be the case in the operating room. Skin fiducials, donut-shaped markers (15 mm diameter, 3 mm thick, 4 mm hole) filled with MR/CT contrast fluid, are glued to the patient prior to scanning. These markers are used for patient registration (see next subsection). Next, the surfaces of essential organs for the surgical procedure at hand are extracted from the images using a semi-automatic segmentation method. A research scientist performs this task with the assistance of the surgeon and sometimes the radiologist. The segmentation method is based on a starting point within the structure/organ and the surface of the structure is determined with a fast-marching level-set algorithm [25]. For an effective and proper extraction of a surface of an organ, input parameters of the segmentation algorithm need some adjustment due to variations in the characteristics of the image modality (CT or MR, contrast imaging or not, etc.). The organ to be segmented (aorta, kidney, tumor, etc.) also influences the settings for these parameters. Next, the registration points (skin fiducials/markers) in the images are marked and saved for quick registration of images in the operating room. Patient registration signifies the process of matching the MR/CT images into physical (tracking) space, i.e., correctly locating them relative to the patient on the operating table [27]. The total time for importing the images, 3D data reconstruction, segmentation and marking of fiducial points in the images is approximately 45 minutes for adrenalectomies. The surgeon and/or radiologist usually spend less than 20 minutes during this data preparation procedure, mainly verifying the segmentations of the tumors and blood vessels.

1.2 Patient Registration in the OR

In the operating room, the preoperative images are registered to the patient using a non sterile pointer, before sterile preparation of the patient. The surgeon places the pointer tip in one skin fiducial at a time and the navigation system samples each of their positions in space. These locations are then matched to the image points found earlier based on a least-square fit approach and the accuracy is calculated [27]. The surgeon can then perform some planning while pointing on the surface of the patient and check the match on the navigation system monitor to verify the accuracy of the registration (Figure 12-3). The patient registration provides the surgeon with interactive random access to the preoperative images, as they are located correctly in space relative to the patient. Next, the fiducials are removed and the patient is prepared for surgery. After insufflation (abdominal cavity is filled with CO_2), the surgeon can plan the procedure in more detail, including the placement of the trocars, by using the navigation system and a sterile pointer. The skin surface of the patient will not match the position of the pointer anymore (due to insufflation), but the retroperitoneum has not shifted and should be correctly located relative to the preoperative images.

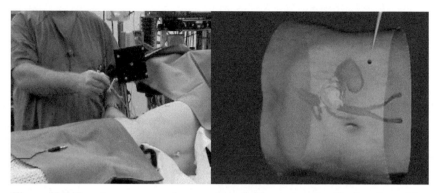

Figure 12-3 Planning surgery using a pointer (left) to select the display view of the segmented preoperative images (right). A graphical representation of the pointer is also seen in the navigation scene (right).

1.3 Navigation and Visualization in the OR

After insufflation and trocar positioning, the laparoscopic pointer with the Doppler device and navigation system is only used in the retroperitoneum. We do not use the navigation system and pointer for organs that are moved or extensively shifted due to insufflation since, in these cases (laparoscopic adrenalectomies, i.e., removal of the adrenal gland), we use preoperatively acquired images for guidance. The accuracy of the rigid LNP is better than 1.5 mm. This means that keeping the tip of the pointer steady and moving the shaft about, results in a maximum scatter of the tip position of 1.5 mm.

The sterile pointer controls the visualizations on the navigation monitor, and the images on the navigation monitor are updated continuously (in real time) according to both position and orientation of the pointer. The navigation system can display the images in different manners; conventional 2D orthogonal slicing (Figure 12-4A), 2D anyplane slicing (Figure 12-4B), surface visualization of segmented structures (models) (Figure 12-4C) or as combinations of these views; the 2D anyplane slice is displayed inside the surface model view (Figure 12-4C3). Moreover, we can use stereoscopic visualization (Figure 12-4D) [23][9][10][11][12] or volume rendering (Figure 12-4E) to further enhance the display of images. With volume rendering, it is possible to remove low/high intensity values from the image data to enhance the visualization for specific structures. By removing low intensity values, only the skeleton and blood vessels (due to CT contrast imaging) are seen as in Figure 12-4E2. For all the methods, crosshairs or a small sphere can be drawn to show the position of the tip of the LNP more clearly. The stereoscopic option can also be used for volume rendering (not shown). Position tracking of the LNP can be turned off to allow manual inspection, e.g. rotation and zooming of the volume (Figure 12-4E3), into positions not physically accessible by means of the LNP alone.

The Doppler instrument is used together with the LNP or with other laparoscopic instruments, prior to cutting to reveal important blood vessels.

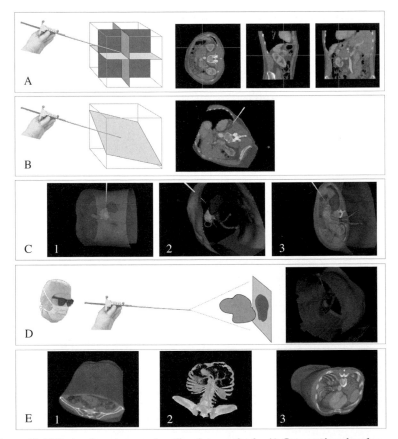

Figure 12-4 Navigation system visualization methods. A) Conventional orthogonal slicing (axial, sagittal, coronal). B) Anyplane slicing. C) Surface model visualization based on segmented structures from the CT/MR images. The surface model view can be combined with the anyplane view as shown in C3. D) Stereoscopic viewing. E) Volume rendering.

Throughout dissection, the Doppler device and the LNP are used regularly to check for blood vessels and to obtain a better overview of the anatomy beneath the organ/tissue surface in the laparoscope image.

2 Intraoperative Imaging

The organs and tissues in the body shift during surgery due to resection, gravity, moving organs out of the way in laparoscopy, opening of the dura in neurosurgery, etc. In neurosurgery, this is known as the brain shift problem. This can only be solved adequately by integrating intraoperative imaging with navigation technology. Several intraoperative imaging modalities have been proposed. These include CT, MRI and ultrasound. Open CT [13][38] and MRI [52][47][36][26][15][50][59] based systems, where the patient is transported into and out of the scanner, have obvious logistic drawbacks that limit the practical number of 3D scans acquired during surgery. Also, repeated use of intraoperative CT exposes both patient and personnel to considerable radiation doses. Thus, the most promising alternatives in the foreseeable future are interventional MRI [3][2][30][48][39] and intraoperative ultrasound [5][58][9][10][11][12][18][19][31]. In an interventional MRI system the surgeon is operating inside the limited working space of the magnet. Choosing speed over quality it is possible to obtain close to real time 2D images defined by the position of various surgical tools in addition to updated 3D maps in minutes without moving the patient. However, these systems require high investments, high running costs, and a special operating room as well as surgical equipment.

Ultrasound, although used by some groups for several years, has just recently gained a broader acceptance in neurosurgery [29] mainly due to improved image quality and relatively low costs. The image quality and user-friendliness of ultrasound have partly been achieved by optimizing and adjusting the surgical setup [53] as well as technical scan parameters in addition to integration with navigation technology [9][10][11][12]. The additional real-time 2D and 3D freehand capabilities, as well as real-time 3D possibilities, may establish intraoperative ultrasound as the main intraoperative imaging modality in future neuronavigation. Ultrasound may be used indirectly in neuronavigation to track the anatomical changes that occur, use these changes to elastically modify preoperative data and navigate according to the manipulated MRI/CT scans [18][19], or the ultrasound images may be used directly as maps for navigation [5][58][9][10][11][12][31][46][51].

2.1 Intraoperative 3D Ultrasound Acquisition

After making a craniotomy, updated high-quality 3D ultrasound maps can be acquired several times during surgery using an integrated ultrasound scanner of a navigation system such as SonoWand® (MISON, Trondheim, Norway). The sensor-frame mounted on the ultrasound probe (5-MHz FPA probe optimized for brain surgery applications) is tracked using the same optical positioning system as previously mentioned (Section 1) during freehand probe movement. A pyramid-shaped volume of the brain is typically acquired by tilting the probe approximately 80 degrees in 15 seconds. The digital images are reconstructed into a regular volume with a resolution of approximately 0.6 mm in all three directions and treated the same way as MRI volumes. The process of ultrasound acquisition, data transfer, reconstruction and display takes less than 45 seconds for a typical ultrasound volume. Repeated 3D scans were performed when needed (as indicated by real-time 2D ultrasound for example). The accuracy of ultrasound-based neuronavigation using the SonoWand system has earlier been evaluated to be 1.4 mm on average [35], and will be valid throughout the operation as long as the dataset used for navigation is frequently updated.

3 Multimodal Imaging in Minimally Invasive Surgery

Image fusion techniques might be beneficial when using the best of both MRI and ultrasound because it is easier to perceive an integration of two or more volumes in the same scene than mentally fusing the same volumes presented in separate display windows. It also gives the user the opportunity to pick relevant and needed information from the most appropriate of the available datasets. Ideally, relevant information should include not only anatomical structures for reference and pathological structures to be targeted (MRI and ultrasound tissue), but also important structures to be avoided, like blood vessels and important functional centers in the brain (MR angiography, ultrasound Doppler, and functional MRI).

3D display techniques are considered to be more user-friendly and convenient than 2D displays, and have shown potential for improving the planning and outcome of surgery [9][11][12][20][45][43][8]. Rendered 3D medical image data and virtual reality visualizations have earlier been reported to be beneficial in diagnosis of cerebral aneurysms as well as in preoperative evaluation, planning and rehearsal of various surgical approaches [17][24][41][40][44][49][16][28][37][55][1]. However, only some studies have been reported where 3D visualizations have been brought into the operating room and have been used interactively for navigating surgical tools down to the lesion [23][56][57]. Additionally, the 3D scene should be continuously updated using intraoperative imaging techniques so as to represent the true patient anatomy for safe and efficient surgery [34].

In the next figures we present some examples of image fusion, or multimodal imaging from neurosurgical cases. Multimodal imaging advantages are not limited to neurosurgery, but apply also to other surgical disciplines such as laparoscopic and endovascular surgery. A Multi-Modal Volume Visualizer (MMVV) was developed for investigating alternative ways to display the image information that is available at the different stages of an operation. We have tested the module using various datasets that have been generated during the treatment of patients with brain tumors and cerebrovascular lesions in the clinic. The neuronavigation system applied during surgery uses both preoperative MR/CT and intraoperative 3D ultrasound [9][10][11][12]. The MMVV scenes were generated after surgery in order to have time to try different visualization approaches. Nevertheless, the application reconstructs the spatial relationship between all the available volumes as seen in the operating room, and makes it possible to explore the optimal integration of preoperative MRI data with intraoperative 3D ultrasound data.

The datasets in Figure 12-5 to 12-8 are MR images (MRI), MR angiography images (MRA), ultrasound tissue images (US), and ultrasound angiography (power Doppler imaging) images (USA). Visualizations are shown as either sliced planes from the reconstructed volumes, surface or geometrically rendered images (GR) or volume-rendered images (VR). The displays focus on the important anatomy of the cases; tumors and blood vessels. Figure 12-5 shows a scene where preoperative and intraoperative images have been fused into the same displays. Figure 12-6 illustrates the problem with brain shift in neuronavigation. The preoperative images no longer match the patient anatomy after opening of the dura. This is seen from the real-time ultrasound images when they are merged with the preoperative MR images in a common coordinate system. Furthermore, Figure 12-6 shows the compensation of the brain shift after the preoperative data have been shifted to match the intraoperative ultrasound images. Figure 12-7 shows ultrasound monitoring of tumor resection. The ultrasound images are merged with MRI slices for better overview. Figure 12-8 shows 3D angiography images from MRI (left) and ultrasound power Doppler (middle and right) during an aneurysm operation.

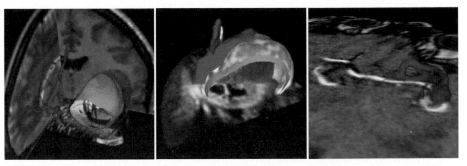

Figure 12-5 Left) Use of updated ultrasound data when available (VR-US vessels in blue as well as an axial US slice) and preoperative MRI data for improved overview. Middle) Visualizing the mismatch between pre- and intraoperative data using a GR-MRI tumor (green) together with a US slice through the same tumor. The VR tumor (white fog) illustrates the greater detail often achieved with volume-rendered display. We can also see a VR-US tumor in red. Right) The mismatch between the preoperative MRA slice through the aneurysm and the intraoperative VR-US-flow aneurysm in red is clearly visible.

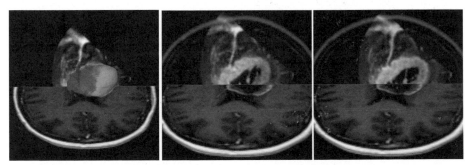

Figure 12-6 Left) The display shows the mismatch between preoperative axial MR slice/GR-MRI tumor (green) and the intraoperative coronal US slice/VR-US tumor (red). The middle and right views show the shift between an axial MR slice and a coronal US slice before (middle) and after (right) manual correction of the shift.

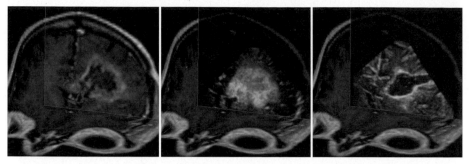

Figure 12-7 The views show multimodal imaging for guiding a tumor operation with resection control. Left) A coronal MRI slice cuts through the target area (VR-US flow in red). The coronal slice is replaced by the corresponding first US slice (middle), and a slice extracted from one of the last 3D ultrasound volumes acquired (right).

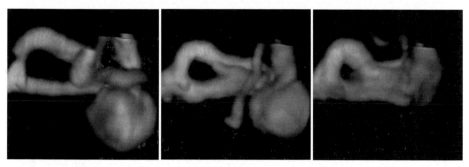

Figure 12-8 3D displays for improved control during an aneurysm operation. Zoom in on the VR-MRA aneurysm (left), and the VR-USA aneurysm before (middle) and after closing of the aneurysm (right).

4 Summary

As mentioned previously, one of the major disadvantages with laparoscopic surgery is the inability to palpate (feel/touch with fingers) organs, and tissue in general, for the surgeon. Another drawback with laparoscopic surgery is the lack of possibility to see beyond surfaces. Researchers have addressed both these disadvantages for quite some time. Laparoscopic tools with embedded force-feedback are under development and researchers have made it possible for the surgeon to see beyond surfaces with augmented reality based on preoperative 3D images. We have also developed and tested a multimodal imaging and navigation system, as described above.

However, even with all this information available, surgeons might need help during the surgical procedure to interpret some of the images available.

Therefore, we have developed the possibility of distributing the 3D intraoperative scene to the radiology department. Both the radiologist and the operator in the operating room are able to interact with the data. By using this collaborative feature it is possible for the surgeon to get expert advice without having the radiologist present in the operating room.

In other words, the surgical navigation system is extended with 3D teleradiology functionality (according to the definition of the American College of Radiology). That is, teleradiology is the electronic transmission of radiological images from one location to another for the purposes of interpretation and/or consultation. 3D reflects that it is possible with this system to distribute a scene containing 3D surface renderings, 3D volume renderings, along with 2D real-time information correctly placed in any of the scenes. The distribution ability incorporated in the surgical navigation system is based on omniORB (http://omniorb.sourceforge.net/), which is fully CORBA (Common Object Request Broker Architecture http://www.omg.org/) compliant.

5 Bibliography

[1] Anxionnat R, Bracard S, Ducrocq X, Trousset Y, Launay L, Kerrien E, Braun M, Vaillant R, Scomazzoni F, Lebedinsky A, Picard L. *Intracranial aneurysms: Clinical value of 3D digital subtraction angiography in therapeutic decision and endovascular treatment.* Radiology 2001; 218: 799-808.

[2] Black PM, Alexander E, Martin C, Moriarty T, Nabavi A, Wong TZ, Schwartz RB, Jolesz F. *Craniotomy for Tumor Treatment in an Intraoperative Magnetic Resonance Imaging Unit.* Neurosurgery 1999; 45: 423-433.

[3] Black PM, Moriarty T, Alexander E, Stieg P, Woodard EJ, Gleason PL, Martin CH, Kikinis R, Schwartz RB, Jolesz FA. *Development and Implementation of Intraoperative Magnetic Resonance Imaging and Its Neurosurgical Applications.* Neurosurgery 1997; 41: 831-845.

[4] Blake CC, Elliot TL, Slomka PJ, Downey DB, and Fenster A. *Variability and accuracy of measurements of prostate brachytherapy seed position in vitro using three-dimensional ultrasound: An intra- and inter-observer study.* Med Phys 2000; 27: 12: 2788-2795.

[5] Bonsanto MM, Staubert A, Wirtz CR, Tronnier V, Kunze S. *Initial Experience with an Ultrasound-Integrated Single-Rack Neuronavigation System.* Acta Neurochir 2001;143:1127-1132

[6] Bucholz RD, Yeh DD, Trobaugh J, McDurmont LL, Sturm CD, Baumann C, Henderson JM, Levy A, Kessman P. *The correction of stereotactic inaccuracy caused by brain shift using an intraoperative ultrasound device.* Lecture Notes in Computer Science Proceedings of the 1997 1st Joint Conference on Computer Vision, Virtual Reality, and Robotics in

Medicine and Medical Robotics and Computer-Assisted Surgery, CVRMed-MRCAS'97, Grenoble, 1997.

[7] Cartellieri M, Kremser J, Vorbeck F. *Comparison of different 3D navigation systems by a clinical "user".* Eur Arch Otorhinolaryngol 2001; 258: 38-41.

[8] Glombitza G, Lamade W, Demiris AM, Göpfert MR, Mayer A, Bahner ML, Meinzer HP, Richter G, Lehnert T, Herfarth C. *Virtual planning of liver resection: image processing, visualization and volumetric evaluation.* Int J Med Inf 1999; 53: 225-237.

[9] Gronningsaeter A, Kleven A, Ommedal S, Aarseth TE, Lie T, Lindseth F, Langø T, Unsgård G. *SonoWand, An ultrasound-based neuronavigation system.* Neurosurgery 2000; 47: 1373-1380.

[10] Gronningsaeter A, Kleven A, Ommedal S, Aarseth TE, Lie T, Lindseth F, Langø T, Unsgård G. *SonoWand, An ultrasound-based neuronavigation system.* Neurosurgery 2000; 47: 1373-80.

[11] Gronningsaeter A, Lie T, Kleven A, Mørland T, Langø T, Unsgård G, Myhre HO, Mårvik R. *Initial experience with stereoscopic visualisation of three-dimensional ultrasound data in surgery.* Surg Endosc 2000; 14: 1074-1078.

[12] Gronningsaeter A, Lie T, Kleven A, Mørland T, Langø T, Unsgård G, Myhre HO, Mårvik R. *Initial experience with stereoscopic visualization of three-dimensional ultrasound data in surgery.* Surg Endosc 2000; 14: 1074-1078.

[13] Grunert P, Müller-Forell W, Darabi K, Reisch R, Busert C, Hopf N, Perneczky A. *Basic principles and clinical applications of neuronavigation and intraoperative computed tomography.* Comput Aid Surg 1998; 3: 166-173.

[14] Gumprecht HK, Widenka DC, Lumenta CB. *BrainLab Vector Vision neuronavigation system: Technology and clinical experiences in 131 cases.* Neurosurgery 1999; 44: 97-105.

[15] Hall WA, Martin AJ, Liu H, Nussbaum ES, Maxwell RE, Truwit CL. *Brain Biopsy Using High-Field Strength Interventional Magnetic Resonance Imaging.* Neurosurgery 1999; 44: 807-814.

[16] Hans P, Grant AJ, Laitt RD, Ramsden RT, Kassner A, Jackson A. *Comparison of three-dimensional visualization techniques for depicting the scala vestibuli and scala Tympani of the cochlea by using high resolution MR imaging.* Am J Neuroradiol 1999; 20: 1197-1206.

[17] Harbaugh RE, Schlusselberg DS, Jeffrey R, Hayden S, Cromwell LD, Pluta D, English RA. *Three-dimensional computer tomograpic angiography in the preoperative evaluation of cerebrovascular lesions.* Neurosurgery 1995; 36: 320-326.

[18] Hata N, Dohi T, Iseki H, Takakura K. *Development of a frameless and armless stereotactic neuronavigation system with ultrasonographic registration.* Neurosurgery 1997; 41: 608-613.

[19] Hata N, Dohi T, Iseki H, Takakura K. *Development of a Frameless and Armless Stereotactic Neuronavigation System with Ultrasonographic Registration.* Neurosurgery 1997; 41: 608-614.

[20] Hayashi N, Endo S, Shibata T, Ikeda H, Takaku A. *Neurosurgical simulation and navigation with three-dimensional computer graphics.* Neurosurgical Research 1999:21.

[21] Herline A, Stefansic JD, Debelak J, Galloway RL, Chapman W. *Technical advances toward interactive image-guided laparoscopic surgery.* Surg Endosc 2000; 14: 675-679.

[22] Herline AJ, Stefansic JD, Debelak JP, Hartmann SL, Pinson CW, Galloway RL, Chapman WC. *Image-guided surgery: preliminary feasibility studies of frameless stereotactic liver surgery.* Arch Surg 1999; 134: 644-650.

[23] Hernes TAN, Ommedal S, Lie T, Lindseth F, Langø T, Unsgaard G. *Stereoscopic navigation-controlled display of preoperative MRI and intraoperative 3D ultrasound in planning and guidance of neurosurgery — New technology for minimally invasive image guided surgery approaches.* Minim Invasive Neurosurg 2002; 46: 129-137.

[24] Hope JK, Wilson JL, Thomson FJ. *Three-dimensional CT angiography in the detection and characterization of intracranial berry aneurysms.* Am J Neuroradiol 1996;17:437-445.

[25] Ibanez L, Schroeder W, Ng L, Cates J. *The ITK Software Guide: The Insight Segmentation and Registration Toolkit.* Edition 1.4, Kitware Inc., New York 2003.

[26] Kaibara T, Saunders JK, Sutherland GR. *Advances in Mobile Intraoperative Magnetic Resonance Imaging.* Neurosurgery 2000; 47: 131-138.

[27] Kaspersen JH, Sølie E, Wesche J, Åsland J, Lundbom J, Ødegård A, Lindseth F, Hernes TAN. *3D ultrasound based navigation combined with preoperative CT during abdominal interventions. A feasability study.* Cardiovasc Intervent Radiol 2003; 26: 347-356.

[28] Kato Y, Sano H, Katada K, Ogura Y, Hayakawa M, Kanaoka N, Kanno T. *Application of three-dimensional CT angiography (3D-CTA) to cerebral aneurysms.* Surg Neurol 1999; 52: 113-122.

[29] Kelly PJ. *Comments to: Neuronavigation by Intraoperative Three-dimensional Ultrasound: Initial Experience during Brain Tumor Resection.* Neurosurgery 2002; 50: 812.

[30] Kettenbach J, Wong T, Kacher DF, Hata N, Schwartz RB, Black PM, Kikinis R, Jolesz FA. *Computer-based imaging and interventional MRI: applications for neurosurgery.* Comput Med Imaging Graph 1999; 23: 245-258.

[31] Koivukangas J, Louhisalmi Y, Alakuijala J, Oikarinen J. *Ultrasound-controlled neuronavigator-guided brain surgery.* J Neurosurg 1993;79:36-42.

[32] Labadie RF, Fenlon M, Cevikalp H, Harris S, Galloway R, Fitzpatrick JM. *Image-guided otologic surgery.* Int Congr Ser 2003; 1256: 627-632.

[33] Lamade W, Vetter M, Hassenpflug P, Thorn M, Meinzer HP, Herfarth C. *Navigation and image-guided HBP surgery: a review and preview.* J Hepatobiliary Pancreat Surg 2002; 9: 592-599.

[34] Lindseth F, Kaspersen J H, Ommedal S, Langø T, Unsgaard G, Hernes T A N. *Multimodal image fusion in ultrasound-based neuronavigation: improving overview and interpretation by integrating preoperative MRI with intraoperative 3D ultrasound.* Comput Aided Surg 2003; 8:2:49-69.

[35] Lindseth F, Langø T, Bang J, Hernes T A N. *Accuracy evaluation of a 3D ultrasound-based neuronavigation system.* Comput Aided Surg 2002; 7:4:197-222.

[36] Martin AJ, Hall WA, Liu H, Pozza CH, Michel E, Casey SO, Maxwell RE, Truwit CL. *Brain Tumor Resection: Intraoperative Monitoring with High-Field-Strength MR Imaging—Initial Results.* Radiology 2000;215:221-228.

[37] Masutani Y, Dohi T, Yamane F, Iseki H, Takakura K. *Augmented reality visualization system for intravascular neurosurgery.* Comput Aid Surg 1998; 3:239-247.

[38] Matula C, Rössler K, Reddy M, Schindler E, Koos WT. *Intraoperative computed tomography guided neuronavigation: Concepts, efficiency, and work flow.* Comput Aid Surg 1998; 3:174-182.

[39] Moriarty TM, Quinones-Hinojosa A, Larson PS, Alexander E, Gleason PL, Schwartz RB, Jolesz FA, Black PM. *Frameless Stereotactic Neurosurgery Using Intraoperative Magnetic Resonance Imaging: Stereotactic Brain Biopsy.* Neurosurgery 2000;47:1138-1146.

[40] Muacevic A, Steiger HJ. *Computer-assisted resection of cerebral arteriovenous malformation.* Neurosurgery 1999;45:1164-1171.

[41] Nakajima S, Atsumi H, Bhalerao AH, Jolesz FA, Kikinis R, Yoshimine T, Moriarty TM, Stieg PE. *Computer-assisted surgical planning for cerebrovascular neurosurgery.* Neurosurgery 1997;41:403-409.

[42] Nelson N, Stock RG. *Prostate Brachytherapy in Patients with Prostate Volumes > 50 cm³: Dosimetric Analysis of Implant Quality.* Int J Radiat Oncol Biol Phys 2000; 46: 5: 1199-1204.

[43] Peters TM, Comeau RM, Psiani L, Bakar M, Munger P, Davey BLK. *Visualization for image guided neurosurgery.* IEEE-EMBC 1995:399-400.

[44] Pflesser B, Leuwer R, Tiede U, Höhne KH. *Planning and rehearsal of surgical interventions in the volume model.* Medicine Meets Virtual Reality IOS Press 2000:29-264.

[45] Psiani LJ, Comeau R, Davey BLK, Peters TM. *Incorporation of stereoscopic video into an image-guided neurosurgery environment.* IEEE-EMBC 1995:365-366.

[46] Regelsberger J, Lohmann F, Helmke K, Westphal M. *Ultrasound-guided surgery of deep seated brain lesions.* Eur J Ultrasound 2000; 12:115-121.

[47] Rubino GJ, Farahani K, McGill D, Wiele B, Villablanca JP, Wang-Mathieson A. *Magnetic Resonance Imaging-guided Neurosurgery in the Magnetic Fringe Fields: The Next Step in Neuronavigation.* Neurosurgery 2000; 46:643-654.

[48] Seifert V, Zimmermann M, Trantakis C, Vitzthum H-E, Kühnel K, Raabe A, Bootz F, Schneider JP, Schmidt F, Dietrich J. *Open MRI-Guided Neurosurgery.* Acta Neurochir (Wien) 1999; 141:455-464.

[49] Soler L, Delingette H, Malandain G, Ayache N, Koehl C, Clemet JM, Dourthe O, Marescaux J. *An automatic virtual patient reconstruction from CT scans for hepatic surgical planning. Medicine Meets Virtual Reality* IOS Press 2000.

[50] Steinmeier R, Fahlbusch R, Ganslandt O, Nimsky C, Buchfelder M, Kaus M, Heigl T, Gerald L, Kuth R, Huk W. *Intraoperative Magnetic Resonance Imaging with the Magnetom Open Scanner: Concepts, Neurosurgical Indications, and Procedures: A Preliminary Report.* Neurosurgery 1998;43:739-748.

[51] Strowitzki M, Moringlane JR, Steudel WI. *Ultrasound-based navigation during intracranial burr hole procedures: experience in a series of 100 cases.* Surg Neurol 2000;54:134-144.

[52] Tronnier V, Wirtz CR, Knauth M, Lenz G, Pastyr O, Bonsanto MM, Albert FK, Kuth R, Staubert A, Schlegel W, Sartor K, Kunze S. *Intraoperative Diagnostic and Interventional Magnetic Resonance Imaging in Neurosurgery.* Neurosurgery 1997;40:891-902.

[53] Unsgård G, Gronningsaeter A, Ommedal S, Hernes TAN. *Brain operations guided by real-time 2D ultrasound: New possibilities as a result of improved image quality — Surgical approches.* Neurosurgery 2002; 51: 402-12.

[54] Unsgård G, Ommedal S, Muller T, Gronningsaeter A, Hernes T A N. *Neuronavigation by intraoperative 3D ultrasound. Initial experiences during brain tumor resections.* Neurosurgery 2002; 50: 804-12.

[55] Vannier MW. *Evaluation of 3D imaging.* Critical Reviews in Diagnostic Imaging. CRC Press 2000; 41:315-378.

[56] Walker DG, Kapur T, Kikinis R, Yezzi A, Zollei L, Bramley MD, Ma F, Black P. *Automatic segmentation and its use with an electromagnetic neuronavigation system.* Abstract presented at the 12th World Congress of Neurosurgery, Sydney, Australia 2001:16-20.

[57] Wilkinson EP, Shahidi R, Wang B, Martin DP, Adler JR, Steinberg GK. *Remote-rendered 3D CT angiography (3DCTA) as an intraoperative aid in cerebrovascular neurosurgery.* Comput Aid Surg 1999;4:256-263.

[58] Woydt M, Krone A, Soerensen N, Roosen K. *Ultrasound-guided neuronavigation of deep-seated cavernous haemangiomas: clinical results and navigation techniques.* Br J Neurosurg 2001;15:485-495.

[59] Yrjänä SK, Katisko JP, Ojala RO, Tervonen O, Schiffbauer H, Koivukangas J. *Versatile Intraoperative MRI in Neurosurgery and Radiology.* Acta Neurochir (Wien) 2002;144:271-278.

13 Biosignal Monitoring and Recording

Thomas Penzel[1], Karl Kesper[1], Heinrich F. Becker[1]

[1]   Department for Internal Medicine, University Hospital of Philipps-University, Marburg, Germany

Biosignal monitoring and recording is the extension of medical investigations taking into consideration the development over time. The usual practice for medical tests is the investigation at one particular time point when the physician sees the patient. Besides the clinical interview the physician checks the pulse, measures blood pressure, takes a blood sample and sometimes urinary sample, and perhaps also measures body temperature and sweating. This collected information is used to develop a diagnosis or if it is not sufficient, to request more investigations. The additional investigations are in many cases functional tests or image-producing examinations. Such examinations can be radiology or ultrasound investigations or endoscopic or angiographic investigations. Functional investigations being requested can be electrocardiography, lung function test or a physical stress test. All these investigations are really point measures even if they involve image generation or a functional test over a short period of time. These point measures are used to generate a medical diagnosis. Based on the diagnosis the physician tries to predict changes over time (e.g. development of a disease or a treatment outcome). In order to verify these predicted changes often a second or a third investigation follows after a couple of days or weeks, again being point measures in essence. This type of measurement is always restricted to a few time points (Figure 13-1).

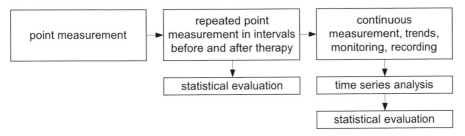

```
┌─────────────────┐   ┌──────────────────────┐   ┌──────────────────────┐
│                 │   │    repeated point    │   │     continuous       │
│ point measurement│──▶│measurement in intervals│─▶│measurement, trends,  │
│                 │   │ before and after therapy│  │ monitoring, recording│
└─────────────────┘   └──────────────────────┘   └──────────────────────┘
                                  │                            │
                                  ▼                            ▼
                      ┌──────────────────────┐   ┌──────────────────────┐
                      │ statistical evaluation│   │  time series analysis │
                      └──────────────────────┘   └──────────────────────┘
                                                             │
                                                             ▼
                                                 ┌──────────────────────┐
                                                 │ statistical evaluation│
                                                 └──────────────────────┘
```

Figure 13-1 Biosignal monitoring and recording marks the move from point measurements to continuous measurement in terms of time. Thus biosignal monitoring means time series analysis in the medical field.

By its nature it cannot give any conclusion about the dynamic behavior of physiological systems. Functional tests are the only and still limited approach to dynamic behavior. To extend the investigations of physiological variables in the time domain is the primary aim of biosignal acquisition or in other terms time series analysis in medicine. By this approach a better understanding of physiological control systems can be achieved. Predictions can be improved by considering the dynamic behavior of physiological regulation.

1   Basics of Monitoring and Recording

During the last few decades biosignal monitoring and recording became essential in many areas of modern medical services. This reflects the recognition of the importance of physiological control systems. The best known case for biosignal monitoring is electrocardiography (ECG). ECG has certainly the longest tradition in biosignal monitoring and recording because it is a strong (amplitude near 1 mV) and relatively robust signal [14]. Electrocardiography can be monitored for diagnostic purposes in a general physician's office with relatively simple and inexpensive devices. It may be recorded with 6 or 12 leads by a cardiologist for a comprehensive diagnosis of specific heart problems (e.g. signs of ischemia or heart attack). This type of ECG is still time limited and it may last a couple of minutes only. This examination can be regarded as a functional investigation which still represents a point measure based on a limited time segment of the continuous signals. In addition to this category of point measures based on functional investigations the ECG may be recorded over much longer periods of time (e.g. 24 hours) in order to detect and possibly explain arrhythmias. This long-term recording allows one to investigate dynamic properties and regulation mechanisms of heart rate for at least one 24-hour period. A 24-hour period is often chosen to obtain information on the circadian changes and the changes observed during sleep compared to daytime activities. Some ECG problems may become manifest only during the sleep period.

In another completely different category of investigations the ECG may be monitored in an operating room or under anesthesia as the primary vital sign to judge patient condition for the attending physician. In this case the continuous monitoring and an optional alarm management is most important. An immediate diagnosis related to the ECG is not done and a recording with permanent storage of the signal is usually not required.

Biosignal recording in medicine is not only restricted to the ECG (Figure 13-2). It includes blood pressure, respiration, electroencephalography (EEG), gastrointestinal variables, and many other parameters [8]. In general biosignals may be derived either from electrical body sources with appropriate amplification (nerves, muscles) or through specific transducers (pressure, flow, tension) which may be simple (piezo elements) or rather sophisticated signal processing systems in (oxygen saturation) themselves.

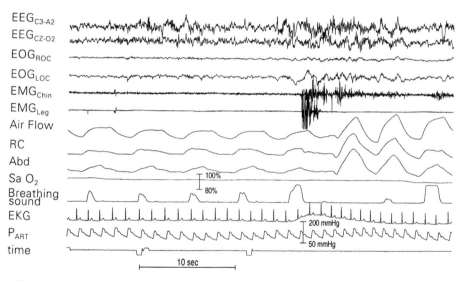

Figure 13-2 The recording of many different physiological parameters is required in several medical settings. This recording example with a multi-parameter recording was acquired in a sleep laboratory. The figure presents a 30-second segment of digital recorded data.

Biosignals may be monitored in acute and intensive care environments or recorded (stored for later analysis) for diagnostic purposes [5]. Applications using the recording of biosignals did increase much in recent years based on the technical possibilities provided by miniaturized and powerful digital recording and processing equipment. The recording of biosignals is now regularly done for diagnostic procedures in cardiology (ECG, blood pressure) and in neurology/neurophysiology (EEG, EMG). Specialty sleep medicine particularly requires the recording of multiple biosignals from different physiological systems (brain, heart, circulation, respiration) due to its interdisciplinary approach [7]. The recording methodology in this context is called cardiorespiratory polysomnography (Figure 13-3).

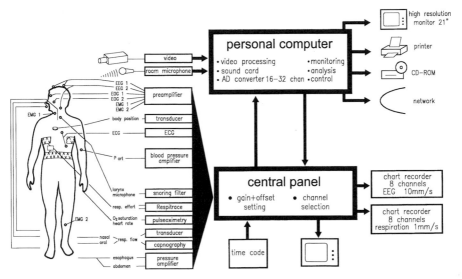

Figure 13-3 Multi-parameter biosignal recording is performed in a sleep laboratory or a neurophysiological laboratory. This includes many options for different signals. All signals are stored digitally by a personal computer. The interface to the amplifiers is usually given through an application software, here denoted as "central panel". Paper chart writers may be used for monitoring purposes and documentation at the same time. For later processing and archiving the possibilities of network access and CD-ROM writing are essential.

The biosignals need careful interpretation by well trained experts in their specific fields of medicine. Thus annotations and expert scorings of the signals recorded are as important as the raw digital data itself. Only through the evaluation of annotations can a human user or a computer algorithm learn the meaning of specific signal patterns. Therefore annotations and visual evaluation as assigned by experts to the recorded signals can be regarded as the key for further signal processing and analysis. Especially in complex settings such as intensive care it is often impossible to judge on the basis of recorded data only without explanatory annotations on recording conditions and actual medical interventions.

2   Signal Acquisition Conditions

Primary focus has to be given to the type of signal derived. Several signals are of electrophysiological origin and are electric by nature (e.g. ECG, EEG). These signals need careful amplification and filtering in order to obtain them with a minimum of artifacts. Other signals need transducers which are close to the physiological variable to be studied (flow, force, tension, movement, biochemical components). The transducers should have high signal-to-noise ratio and should be efficient in terms of power consumption. If possible sensors should be placed non-invasively on the skin. This issue implies the aspect of single or multiple use sensors as well as sterilization issues for the sensor.

All acquisition of raw physiological signals is dependent on the settings of amplification and filtering. This determines signal-to-noise ratio for the information obtained. Despite similar settings, the resulting signals recorded by equipment from different manufacturers often differ. This is due to different implementation of sensors, amplifiers and filters by different manufacturers. Signal-to-noise ratio in low-voltage signals such as brain waves is especially sensitive to the implementation of amplifiers and the specific circuits chosen. Therefore the resulting data are often device dependent and the device specification has to be documented with the data.

As different signal channels are interpreted together the inter-signal synchronization is also important and must be thought of when selecting the recording equipment (or even the analog-digital converters) used throughout the study. Inter-signal synchronization becomes a serious problem when different data are recorded using different devices with independent clocks. This is the case in sleep recordings and parallel recording of long-term ECG, long-term blood pressure, or activity using a wrist-worn actigraph. In intensive care it is very common to record data with different devices in parallel. Besides the bedside vital signs monitor this may be a ventilator, infusion pumps, and a fluid management system. For exact evaluations one has to guarantee that the start time of the different devices matches and one has to correct for a drift between clock rates of the devices. Differences of one minute over a 24-hour period are commonly observed. For normal clinical service this time shift is not important but for scientific studies looking for causal relationships this is important.

Sampling rates must be chosen in such a way that the signals can be reproduced in sufficient quality and that the requirements of subsequent signal analysis are covered. The specifications are appropriate for intensive care, cardiology, neurology and for polysomnographic recordings are presented in Table 13-1.

Table 13-1 Requirements for digital biosignal recording are specified for some major areas of monitoring and recording. The digital amplitude resolution is chosen according to the measurement precision of the underlying instrument (n. a. = not applicable) [7].

function	signal	optimal sampling rate	digital resolution
neurophysiology	electroencephalogram	200 Hz	0.5 µV/bit
	electrooculogram	200 Hz	0.5 µV/bit
	electromyogram	200 Hz	0.2 µV/bit
respiration	oro-nasal airflow	25 Hz	n.a.
	respiratory movements	25 Hz	n.a.
	esophageal pressure	100 Hz	0.5 mmHg/bit
	capnography	25 Hz	0.1%/bit
	oxygen saturation	1 Hz	1 %/bit
	transcutaneous pO_2, pCO_2	1 Hz	0.1 mmHg/bit
	breathing and lung sounds	5000 Hz	n.a.
cardiovascular	ECG	250 Hz	10 µV/bit
	heart rate	4 Hz	1 bpm
	blood pressure	100 Hz	1 mmHg/bit
auxiliary	body temperature	1 Hz	0.1 ° C/bit
	body position	1 Hz	n.a.
	esophageal pH	1 Hz	0.1 pH/bit

It has to be considered that the sensor and transducer specific characteristics are very important in respiration recording if subsequent comparisons of analysis results are made. The gold standard methodology consists of pneumotachography for quantitative airflow and esophageal pressure for quantitative respiratory effort. Both methods pose some discomfort on the patient and for long-term recording less intrusive and semi-quantitative methods are preferred. For respiratory movement recording, piezo transducers, pneumatic belts, impedance and inductive plethysmography are used as alternatives. The resulting waveforms have completely different signal characteristics, so that no uniform analysis of respiration can be implemented. For respiratory airflow different kind of thermistors, thermocouples and nasal pressure sensors are in use. The pressure sensors deliver a signal which has a quadratic relation to actual airflow. This must be corrected prior to further analysis. Thereafter the differences between the resulting waveforms are smaller than the differences found for respiratory movement signals.

For oxygen saturation pulse oximetry devices from different manufacturers were used. Pulse oximeters use different settings for the averaging of pulses and different algorithms when calculating oxygen saturation, based on reflected or transmitted light in several wavelengths. The signal finally recorded is not the raw signal used by the oximeter but the result of a signal processing algorithm used in feature extraction.

3 Signal Processing Algorithms

The application of signal processing methods and the development of new methods is one of the most important tasks in biosignal monitoring and recording. Signal processing methods have been developed to extract heart rate from the ECG, to detect and to classify arrhythmias, and to derive more information such as respiration, physical and mental stress signs [14]. Signal processing may help to derive a medical diagnosis or may help to simplify the monitoring task during anesthesia by giving alarms in case of abnormalities of the ECG waveform or of the heart rate as the result of a real-time analysis. Biosignal monitoring is therefore the application of general methods developed for time series analysis and signal processing to the biological and specifically to the medical field.

Biosignal processing implies filtering of the digital acquired signals and continues with feature extraction in the time domain and the frequency domain. New algorithms apply concepts derived from statistical physics in order to detect and characterize non-linear processes underlying the physiological variations [6]. Again the ECG and heart rate play a pioneering role in applications of biosignal processing [1]. Many of the methods are also applied to EEG signals and in recent years to more signals mentioned earlier.

The analysis of the heart rate is often done using frequency domain methods. Fourier transform and alternative methods to estimate spectral power had been applied and specific frequencies had been identified as reflecting physiological information. The low-frequency component (0.04 – 0.15 Hz) of the heart rate power spectrum has been attributed to baroreflex sympathetic control of blood pressure. The high-frequency component (0.15 – 0.4 Hz) has been attributed to the respiratory rhythm and is believed to be related to parasympathetic control of heart rate [1], [13]. The very low frequency component (< 0.04 Hz) has not been related to physiological rhythms with much success. There are still different hypotheses to be tested. Some parts of these very low frequency components are related to specific disorders, such as obstructive sleep apnea characterized by respiratory cessations with a one-minute rhythmicity during sleep. The identification of this specific rhythm can be used as a diagnostic approach for a disorder having its causes in sleep and respiration [10]. In this case the analysis of heart rate can serve as an indirect diagnostic tool based on signals much easier recorded than sleep and respiration itself (Figure 13-4).

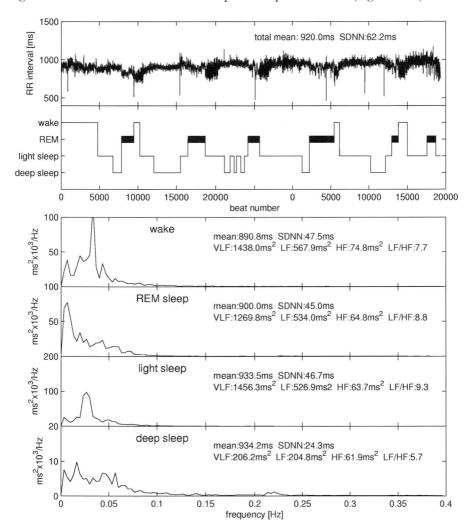

Figure 13-4 A frequency analysis of heart rate variability can help to identify a specific sleep disorder known as sleep apnea. This disorder is characterized by respiratory cessions with a one-minute periodicity. This periodicity is found in the power spectra of heart rate again. To apply the power spectra successfully it is necessary to analyze heart rate for the different sleep stages separately [10].

Statistical physics methods start with the assumption of random processes and underlying processes controlling the random behavior. These underlying processes may influence the correlation within the time series. Correlation within a time series is also investigated using autocorrelation analysis. But biological time series often bear additional influences over short or long terms which can be denoted as trends [12]. A detrended fluctuation analysis can first remove the trends and then investigate the correlation behavior within the time series [6]. This was done for heart rate time series again [6].This type of analysis could reveal that one important contribution to correlation behavior during sleep are the different sleep stages [2]. This uncovered that the different sleep stages really go along with different regulation of the physiological functions. These differences are so characteristic that they are now used to differentiate the sleep stages based on heart rate analysis. This approach marks the transition from data analysis to models and then a prediction of physiological regulation. The prediction in this case still needs validation studies in order to show that it is reliable under well described conditions.

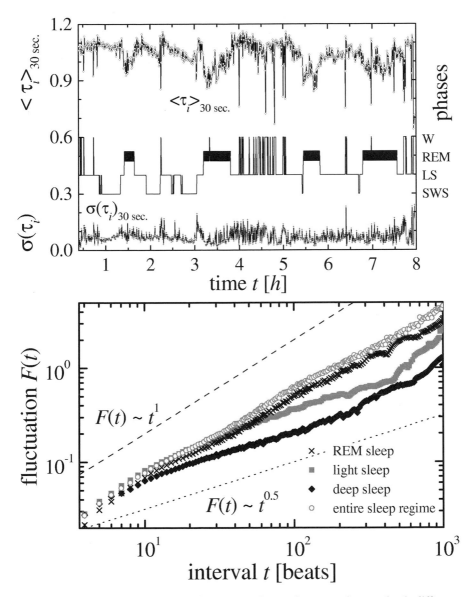

Figure 13-5 A correlation analysis of heart rate fluctuations reveals completely different beat-to-beat correlation for the different sleep stages. This difference is consistent over a wide range of heart beats and therefore is regarded as a reliable finding [2].

4 Multi-parameter Biosignal Database

As a case study for a biosignal database the European project SIESTA is introduced here [4], [9]. Sleep recordings in sleep laboratories are performed in order to objectify sleep disorders after having evaluated the subjective symptoms of insomnia ("I cannot sleep") and hypersomnia ("I am always tired and I do fall asleep even when trying to stay alert"). In order to objectify a sleep disorder diagnosis a sleep recording must be done in a sleep laboratory. Biosignals reflecting neurophysiological, respiratory and cardiac activities are recorded for 8-10 hours during the night. During the recording, the signals are also monitored, thus allowing the attending personnel to take notes on movements, talking during sleep or other events being of possible relevance. After recording the raw data are evaluated by sleep experts using rules developed by a committee chaired by A. Rechtschaffen and A. Kales in 1968. These traditional rules are based on chart recordings of electroencephalography, electrooculography and electromyography in 30-second epochs. This visual scoring of sleep signals results in four non-REM (rapid eye movement) sleep stages 1 and 2 being light sleep, 3 and 4 being deep sleep, and REM sleep. Wakefulness and body movements are also scored and noted. This visual scoring is still state of the art in the evaluation of polygraphic sleep recordings today. Several limitations of this traditional paper-oriented approach became apparent in the last 30 years and led to multiple approaches to use computer-based sleep analysis in order to overcome the limitations. The SIESTA project was initiated in 1997 to acquire a large reference database of sleep recordings from healthy volunteers covering different age groups and also patients with sleep disorders selected according to their highest prevalence [4]. The aims of this multi-center study were:

- to develop an enhanced computer-based system for analyzing polysomnographies in a reliable, reproducible way based on a small temporal resolution and a high amplitude resolution,
- to obtain an increased understanding of the contribution of well defined and computed variables to sleep analysis,
- to achieve an improved description of sleep for subjects that do not fall into the categories of Rechtschaffen and Kales – e.g. elderly persons, patients with sleep disorders,
- to compile a sleep scoring manual with the definitions of the procedures and terms developed in the SIESTA project.

5 Biosignal Database Quality

In order to have a systematic access to recorded signals and the annotations, rules were settled in the study protocol, with minimum criteria for the signals recorded by all partners in a multi-center study. In the SIESTA project all signals were either directly recorded using the EDF format or they were converted into the EDF format with the local equipment [3], [15]. One file containing the continuously recorded signals was produced per sleep recording.

Having acquired the data, a thorough quality control first checked the formal criteria of the signal database [11]. It was advantageous that only one data file of biosignals for each recording had to be checked. The check tested the contents of the fields in the global header and the signal headers according to the EDF file format definition. The fields were checked in terms of correct characters and the order of signals was checked by interpreting the labels in the signal headers. The set of labels was previously defined in the study protocol of the SIESTA project. Some typing errors could be corrected automatically whereas others such as a shuffled order of signal channels needed visual inspection prior to corrections.

The digitized raw signals were tested using a histogram analysis in order to identify signal characteristics, technical failures and artifacts. The bin-width of the histograms was chosen to be the quantization of the analog-digital converter (ADC). In case of a 16-bit signed integer number, as used in the EDF format, the histogram H(i) had bins in the range $-32768 \leq i \leq 32767$.

The final check of the signal quality is the visual inspection of the signals by an expert. During the inspection phase quality related annotations can be added to the database. Signal artifacts and biological artifacts were noted. Polygraphic recordings may be superimposed by many different types of non-cortical sources. In order to describe the sleep process, these non-cortical sources must be removed, or at least detected. Nine types of artifacts (EOG, ECG, muscle, movement, failing electrode, sweat, 50 Hz, breathing, pulse) were visually identified. Different artifact detection methods (least mean squares algorithm, regression analysis, independent component and principal component analysis, etc.) are able to remove technical and signal artifacts. They were tested on recordings with the annotated artifacts. After validating different artifact processing algorithms, adaptive FIR filtering, regression analysis and template removal were recommended to minimize the ECG interference, 50 Hz notch filtering for minimizing the line interference, adaptive inverse filtering for muscle and movement detection and combined overflow and flat line detector for failing electrode artifacts.

6 Biosignal Archiving Considerations

Signal data need storage space. Digital storage space becomes low in terms of cost and is also more condensed in terms of physical volume dimensions. Using the signal specifications given in Table 13-1 a digital recording of one night of sleep with 16 channels being recorded for eight to ten hours requires approximately 130 megabytes of digital memory. A recordable CD-ROM can hold four recordings of this size. The database of sleep recordings produced by the SIESTA project consists of 200 healthy volunteers and 100 patients with selected sleep disorders [4]. Each subject was recorded for two nights resulting in 600 recordings. This equals approx. 150 CD-ROMs. In order to have an easy and systematic access to all data files and all information a database which holds all data recorded and the related files was installed. The database holds all medical information on the subjects, file information about the available data, technical reports and signal information with artifact annotations, quality annotations and interpretation results. The database with the large signal data files resides on a central server. Today DVDs are an alternative to CD-ROMs in order to reduce the number of separate disks. With these technical advances archiving and accessing a database of biosignals can be done in a convenient way.

7 Summary

Biosignal monitoring and recording are an integral part of medical diagnosis and treatment control mechanism. These methods mark the transition from point oriented measures to continuous measures in medicine. This transition is much more appropriate to the dynamics of physiological regulation in health and disease. Modern approaches for sensor technology, for new analysis algorithms and for database technologies help to move this emerging area forward. Technical advances originating in computer technology, in consumer electronics and microtechnology can support these technological advances.

8 Bibliography

[1] Akselrod S, Gordon D, Ubel FA, Shannon DC, Barger AC, Cohen RJ: Power spectrum analysis of heart rate fluctuations: a quantitative probe of beat-to-beat cardiovascular control. Science 213: 220-222, 1981.
[2] Bunde A, Havlin S, Kantelhardt JW, Penzel T, Peter JH, Voigt K: Correlated and uncorrelated regions in heart-rate fluctuations during sleep. Phys. Rev. Lett. 85: 3736-3739, 2000.

[3] Kemp B, Värri A, Rosa AC, Nielsen KD, Gade J: A simple format for exchange of digitized polygraphic recordings. Electroencephalography and Clinical Neurophysiology 82: 391-393, 1992.

[4] Klösch G, Kemp B, Penzel T, Schlögl A, Gruber G, Herrmann W, Rappelsberger P, Trenker E, Hasan J, Värri A, Dorffner G: The SIESTA project polygraphic and clinical database. IEEE Engineering in Medicine and Biology 20 (3): 51-57, 2001.

[5] Korhonen I, Ojaniemi J, Nieminen K, van Gils M, Heikelä A, Kari A: Building the IMPROVE data library. IEEE Engineering in Medicine and Biology 16: 25-32, 1997.

[6] Peng CK, Havlin S, Stanley HE, Goldberger AL: Quantification of scaling exponents and crossover phenomena in nonstationary heartbeat time-series. Chaos 5: 82-87, 1995.

[7] Penzel T, Brandenburg U, Fischer J, Jobert M, Kurella B, Mayer G, Niewerth HJ, Peter JH, Pollmächer T, Schäfer T, Steinberg R, Trowitzsch E, Warmuth R, Weeß HG, Wölk C, Zulley J: Empfehlungen zur computergestützten Aufzeichnung und Auswertung von Polygraphien. Somnologie 2: 42-48, 1998.

[8] Penzel T, Brandenburg U, Peter JH: Langzeitregistrierung und Zeitreihenanalyse in der Inneren Medizin. Internist 38: 734-741, 1997.

[9] Penzel T, Kemp B, Klösch G, Schlögl A, Hasan J, Värri A, Korhonen I: Acquisition of biomedical signals databases. IEEE Engineering in Medicine and Biology 20 (3): 25-32, 2001.

[10] Penzel T, McNames J, de Chazal P, Raymond B, Murray A, Moody G: Systematic comparison of different algorithms for apnoea detection based on electrocardiogram recordings. Med. Biol. Eng. Comput. 40: 402-407, 2002.

[11] Schlögl A, Kemp B, Penzel T, Kunz D, Himanen S-L, Värri A, Dorffner G, Pfurtscheller G: Quality control of polysomnographic sleep data by histogram and entropy analysis. Clin. Neurophysiol. 110: 2165-2170, 1999.

[12] Taqqu MS, Teverovsky V, Willinger W: Estimators for long-range dependence: an empirical study. Fractals 3: 785-798, 1995.

[13] Task force of the European Society of Cardiology and the North American Society of Pacing and Electrophysiology: Heart rate variability. Standards of measurement, physiological interpretation, and clinical use. Circulation 93: 1043-1065, 1996.

[14] Tompkins WJ: Biomedical Digital Signal Processing. Englewood Cliffs, Prentice-Hall, 1993.

[15] Värri A, Kemp B, Penzel T, Schlögl A: Standards for biomedical signal databases. IEEE Engineering in Medicine and Biology 20 (3): 33-37, 2001.

14 Enhancing Medical Education through Telelearning

Mariusz Duplaga[1], Krzysztof Juszkiewicz[3], Bartosz Kwolek[2], Mikołaj Leszczuk[3], Zdzisław Papir[3], Paweł Rzepa[2], Krzysztof Zieliński[2]

[1] Collegium Medicum, Jagiellonian University, Kraków, Poland
[2] Department of Computer Science, AGH University of Science and Technology, Poland
[3] Department of Telecommunications, AGH University of Science and Technology, Poland

The state-of-the-art in medicine changes quickly. This imposes continuous pressure on health professionals to update their skills and knowledge. Keeping track of ongoing changes in medical doctrine may be impossible for many of them, especially if one considers the trends for a growing load of clinical work and complex reimbursement process in numerous countries.

Established methods of continuing education offered to health professionals appear frequently ineffective for keeping clinical competences up-to-date.

Quite often these traditional approaches to postgraduate medical education do not seem to be cost-effective as they require accessibility from health professionals at a particular time and place. Many traditional ways of updating medical knowledge offered to health professionals fail due to lack of coherence with everyday experience.

In the ideal situation, medical postgraduate education should be a seamless part of the clinical environment. Furthermore, access to upgrading clinical skills and knowledge should be ubiquitous; not bound to a specific time or place. Such requirements are fulfilled by a new approach to education, so-called distance learning. Distance learning could be described as "the acquisition of knowledge and skills through mediated information and instruction, encompassing all technologies and other forms of learning at a distance" [45]. The term distance learning does not have one, simple and concise definition widely accepted throughout the scientific and commercial world. Different authors reveal numerous approaches when shaping the definition of distance learning, however, most of them accept the following attributes:

- separation of teacher and student in time, in distance, or both,
- two-way communication (including e-mail, teleconferences, newsgroups, chat-rooms) that allows teacher and student to cooperate in a synchronous or asynchronous way,
- use of video, audio, computer, multimedia communication or traditional printed materials mixed together.

Distance learning offers a number of advantages to clinicians. It removes barriers to learning resulting from time and place, allowing clinicians to access educational resources in their work or home environment. Of course, distance education requires the use of dedicated instructional delivery systems, which will serve as a connection between health professionals and educational resources.

1 Importance of Medical Studies — What Is Specific in Them

Internet development incited high expectations about the access to digital resources. This phenomenon was also mirrored in the healthcare domain where both health professionals and patients expect the ability to access high quality educational, multimedia-based resources online. Simultaneously, persistent pressure on clinicians to maintain professional development and lifelong medical education has a great impact on the search for efficient tools of information sharing in this environment. It is also obvious that digital recordings of medical procedures e.g. endoscopic diagnostic and therapeutic techniques may be used as real-life educational resources for physicians in training. The educational and training processes may be considerably enhanced through the use of huge volumes of recordings obtained by diagnostic and therapeutic procedures that were performed in healthcare institutions. This potential is not fully appreciated, even if there were many initiatives focused on the reutilization of "everyday practice" resources for educating and training after appropriate preparation of the data.

The flood of information and access to huge resources would not be possible without the use of digital libraries. Digital library may be defined as the electronic extension of functions users typically perform and the resources they access in a traditional library [48]. However, the concept of digital library extends access to resources, which are available in other types of repositories like video recordings or museum objects. The process of shifting from text and image-based systems to audio and video is continuous.

Development process of a medical digital video library should include all the steps necessary for digital library preparation. They cover conversion of content from physical/analog to digital form, extraction, creation of metadata, indexing information describing the content, storage of digital content and metadata in multimedia repository, establishment of client services for the browser, content delivery via file transfer or streaming media, access through a browser or dedicated client and establishing access via network. The implementation of a digital video library requires the development of a medical virtual learning environment for health professionals.

Miron and Blumenthal described an approach to conversion of analog video to digital data implemented in surgical ophthalmology unit [27].

Digital video may be used in these areas of medical education where the traditional approach was not successful. Hamilton et al. explored the application of digital video integrated with computer-assisted learning system allowing for the study of post-natal human development. The behavior patterns of children between 6 weeks and 12 months of age were recorded on VHS tape and then digitalized, edited and integrated with computer-assisted learning system which could be accessed through network [15].

The common feeling of many clinicians about performing invasive procedures, and particularly surgeons, is that many extremely interesting materials cannot be recorded during everyday activities and shown afterwards. Kumar and Pal described a cost-effective and timesaving approach to recording digital video during cardiac surgery procedures. They used a special video camera mounting arm installed in the operating room [21].

The technology of Internet streaming of video resources was appreciated by medical educators who perceived it as a possible enhancement of the educational process [34].

The results of the use of streaming video for additional education was tested by Green et al. [13]. These authors evaluated student nurses' reactions to streaming videos supporting a Life Sciences module. The students were able to view online e-learning sessions with integrated streamed video. E-learning resources were available to them through Blackboard, a Virtual Learning Environment. Of the 656 students who entered e-learning resources online, more than half browsed the video streams. From this group, about 60% appreciated viewing the videos, but only 25% confirmed that they were able to learn from them [13]. The usefulness of online video resources for continuing professional development was also evaluated by other authors [33]. It is frequently underlined that the use of video on-demand resources can overcome barriers to learning [39]. Such a barrier is considerable distance between healthcare facilities from main medical educational center. The continuing medical education resources may be delivered to health professionals working in rural or peripheral medical facilities as interactive video courses or in asynchronous mode. This latter option is particularly important for clinicians who can review available material at a convenient time. The access to online health databases including digital video library may be important for tracing continuous medical education [49]. The capabilities of streaming video were appreciated by the editors of Annals of Thoracic Surgery who since 1998 have added online video clip adjuncts to papers published [14]. Adding the video imaging improves the impact of training on healthcare professionals. Lavitan et al. studied the effects of video viewing before undertaking practical interventions in a group of paramedic trainees. The success rates among trainees who, apart from traditional training courses, were given the opportunity to see videos on intubation were higher than in a trainee group not given that opportunity [22].

Leung et al. described the use of streaming audio and video technology with the objective of enhancing emergency physician education. In this case, lectures were recorded with digital camera recorder in a soundproof studio. Both high- and low-bandwidth options were available to optimize the viewer's Internet connection. The RealPlayer software was used for playback. The authors underlined the advantages of such approach to medical education relying on a flexible online learning experience and the fact that education process may be realized at the convenience of the clinicians undertaking the course [24]. In some settings, "orientation video" is made available through the Web in order to improve access and compliance with the department of emergency for residents and students beginning training in this unit [12].

University of Kentucky streaming video technology was used to develop a web-cast model to allow institutions to broadcast live and prerecorded surgeries, conferences and courses in real time over networks. Gandsas et al. focused on the broadcast of prerecorded laparoscopic paraesophageal hernia repair to a national and international audience using desktop computers enabled with off-the-shelf, streaming software and standard hardware [11]. The use of medical digital video library is usually accompanied by other tools allowing discussion about course materials. Such approach was applied by Wiecha et al. who enabled students' evaluation of online modules to reinforce course aims and concepts in discussion groups [47].

The European Institute of Telesurgery (EITS) founded in 1994 supports the use of education resources for surgeons. The Institute was determined to develop new computer and training technologies in surgery. Its foundations were the result of the expectations of the surgery community related to access of the surgery site created by surgeons and targeted for surgeons and their patients.

The diffusion of surgical knowledge was carried out through the use of videos and 3D animated computer graphics [26].

Some authors put particular focus on limitations related to low-bandwidth connections to the digital video library [38]. "This issue becomes a real problem when one considers the phenomenon of digital divide" occurring in many areas of the world which hampers the access of health professionals in numerous developing countries.

2 Computer-Based Training Standards and Standardization Organizations

Today distance learning software is being written by an extensive number of parties using very diverse tools or authoring systems. Many of the systems' components can't cooperate with each other, some of them require little effort to force teamwork, and others collaborate without any difficulties. The need for systems to be brought together resulted in establishment of many standardization organizations, including the following.

2.1 AICC

The Aviation Industry CBT (Computer-Based Training) Committee (AICC) [3] develops guidelines for the aviation industry in the development, delivery, and evaluation of CBT and related training technologies.

The AICC generates and distributes three different types of documents. The first type of documentation includes the AICC Guidelines and Recommendations (AGR). AGRs represent the official voice of the AICC with respect to a designated area. All AGRs have been formally voted upon and approved by the general voting membership of the AICC. Technical reports are the second type of documentation. They typically contain the technical detail underlying an AGR. White papers and working documents are the third type of documentation. All the publications are available on the AICC web page.

The areas of AICC interest include guidelines for courseware delivery stations, digital audio, operating/windowing system, digital video and user interface, peripheral devices, and interoperability with other CBT systems. The AICC has developed a free automated testing program for verifying conformance with file-based and Web-based computer managed instruction systems and CBT courseware.

2.2   ADL

The Advanced Distributed Learning (ADL) Initiative [2], sponsored by the Office of the Secretary of Defense (OSD), is a collaborative effort between government, industry and academia to establish a new distributed learning environment that permits the interoperability of learning tools and course content on a global scale. The ADL Initiative is evolving the development and implementation of ADL specifications and guidelines such as the Sharable Content Object Reference Model (SCORM). The SCORM is a reference model that defines the interrelationship of course components, data models and protocols so that learning content objects are sharable across systems that conform with the same model. The SCORM applies current technology developments to a specific content model by producing recommendations for consistent implementations by the vendor community. It is built upon the work of the AICC, IMS, IEEE, ARIADNE and others to create one unified "reference model" of interrelated technical specifications and guidelines designed to meet DoD's high-level requirements for Web-based learning content. The SCORM includes aspects that affect learning management systems and content authoring tool vendors, instructional designers and content developers, training providers and others.

2.3   IMS

IMS Global Learning Consortium [19] develops and promotes the adoption of open technical specifications for interoperable learning technology. The scope for IMS specifications, broadly defined as "distributed learning", includes both online and off-line settings, taking place synchronously or asynchronously. This means that the learning contexts benefiting from IMS specifications include Internet-specific environments as well as learning situations that involve off-line electronic. The learners may be in a traditional educational environment, in a corporate or government training setting or at home.

2.4   ARIADNE

The ARIADNE Foundation's [4] main goals are the following:
- foster cooperation between educational bodies through the setup and exploitation of a truly European Knowledge Pool,
- keep social and citizenship aspects dominating education, combat an evolution towards making it a mere marketable item,
- uphold and protect multilingualism and the use of national/regional languages in education,

- define by international consensus what aspects of ICT-based formation should be standardized and what should be left local.

2.5   MedBiquitous

All of the bodies mentioned earlier do not target a proprietary educational area but produce standards for general learning. The MedBiquitous Consortium [42] is an organization whose mission is to develop Internet technologies for global communities of physicians and other medical professionals that advance professional education and expertise, facilitate collaboration, and raise the level of patient care. Again, it does not reinvent the wheel. MedBiquitous is working with ADL to customize SCORM standards to make them more useful for medicine. MedBiquitous customizations would allow educators to indicate a module's subject using a medical terminology, tie modules to objectives or competencies within a medical curriculum, disclose financial relationships of module authors up front and indicate the number of CME (Continuing Medical Education) credits awarded per module.

2.6   Other CBT Standardization Organizations

There are many other standardization organizations in the world such as ALIC[1], EdNA[7], IEEE LTSC, OKI [28], SIF [43], WSLT[5]. The ones described before are only examples that seem to be the most recognized. All of the organizations do not try to define they own prescriptions for distance learning systems. They do not compete but rather collaborate and complement one another in order to specify worldwide standards accepted by a majority of industry and academia. AICC, IMS, IEEE LTSC are for example the active members of the ADL Initiative and influence its standards.

3   Requirements of Distance Learning Platform for Medicine

Distance learning platform development must be guided by the requirements defined by its users, therefore the groups of users that benefit from the medical platform must first of all be specified. The following groups of system clients can be identified:

- learners participating in regular courses, either medical school students or professionals who improve their skills during continuing medical education process,
- clinicians wanting to consult an evidence as it arises with an evidence base or an expert either online or another way,

- teachers and consultants acting as expert educators,
- contributors who fill the platform with educational material of proper quality.

A medical platform must present for all of those users various features covering different aspects of the platform, including interaction between participants, access to the platform, tools for preparing educational material that should be stored and delivered for learners, etc.

Summarizing, the requirements can be specified as follows:
- Ability to collaborate between all members, using both synchronous and asynchronous communication,
- Adapting the educational resources structure to suit the needs of the learner,
- Building an adjustable graphical end-user,
- Delivering means of annotation and searching through multimedia medical records,
- Delivering user-friendly and adaptable authoring tools for producing and managing adjustable educational materials and portable multimedia environment,
- Enabling authentication, authorization and information confidentiality allowing multilevel access to educational data per user or role basis supporting author copyrights and methods for storing medical data,
- Enabling personalization mechanisms allowing one to customize the students' learning environment,
- Enabling possibility of storing properly instrumented data for any platform user,
- Enabling tools for evidence anonymity through hiding of personal data kept in medical resources,
- Ensuring compatibility with external system offering medical materials by conforming to distance learning standards,
- Ensuring instruments for storing and delivering static and dynamic digital data with diagnostic and reference quality,
- Introducing mechanisms that allow one to individually monitor, support, and assess learning progress.

To make this vision of a medical platform a reality will require the support of collaborative technologies:
- high-speed computer networks for transferring images of diagnostic quality,
- huge-capacity storage devices for storing high-quality recordings,

- modern end-user personal equipment allowing adjustable display of medical data,
- high-performance computing servers for analyzing, searching and processing medical data.

All of these technologies are present in the market nowadays and are able to leverage a flexible, powerful environment capable of running a high-quality distance learning platform for medicine.

4 Overview of Existing Distance Learning Platforms

Distance learning is becoming a strategic issue for numerous commercial and educational organizations. Many leading corporations have implemented Learning Management Systems (LMS) to answer needs in distance education. Moreover, quite a few non-commercial systems have spread simultaneously and tried to attract a broad learning audience. The following are examples of the most popular distance learning platforms for medicine.

4.1 Pathlore LMS 6

Pathlore [31] Learning Management System (LMS) is a single, integrated presence based on standard technology platforms that enables assessment, planning, delivery and management of organizational learning. Pathlore LMS enables appropriately combined instructor-led, online and virtual classrooms; it has multiple interface options (web and phone) that give the flexibility to reach learners on their terms. Pathlore LMS is AICC Certified and SCORM 1.2 Certified. Pathlore LMS provides flexible and collaborative functions allowing content managers to integrate training material or courseware created with most standard authoring tools, easily support third-party packaged courseware and use any courseware that complies with either AICC or SCORM standards.

Pathlore has been deployed in more than 100 hospitals and health networks, as well as pharmaceutical companies and other organizations. Pathlore customers include SSH Healthcare, Advocate Health Care, Affinity Health Systems, Bayer Corporation, Solvay, Merck Corporation and others.

4.2 THINQ TrainingServer

The THINQ [44] TrainingServer LMS is a learning platform that allows one to initiate, manage and track all learning-related activities through an organization.

The THINQ LMS offers a highly configurable learner interface that can be modified to include new fields, layouts and branding in one or multiple languages. THINQ LMS manages personalized learning plans, tracks required certifications, assesses skills and competencies, views skill gaps, collaborates with peers, launches and tracks e-learning courseware, enrolls and participates in instructor-led and blended learning programs.

The THINQ LMS can be accessible to learners with disabilities, in compliance with American regulation Section 508. The THINQ LMS is SCORM 1.2 RTE Level 3 Certified.

THINQ solutions gained a competitive share in a healthcare and pharmaceutical market. The THINQ LMS is helping to deliver and track the managerial training content for CVS/pharmacy, Empire Blue Cross/Blue Shield, IMS Health, Kennedy Health System, Pfizer, Siemens Medical, Smith & Nephew and others. Similarly to Pathlore, THINQ has been listed as a "leader" in Gartner Learning Management System Magic Quadrants.

4.3 IBM Lotus® LMS

The Lotus Learning Management System is a scalable, flexible platform for managing both classroom-based and online learning activities, resources, curricula and catalogs across an enterprise. Lotus Learning Management System software helps maximize value for various modes of training delivery — self-paced learning, virtual learning and collaboration or physical classrooms.

With Lotus Learning Management System software, subject matter experts (SME) can create their own custom courseware, including audio or video and links to external resources, including Web sites and reference databases. Lotus Learning Management System software also supports a vast library of SCORM- and AICC-compliant coursewares.

A share in the distance learning marketplace are trying to gain freeware, open source e-learning environments as well. They are quickly evolving and transform to advanced multimedia environments. The sample — .LRN [25] — capabilities include course management, online communities, learning management, and content management applications.

In the context of expenses for installation, maintenance and support for medical distance learning environments a use of Application Service Provider model seems to be a very interesting solution. One of the companies supplying ASP solutions for distance learning, GeoLearning Inc. [11] claims that "Designed to launch, track and manage online training for mid-size organizations,

GeoExpress can be implemented in 30 days or less for only $49 per user, including ASP hosting, security and technical support." Their product, GeoExpress, is based on web technologies and thus GeoExpress users need only access to a Web browser equipped computer with Internet access. GeoLearning does not boast about any deployments in healthcare, but the model it follows is really interesting and it is very likely to attract many other corporations.

5 Case Studies

Generally, all the existing solutions are well adopted for common situations. There is need to develop dedicated application, when considering specific medical conditions. Such development can be presented as case studies.

5.1 Medical Digital Video Library

Digital Video Library usually is not a homogeneous product. Typically, one deals with integration of several modules (components). Each of them executes some specified task; very often resolving some particular, conceptual problem, and only seamless interworking of modules gives the final product, the DVL [17]. Since the area of research is fast developing [37] and is (at the time of writing) more than four years old, the authors propose an extension of the concept of DVL, see Figure 14-1.

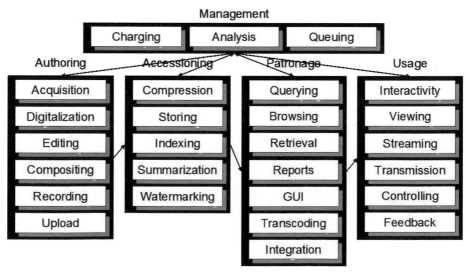

Figure 14-1 Main components of DVL along with subsystems.

Interesting modules, being the authors' (partly or completely) innovationed approaches, which are described in this section are: automatic content segmentation module, media streaming and video quality adaptation module, video uploading, handling and format conversion module, back-office database subsystem, GUI (Graphical User Interface) module as well as quality feedback module.

Automatic content segmentation

The natural, obvious and intuitive criterion of a shot change is a sudden peak of the difference between successive frames. The method of analysis of that difference would be correct, if the "threshold" could be set unambiguously (all frame-pairs having a difference larger than some value would be considered a shot change).

Therefore, a more sophisticated algorithm was developed. The key issue is now not the difference but the difference between the current and the previous difference [1].

The aforementioned algorithm for content segmentation has been applied to medical videos, recorded during endoscopic examinations. Such pictures consist of a fast moving area (the main picture), several textual fields as well as many black areas.

Most of the endoscopic recordings are not full-screen videos, but the visible area consists of fields, from which only about 30% are occupied by a fast moving picture (e.g. *fps* ratio of 25). The rest is a black background, usually containing slowly changing control captions (examination number, patient's first name/last name, date and time of the examination, patient's birth date, patient's age, diagnosis); see Figure 14-2.

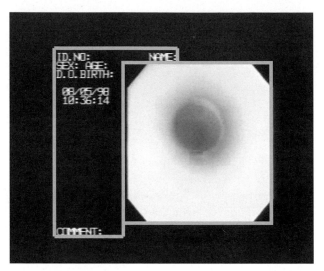

Figure 14-2 Example frame of bronchofiberoscopic recording.

The authors found that analysis of the main picture is not enough. Therefore, a modification has been developed, causing the algorithm to rely on two defined picture areas: the first one – the main picture and the second one – the area displaying information captions. Then, only a simultaneous cut detection in both areas indicates a new video segment [9].

Media streaming and video quality adaptation

New possibilities of stream transmission (streaming) have appeared along with elaborating protocols specially for stream media: Real Time Streaming Protocol (RTSP) and Real Time Protocol (RTP), described in [35], [36].

For convenience, functionality of real-time transport has been divided into two protocols: content transport, carried over RTP protocol, and control messages, carried over RTP Control Protocol (RTCP), on which multimedia architecture in IP networks is based.

The RTP was designed as an end-to-end transport protocol that is suitable for both unicast and multicast transmission of real-time data, such as interactive audio or video, by providing sequence numbering, time stamping, and payload type identification. RTP is typically based on UDP (User Datagram Protocol) to utilize its multiplexing and check-sum services. It is used by most video servers such as Darwin Streaming Server and Helix Universal Server.

One of the main elements on which the architecture of a live video system is based is the video server. The main components of the video server include a video pump (streaming server) for real-time video stream retrieval and an application server high-level control/management entity. The application server allows a user to select content and is responsible for forwarding the playback control commands such as pause and resume to the video pump. With the aim of programming interface, the application server launches the video pump on a remote machine. One of the commonly accessible solutions for a streaming server is Helix DNA Server. It is a universal delivery engine supporting the real-time packetization and network transmission of any media type to any device. Its advantage is that it allows connecting up to 64,000 viewers [16].

The client-side platforms (as in the case of typical MDVL client) may be composed of workstations, PCs (Personal Computers), mobile terminals, or stand-alone set-top-boxes. The video is delivered to the client directly by the server through the video pump. It is needed to implement some software for playing streaming, e.g. Real Player [32]. However, for integration with the whole system, the Web server provides interface, which uses and realizes functions of video streaming player, as the most often manner of communication with users who access the system over the Web. It is based on active and dynamic WWW (World Wide Web) sides. Thanks to this, it is additionally possible and necessary to introduce authorization of access to different levels of confidentiality to the medical streams. User authentication can be performed by entering username/password information under the SSL (Secure Socket Layer) session encryption. Clients with suitable network access can choose from a number of streams that are transmitted using multiple unicast (splitter) or – in the future – multicast mechanisms (IP-Multicast) [8].

Video uploading, handling and format conversion

Granted users (administrators) can upload video content to the Medical Digital Video Library. There are two methods of content uploading. The first method requires some computer skills and it is intended for and currently used by system creators. The administrator has to upload appropriate MPEG-1 files to the mass storage server (using File Transfer Protocol, Network File System or similar). If the source content exists only in the DICOM format (e.g. it is retrieved from some medical digital imaging device), there exists a special custom-made script, converting DICOM files to MPEG-1, trying to execute the process with the highest possible quality (since obviously MPEG-1 introduces some quality limitations, compared to DICOM).

The second method of uploading the content to the Medical Digital Video Library does not require any advanced computer skills and it is intended for system administrators, having only a medical background (i.e. doctors). All the operations are executed automatically. Uploading does not require any sophisticated tools; only standard Web browser is required.

Back-office database subsystem

All the information about uploaded video files is stored in a database system based on MySQL database engine. The information is divided into functional tables. One of them includes properties of video files such as file name and location, picture dimensions and duration given in seconds. They are added automatically after first use of a given file, stored on disk.

The whole description of each object available in video library is saved in the second table. There one can find the reference to originating film, the start and end points, object duration, and all medical needed descriptions such as title, procedures, name of disease, etc.

The virtual object description is enough for its presentation by the video server. However, for the best video server performance, there is a strong need for objects to be created as a disk file. Presentation of more complex objects can be realized using the SMIL multimedia standard, based either on disk file or on the virtual list residing in database storage system. Possibility of presentation of virtual only objects is very useful in case of long time creation of the appropriate disk file.

GUI (Graphical User Interface)

The main purpose of the GUI is to facilitate access to the resources of the library as well as management of its content. Though a regular user usually is confined to searching and watching the content he is concerned with, the user who maintains and manages the library (super-user/administrator) is able to perform a much greater number of operations. Because he does not have to have knowledge of all technical aspects of the system it is advisable for the maintenance to be simple and intuitive.

The aesthetics of the design is also of some importance.

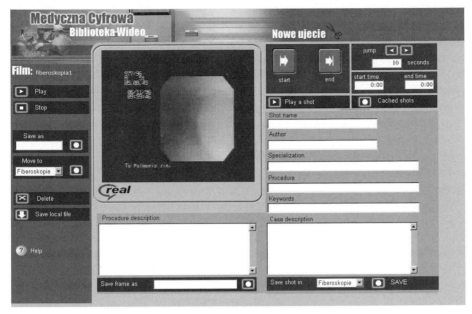

Figure 14-3 GUI (Graphical User Interface).

The super-user has a few panels at his disposal that enable (among other things): classification of the content, creation of the takes (short fragments of source video file), creation of sequences of takes and entering a full description of them. Figure 14-3 is a screenshot showing the tool for creating the takes. In the left part of the screen the buttons connected with operations on a chosen video file are gathered, e.g. opening the file, moving to another directory or downloading to local hard disk. In the middle there is a window where the video can be played. On the right side one can find the editing panel – a tool that makes easier editing of given material. A take can be created in two ways:

- by entering explicitly in appropriate fields the time of the beginning and ending of a shot,
- with the use of "beginning of shot," "end of shot" buttons when the video is played.

Then the chosen fragment of the video can be described by entering all necessary information in fields of the form. The process comes to an end when the created take is recorded in specified directory of the library.

Quality feedback

The quality of motion pictures (perceived QoS) presented in the Medical Digital Video Library is continuously monitored using the modified Mean Opinion Score method. The method was first proposed for measuring quality of telephony services [20]. It can be adapted to the requirements of motion picture quality measurement [18]. The authors selected the following three scales:

Table 14-1 Quality scales

Mark	Watching effort	Watching quality	Degradation category
5	complete relaxation possible; no effort required	excellent	invisible
4	attention necessary; no appreciable effort required	good	visible, but not annoying
3	moderate effort required	fair	slightly annoying
2	considerable effort required	poor	annoying
1	no meaning understood with any feasible effort	bad	very annoying

The users are asked answer to the above-mentioned questions after watching the video. Appropriate statistics allow for tuning encoding parameters and other aspects of MDVL in order to satisfy the users.

5.1.2   Integration of Modules

The Medical Digital Video Library is currently being integrated from several components. The whole application is distributed among several machines, see Figure 14-4.

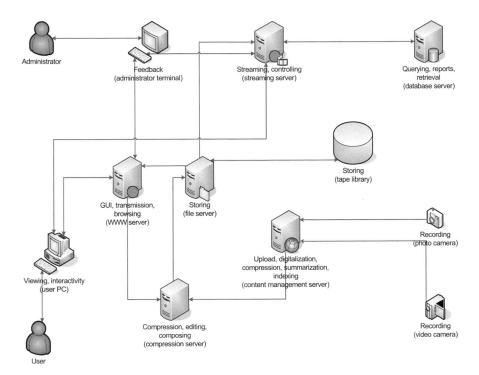

Figure 14-4 MDVL architecture.

To begin, the MDVL is fed by analogue (Super)-VHS tapes, played by video cassette player. The tapes are digitalized using encoding station (personal computer plus Optibase encoding card). Currently, only pre-recorded content is supported; however, in the future live events will be available as well.

A different machine, running the authors' software, segments the content, provides some preliminary indexing and executes some other preprocessing tasks (like anonymization, picture cropping). The content is then stored in high-quality (average bandwidth of around 5 Mbit/s) MPEG-1 video files (audio track is not necessary).

The next stage is adaptation of the content to several access bandwidths that can be expected from users. Therefore, the files are converted at the second encoding station (PC-based) to the RealMedia SureStream format. In addition, the later browsing process is faster in case of RealMedia content.

The content itself is streamed from another machine, Sun Solaris server, running RealNetworks Helix DNA Server. This software is an efficient and free (open-source) solution for video streaming over IP networks. The streamed content can then be received at users' computers, using free and popular players (RealPlayer family) or by plug-ins running as a part of a Web-based application.

The latter solution has been chosen for the case of MDVL, since the generic RealPlayer does not provide advanced and customized features, like searching, annotating and browsing. The Apache Server, running on another Sun Solaris machine, serves the Web-based application.

5.2   VVFS — Virtual Video File System

This case study describes an effort made in the Department of Computer Science of AGH-UST concerning improving video server scalability with the Virtual Video File System (VVFS) concept. VVFS aims to fill a gap in the currently available multimedia software by combining a low-cost software video server running on a UNIX workstation with massive storage. It is intended to be a system which improves video server functionality and scalability. The presented concept is rather general in nature, but it has been implemented using the Oracle Video Server [29][30] and the UniTree Storage System [46].

5.2.1   VVFS Concepts

The VVFS logical structure is a hierarchical tree. The basic node is a directory. There is one root directory without a parent directory. Every directory (excluding root) has exactly one parent directory. Every directory contains 0 or more file system units, such as directories, files or links. Every file corresponds to exactly one film. Aside from multimedia content, it contains definable properties, such as short film descriptions, lists of authors, etc. Every file has its owner and a set of access rights.

Links are provided to ease the management of large film databases. There are two types of links: links to files and links to directories. There is no distinction between hard and symbolic links, as in UNIX-like file systems. Links in the VVFS share selected features of hard and symbolic links.

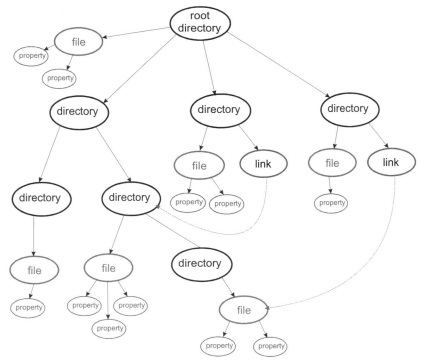

Figure 14-5 File system logical structure.

5.2.2   System Functionality

Unauthorized access is prevented through the use of passwords. The most important task of the VVFS is providing functionality for a multimedia database. The solution is a file system which combines the advantages of UNIX-like systems with additional special features. Thanks to the links mechanism, the same films can be accessed from various directories, which may be user-based, subject-based and so on. A film is more than just a multimedia stream stored in a file — it also has properties, such as a short description or additional meta-information, helpful in operating a large video library.

Another important aspect of the system is support for the hierarchical storage. Films may be archived on an FTP server when not used. Such a solution dramatically reduces hardware costs. A high-speed, expensive video server storage can keep only those multimedia materials that are requested by the users whilst the full content of the multimedia database can be stored on an FTP server and uploaded to the video server on demand. In order to reduce waiting for the video to be uploaded the request mechanism has been introduced. If a user requests a film early enough, there is a great probability that the file will be available when needed. In this case any transfer is scheduled by the system. Users are not directly involved in the transfer process, so the overall system convenience increases.

5.2.3   Physical Architecture

The physical configurations of VVFS may be set up according to a particular hardware and network configuration. All the system components, including external units, such as a video server and an FTP server may work on the same physical machine, although the purpose of such a configuration is questionable. The common scenario is when a video server resides on one physical server, an FTP server occupies another and the VVFS system is placed on another one.

VVFS cooperates with external systems which are described below. The particular implementations used in projects are given in parentheses.

Video Server (Oracle Video Server) This is a high-performance video server. It is used by the system for the purpose of playback and recording of films. The native file system for the Oracle Video Server is a **Media Data Store (MDS)**, which is optimized for fast transfers, but definitely not for user convenience. It doesn't support directories. All the files are stored in the same namespace. Fortunately, the system conceals the MDS nature from the user while preserving its advantages.

Data Server (Oracle Data Server) The Oracle Data Server is a high-performance, advanced relational database engine. It is used by the system to store meta-data: such as file system properties, video properties.

FTP Storage Server (UniTree) UniTree is a hierarchical storage system. It may cooperate with high-capacity storage devices, like magnetic tapes. Its disadvantage is longer access time when compared with other FTP servers.

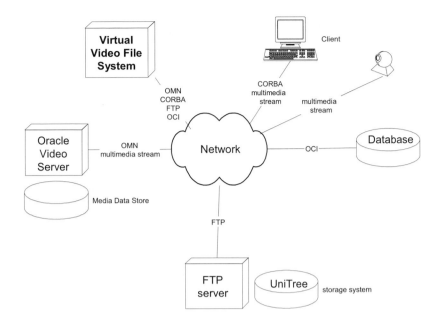

Figure 14-6 VVFS physical model.

5.2.4   User Interface

The VVFS system has been equipped with stand-alone Java client application that provides a GUI to manipulate the system. It is intended to be used both by ordinary users and administrators. Some functions are available only for administrators.

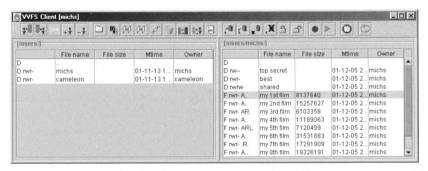

Figure 14-7 Client application (main window).

The main window of the client application is shown in Figure 14-7. Two panels allow exploration of the file system in a manner similar to working with popular file commanders. The vertical splitting line can be moved left or right for user convenience. The current directory for each panel is shown in its top left-hand corner.

The top toolbar contains buttons to execute various operations. Most operations are associated with pop-up windows. An example is the property view/edit window shown in Figure 14-8.

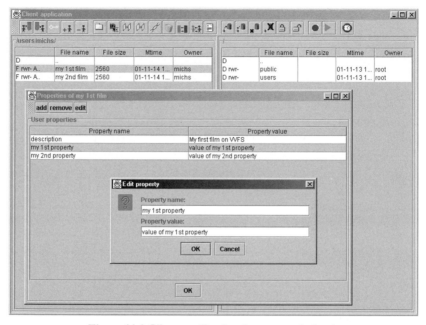

Figure 14-8 Client application (property window).

6 Summary

This chapter has analyzed the importance of specific medical studies and computer-based support for them. Main standardization organizations were presented, such as AICC, ADL, IMS and others. Some distance learning platforms were described including two case studies of solutions from AGH University of Science and Technology.

7 Bibliography

[1] *About ALIC – Advanced Learning Infrastructure Consortium*, http://www.alic.gr.jp/eng/

[2] *ADL – Advanced Distributed Learning Initiative*, http://www.adlnet.org/

[3] *AICC – The Aviation Industry CBT Committee*, http://www.aicc.org/

[4] *ARIADNE Foundation*, http://www.ariadne-eu.org/

[5] *CEN Learning Technologies Workshop* http://www.cenorm.be/
[6] *IEEE LTSC – Learning Technology Standards Committee*,
     http://ltsc.ieee.org/
[7] *Welcome to EdNA Online*, http://www.edna.edu.au/
[8] Duplaga M., Juszkiewicz K., Leszczuk M., Szczepanski D.: *Browsing Medical Digital Video Library with Internet-Based Point-to-Multipoint Live Streaming Support*, 1st International Conference on E-health in Common Europe (Krakow, Poland)
[9] Duplaga M., Leszczuk M., Papir Z.: *Fast Algorithms for Segmentation of Medical Video Content as a Repository of Structured Multimedia Content*, IWSSIP'04 (Poznań, Poland)
[10] Gandsas A., McIntire K., Palli G., Park A.: *Live streaming video for medical education: a laboratory model.* J Laparoendosc Adv Surg Tech A 2002; 12(5): 377-382
[11] GeoLearning Inc. http://www.geolearning.com
[12] Gisondi Michael A., Mahadevan Swaminatha V., Sovndal Shannon S., Gilbert Gregory H.: 19 *Emergency Department Orientation Utilizing Web-based Streaming Video.* Academic Emergency Medicine 2003; 10(8): 920
[13] Green S.M., Voegeli D., Harrison M., Phillips J., Knowles J., Weaver M., Shephard K.: *Evaluating the use of streaming video to support student learning in a first-year life sciences course for student nurses.* Nurse Education Today 2003; 23: 255-261
[14] Greene P.S.: *Streaming Video for The Annals Internet Readers.* Ann Thorac Surg 1998; 65: 1188-1189
[15] Hamilton N.M., Frade I., Duguid P., Furnace J., Kindley A.D.: *Digital video for networked CAL delivery.* J Audiovisual Media in Medicine 1995; 18(2): 59-63
[16] Helix Community: *Helix DNA* Server. http://www.helixcommunity.org
[17] Hunter J., Witana V., Antoniades M.: *A Review of Video Streaming Over Internet*, Technical report DSTC TR97-10, August 1997
[18] IDMS/PROMS'2002 Tutorial - *Internet Multimedia (streaming media)*, November 26 2002, Henning Schulzrinne, Columbia University, USA
[19] *IMS Global Learning Consortium* http://www.imsglobal.org
[20] *ITU-T P.830* (02/96)
[21] Kumar S.A., Pal H.: *Digital Video Recording of Cardiac Surgical Procedures.* Annals of Thoracic Surgery 2004; 77(3): 1063-1065
[22] Lavitan R.M., Goldman T.S., Bryan D.A., Shofer F., Harlich A.: *Training With Video Imaging Improves the Initial Intubation Success Rates of Paramedic Trainees in an Operating Room Setting.* Ann Emerg Med 2001; 37:46-50
[23] Leszczuk M., Papir Z.: *Accuracy vs. Speed Trade-Off in Detecting of Shots in Video Content for Abstracting Digital Video Libraries*, in Protocols and Systems for Interactive Distributed Multimedia, F. Boavida, E. Monteiro, J. Orvalho (editors), pp. 176-189, Springer-Verlag, 2002

[24]Leung J., D'Onofrio G., Duncan B., Trepp R., Vasques N., Schriver J.: *Apply Streaming Audio and Video Technology to Enhance Emergency Physician Education.* Acad Emerg Med 2002; 9(10): 1059

[25]*LRN Consortium* http://dotlrn.org

[26]Malassagne Be., Mutter D., Leroy J., Smith M., Soler L., Marescaux J.: *Teleeducation in Surgery: European Institute for Telesurgery Experience.* World Journal of Surgery 2001; 25: 1490-1494

[27]Miron H., Blumenthal E.Z.: *Bridging analog and digital video in the surgical setting.* J Cataract Refract Surg 2003; 29: 1874-1877

[28]*Open Knowledge Initiative* http://web.mit.edu/oki

[29]Oracle Corporation. Oracle Video Server TM Developers Guide, 3.0 edition, 1998.

[30]Oracle. Oracle R Media Net Developer's Guide, 3.3 edition, 1997

[31]*Pathlore* http://www.pathlore.com

[32]RealNetworks.com: *Real One Player.* http://www.real.com/realone/index.html

[33]Reynolds P.A., Mason R.: *On-line video media for continuing professional development in dentistry.* Computers and Education 2002; 35(1): 65-98

[34]Rosser J., Herman B., Ehrenwerth C.: *An overview of video streaming on the Internet and its application to surgical education.* Surg Endosc 2001; 15: 624-629

[35]Schulzrinne H., Casner S., Frederick R., Jacobson V.: *RTP: A Transport Protocol for Real-Time Applications* (RFC 1889)

[36]Schulzrinne H., Rao A., Lanphier R.: *Real Time Streaming Protocol* (RFC 2326)

[37]Smith J.R.: *Digital Video Libraries and the Internet,* IEEE Communications Magazine, January 1999, pages 92-97

[38]Stringer J.K.: *Video streaming: pushing a swimming pool through a straw.* J Biocommun 2001; 28(1): 12-14

[39]Strom J.: *Overcoming Barriers for Teaching and Learning.* Int Symp Educational Conferencing, Banff, Canada, May 30 – June 1 2002 http://www.clickandgovideo.ac.uk/Jim_barriers.htm

[40]Sun Microsystems, *e-Learning Applications Infrastructure,* http://www.sun.com/products-n-solutions/edu/whitepapers/pdf/eLearning_Application_Infrastructure_wp.pdf

[41]Sun Microsystems, *e-Learning Interoperability Standards,* http://www.sun.com/products-n-solutions/edu/elearning/eLearning_Interoperability_Standards_wp.pdf

[42]*The MedBiquitous Consortium* http://www.medbiq.org

[43]*The Schools Interoperability Framework* http://www.sifinfo.org

[44]*THINQ* http://www.thinq.com

[45]*United States Distance Learning Association* http://www.usdla.org

[46] *UniTree User Guide* Release 2.0. http://www.cyf-kr.edu.pl/ack/unitree/UT-ug/usertitl.html

[47] Wiecha J.M., Gramling R., Phyllis J., Vanderschmidt H.: *Collaborative e Learning Using Streaming Video and Asynchronous Discussion Boards to Teach the Cognitive Foundation of Medical Interviewing: A Case Study.* J Med Internet Res 2003; 5(2): e13

[48] Wright C.D. *Digital Library Technology Trends.* White Paper. Sun Microsystems Inc.

[49] Zollo S.A., Kienzle Michael G., Henshaw Zak, Crist Louis G., Wakefield Douglas S.: *Tele-Education in a Telemedicine Environment: Implications for Rural Health Care and Academic Medical Centers.* J Med Syst 1999; 23(2): 107-122

15 Acronyms

2D — two-dimensional
3D — three-dimensional
6WINIT — Pv6 Wireless INternet IniTiative
ACL — Access Control List
ACR — American College of Radiology
ACR-NEMA — American College of Radiology - National Electrical Manufacturers Association
ADC — Analog-Digital Converter
ADL — Advanced Distributed Learning
ADL — *open*EHR Archetype Description Language
ADSL — Asymmetric Digital Subscriber Line
ADT — Admit Discharge Transfer
AGR — AICC Guidelines and Recommendations
AICC — The Aviation Industry CBT Committee
AIDS — Acquired Immune Deficiency Syndrome
ANSI — The American National Standards Institute
ASHA — American Speech-Language-Hearing Association
ASP — Application Service Provider
ASTM — American Society for the Testing of Materials
ATM — Asynchronous Transfer Mode
AVI — Audio Video Interleaved
BLS — U.S. Department of Labor's Bureau of Labor Statistics
BRA — Basic Rate Access
CAS — Clinical Appointment System
CBAC — Context-Based Access Control
CBT — Computer-Based Training
CC — Common Criteria
CCITT — Committee Communication International Telephone and Telegram
CDA — Clinical Document Architecture
CDA — HL7 Clinical Document Architecture
CDMA — Code Division Multiple Access
CEN — Comité Européen de Normalisation (European Committee for Standardization)
CHESS — Comprehensive Health Enhancement Support System
CM UJ — Collegium Medicum Jagellonian University

CME — Continuing Medical Education

COM — Component Object Model

CORBA — Common Object Request Broker Architecture

CORBAmed — the division of CORBA that is devoted to the domain of healthcare

CPE — Customer Premises Equipment

CPR — Computer-based Patient Record

CPRI — Computer-based Patient Record Institute

CRT — Cathode Ray Tube

CT — Computed Tomography

CTCPEC — Canadian Trusted Computer Product Evaluation Criteria

CUI — Unique Concept Identifier

dB — Decibel

DCOM — Distributed Component Object Model

DDB00 — Malcolm Duncan's Diseases Database 2000

DICOM — Digital Imaging and Communications in Medicine

DIMDI — German Institute for Medical Documentation and Information

DoD — Department of Defense

DRGs — Diagnostic Related Groupings

DSL — Digital Subscriber Line

DVL — Digital Video Library

ECG — Electrocardiogram

EDGE — Enhanced Data Rate for Global Evolution

EDGE   Enhanced Data Rates for GSM Evolution

EDI — Electronic Data Interchange

EDIFACT — Electronic Data Interchange for Administration Commerce and Transport

EEG — Electroencephalography

EFMI — European Federation for Medical Informatics

EHCR — Electronic Healthcare Record Communication

EHCR Support Action — Electronic Healthcare Record Support Action project

EHR — Electronic Health Record

EHRcom — ENV 13606

EIRP — Effective Isotropic Radiated Power

EITS — The European Institute of Telesurgery

EJB — Enterprise Java Beans

ENV — European Prestandard

FHCR — Federated Healthcare Record

FPS — Frames Per Second

FTP — File Transfer Protocol

GEHR — Good European Health Record project

GINA — Global Initiative For Asthma

GOLD — Global Initiative For Chronic Obstructive Lung Diseases

GP — General Practitioner
GPRS — General Packet Radio Service
GPS — Global Positioning System
GR — Geometrically Rendered Images
GSM — Global System for Mobile Communication
GUI — Graphical User Interface
HIPAA — The Health Insurance Portability and Accountability Act
HIS — Hospital Information System
HISA — Health Information Systems Architecture
HIV— Human Immunodeficiency Virus
HL — Hearing Level
HL7 — Health Level Seven
HMD — HL7 Hierarchical Message Definition
HSCSD — High Speed Circuit Switched Data
HSCSD — High Speed Circuit Switched Data
HTML — HyperText Markup Language
HTN — Health Telematic Network
HTTP — HyperText Transfer Protocol
HTTPS — Hyper Text Transfer Protocol with Secure Sockets Layer
HU — Hounsfield Units
ICD — International Classification of Diseases
ICD-10 — The Tenth Revision of the International Statistical Classification of Diseases and Related Health Problems
ICD10AM — the Australian Modification of ICD10
ICD-9-CM — International Classification of Diseases, Ninth Revision, Clinical Modification
ICP — Integrated Care Pathway
ICPC2E — International Classification of Primary Care 2nd Edition
ICPC2P — International Classification of Primary Care, Version 2-Plus, Australian Modification
ICPM — International Classification of Procedures in Medicine
ICPM-DE — International Classification of Procedures in Medicine, Dutch Extension
ICT — Information and Communication Technology
IEEE — Institute of Electrical and Electronics Engineers
IGS — Image-guided Surgery
IHE — Integrating the Health Environment
IMS — IMS Global Learning Consortium
IP — Internet Protocol
ISDN — Integrated Services Digital Network
ISM — Industry, Science and Medical
ISO — International Standards Organisation

ISO TC/215 — CEN Technical Committee responsible for health interoperability standards
ISO TS — ISO draft Technical Specification
IST — Information Society Technologies
ITSEC — Information Technology Security Evaluation Criteria
J2EE — Java 2 Platform, Enterprise Edition
JMX — Java Management Extensions
JPEG — Joint Photographic Experts Group
KCT — Krakow Centre of Telemedicine
LAN — Local Area Network
LED — Light Emitting Diode
LGOB — Loudness Growth in half-Octave Bands
LIS — Laboratory Information System
LMDS — Local Multipoint Distribution System
LMS — Learning Management Systems
LNP — Laparoscopic Navigation Pointer
LRT — Long Running Transaction
LSB — Least Significant Byte
MAC — Media Access Control
Mb — Megabits
MDS — Media Data Store
MDVL — Medical Digital Video Library
MEDICL — Medical Diagnosis and Computer-aided Learning
MEDLINE — life sciences and biomedical bibliographic information search engine
MENiS — Polish Ministry of Education and Sport
MeSH — Medical Subject Headings
MIT — Massachusets Institute of Technology
MMVV — Multi-Modal Volume Visualizer
MOS — Mean Opinion Score
MPEG-1 — Moving Pictures Experts Group coding standard
MR — Magnetic Resonance
MRA — MR Angiography Images
MRI — Magnetic Resonance Imaging
MTHICD9 — NLM-generated entry terms for ICD-9-CM
NEMA — National Electrical Manufacturers Association
NFS — Network File System
NHS — National Health Service
NHS CCC — National Health Service Centre for Coding and Classification
NIC — Network Interface Card
NLM — The National Library of Medicine
NMR — Nuclear Magnetic Resonance
NPfIT — The National Programme for IT

OASIS — Organization for the Advancement of Structured Information Standards

OFDM — Orthogonal Frequency Division Multiplexing

OMG-HDTF — Object Management Group Health Domain Task Force

*open*EHR — *open*EHR Foundation

OR — Operating Room

OSD — Office of the Secretary of Defense

OSI — Open Systems Interconnection

OSI/ISO — Open Systems Interconnection by International Organization for Standardization

PACS — Picture Archiving and Communication System

PAN — Personal Area Network

PC — Personal Computer

PCS — Patient Classification Systems

PDA — Personal Digital Assistant

PHI — Protected Health Information

PKI — Public Key Infrastructure

POC — Point-of-Care

POCCIC — Point-of-Care Connectivity Industry Consortium

POCIS — Point-of-Care Information System

POTS — Plain Old Telephone Service

PSTN — Public Switched Telephone Network

PubMed — National Library of Medicine's search service

QoS — Quality of Service

R&D — Research and Development

RAD — Resource Access Decision

RADIUS — Remote Access Dial-In User Service

RBAC — Role-Based Access Control

RC4 — Rivest Cipher 4

Read Code — Clinical Terms Version 3

REM — Rapid Eye Movement

RIM — HL7 Reference Information Model

RIS — Radiological Information System

RMI — Remote Method Invocation

RMIM — HL7 Restricted Message Information Model

RSA — Rivest, Shamir, Adleman

RTCP — Real Time Control Protocol

RTP — Real Time Protocol

RTSP — Real Time Streaming Protocol

SAML — Security Assertion Markup Language

SCORM — Sharable Content Object Reference Model

SCP — Service Class Provider

SCU — Service Class User

SDO — Standards Development Organisation
SDT — Speech Detection Threshold
SME — Subject Matter Expert
SMIL — Synchronized Multimedia Integration Language
SMS — Short Message Service
SNOMED — Systematized Nomenclature of Human and Veterinary Medicine
SOA — Service-Oriented Architecture
SOAP — Simple Object Access Protocol
SOSA — Service-Oriented Security Architecture
SPL — Sound Pressure Level
SRT — Speech Reception Threshold
SSID — Service Set Identifier
SSL — Secure Socket Layer
SSO — Single Sign-On
SVT — Supra-Ventricular Tachycardia
TC/251 — Technical Committee 251
TCP — Transmission Control Protocol
TCP/IP — Transmission Control Protocol over Internet Protocol
TCSEC — Trusted Computer System Security Evaluation Criteria
TDM — Time Division Multiplexing
TTP — Trusted Third Party
UBAC — User-Based Access Control
UDDI — Universal Description, Discovery, and Integration
UDP — User Datagram Protocol
UML — Unified Modeling Language
UMLS — Unified Medical Language System
UMTS — Universal Mobile Telecommunications System
UNII — Unlicensed National Information Infrastructure
US — Ultrasound Tissue Images
USA — Ultrasound Angiography Images
VHS — Video Home System
VoIP — Voice over Internet Protocol
VPN — Virtual Private Network
VR — Volume Rendered Images
VVFS — Virtual Video File System
WAN — Wide Area Network
WAP — Wireless Application Protocol
WCDMA — Wideband Code Division Multiple Access
WEP — Wired Equivalent Privacy
WHO — World Health Organization
WHOART — WHO Adverse Reaction Terminology
WLAN — Wireless Local Area Network
WSDL — Web Services Description Language

WWAN — Wireless Wide Area Network
WWW — World Wide Web
XDS — Cross-Document Sharing
xDSL — a family of Digital Subscriber Line techniques
XML — Extensible Markup Language
XrML — Extensible Rights Markup Language

Index

identity or credential subsystem, 69

information flow control subsystem, 69

security audit subsystem, 67

solution integrity subsystem, 68

communication technologies. *See also* telecommunication network

wireless networks, 85–89

mobile e-health services, 88

PAN, 86

SSID, 90

WLAN, 86

WWAN, 86

communication, interactive and multimedia, 54

Compaq iPAQ, 87

compositional context, 151

computer-based patient record, 142

recommendations, 142

consultant station, 57. *See also* Internet environment; Konsul

DICOM, 57

FTP, 57

non-interactive consultations, 56

context-based access control, 76

Continuing Medical Education, 305, 308

control systems, 187

CPE. *See* customer premises equipment

CPR. *See* computer-based patient record

Coding Scheme (CS), 104

credential subsystem, 69

Common Criteria, 69

CSD. *See* Circuit Switched Data

CUI. *See* unique concept identifier

customer premises equipment, 33

data rate

EDGE, 28

data server (oracle data server), 322

data value context, 152

decision support systems, 182–203

artificial intelligence, 185

expert systems, 185, 186–187

knowledge-based system, 185

logical decision support systems, 198–202

probabilistic decision support systems, 191–192

design systems, 187

DIABCARD, 130

diagnostic systems, 187

Digital Imaging and Communications in Medicine (DICOM), 95, 102, 118, 126, 210–211, 275. *See also* Konsul; TeleDICOM

FPImage distribution, 57

image processing, 6

Digital Subscriber Line, 30, 206

Digital Video Library, 312. *See also* telelearning

distance learning platforms, 310

requirement, 308

medical education enhancement, 302

medical studies, 303

digital library, 303

digital video, 304

Internet streaming, 304

standardization organizations, 306

ADL, 307

AICC, 306

ARIADNE, 307

CBT, 308

IMS, 307

MedBiquitous, 308

discriminant analysis, 196. *See also* decision support system; expert system

distance learning platforms, 310

coherence control subsystem,
188, 189
explanation subsystem, 188,
189
inference engine, 188, 190
information acquisition
subsystem, 188, 189
knowledge acquisition
subsystem, 188–189
knowledge base, 187, 188
learning subsystem, 188, 190
user interface subsystem, 188,
189
explanation subsystem, 188, 189.
See also decision support system;
expert system
FDD, 32. *See also* TDD; UMTS
federation approach, 160. *See also*
EHR
FHCR (Federated Healthcare
Record)
federation schema, 161
fibreoptic networks, 26–27. *See also*
access techniques
point-to-point connections, 27
security aspects, 27
frame-based expert systems, 200.
See also decision support system;
expert system
object-oriented programming, 200
static knowledge, 200
FTP Storage Server (UniTree), 322
GALEN, 113, 130
General Packet Radio Service, 28,
103, 104, 106. *See also* EDGE;
GSM; HSCSD
CS-1, 104
CS-2, 104
data rate, 28
GPRS Support Node (GGSN),
108
QoS, 28

transmission bearer, 104

geometrically rendered, 280

GGSN (GPRS Support Node), 107,
108
glaucoma, 123–125. *See also*
TOSCA
data dictionary for, 125
terminology version, 123
Global System for Mobile (GSM)
Communications, 27–28, 40, 103
CSD, 103
data transmission, 27
EDGE, 27
GPRS, 27, 103
HSCSD, 27, 103
POTS, 27
SMS, 27
telemedical services, 27
electrocardiogram, 27
third generation services, 104
EDGE, 104
UMTS, 104
GPRS. *See* General Packet Radio
Service
GR. *See* geometrically rendered

Graphical User Interface (GUI), 313,
316
Health Information Systems
Architecture, 208
Health Level 7, 209. *See also* ISO
reference model; telematics
networks, health
domain tables and coded
attributes cross-reference
tables, 122
external domain, 122
vocabulary domain values table,
122
health portals, 48. *See also* Internet
environments; medical portals

software platform and operating system, 36
software router, 36
UMTS, 32
ISM
  frequency bands, 92
ISO reference model, 121
  HL7, 121
ISP, 26
IT-enhanced healthcare
  e-health, 11–14
KAMATO (Knowledge Acquisition and Management Tool). *See also* TOSCA
  terminology module, 128, 129
  UMLS, 127
KCT. *See* Krakow Centre for Telemedicine
Kerberos, 91. *See also* WLAN
knowledge acquisition subsystem, 188–189. *See also* decision support system; expert system
knowledge-based system, 185. *See also* decision support system; expert system
knowledge representation, 190, 200
  logical expert system, 190
  probabilistic expert system, 190
Konsul, 56–58, 57. *See also* telecare
  architecture, 57
    acquisition station, 57
    system server, 57
Krakow Centre for Telemedicine, 55
Laboratory Information System, 207
LAN, 90. *See also* IP network; telecare
  data security, 26
  distributed geographical region, 26
laparoscopic navigation pointer,
laparoscopic surgery, 272–274
  intraoperative imaging, 278

minimally invasive surgery, 279
MR/CT images, 275
multimodal imaging, 279
navigation and visualization in the OR, 276
patient registration in the OR, 275
preoperative segmentation and imaging, 275
Learning Management Systems, 310
learning subsystem, 188, 190. *See also* decision support system; expert system
LGOB (Loudness Growth in half-Octave Bands), 231, 235, 236. *See also* hearing screening
LIS (Laboratory Information System), 207
LMDS (local multipoint distribution system), 30, 32–33, 32
  access techniques, 33
    CDMA, 33
    FDMA, 33
    TDMA, 33
  benefits of, 33
  disadvantages of, 33
  distribution, 33
  multipoint, 33
  network architecture, 33
    base station, 33
    CPE, 33
    fibre-based infrastructure, 33
    NOC, 33
  transport methodologies, 33
    ATM, 33
    IP, 33
LMS (Learning Management System), 310
LNP. *See* laparoscopic navigation pointer
local multipoint distribution system, 32, 33

Organization for the Advancement
of Structured Information
Standards (OASIS), 77
OSI network, 90
OSI/ISO, 50
outer TCP/IP networks, 26
packet-based communication, 205.
See also telematics networks,
health
ADSL, 206
DSL, 206
TCP/IP, 206
UDP/IP, 206
PACS (Picture Archiving and
Communication Systems), 95–96,
103, 207. *See also* HIS; RIS;
wireless communication
technology
PANs (personal area networks), 86,
96, 97. *See also* Bluetooth
Pathlore LMS 6, 310. *See also*
telelearning
PCS (patient classification systems),
114
PDA (personal digital assistant), 96,
100, 222. *See also* CAS
Picture-Archiving and
Communication System, 207
PKI, 103
planning systems, 187
POCIS (Point-of-Care Information
System), 50, 53. *See also*
POCCIC
POCs (Point-of-Care), 49–51, 96
applications for, 49
integration with hospital system,
51
POCCIC, 50
POCIS, 50
polygraphic recordings, 299
portal technologies, 53–54
access to resources, 53

medical systems, 54
POTS (Plain Old Telephone
Service), 27
PRA (Primary Rate Access), 25
predicate calculus, 202. *See also*
decision support system
prediction systems, 187
Primary Rate Access, 25
probabilistic decision support
systems, 191–192. *See also*
decision support system; expert
system
Bayesian decision support
systems, 192
Bayes' formula, 193
MEDICL, 194, 195
optimal decision function, 194
predictive value positive, 193
predictive value negative, 193
sensitivity (*SE*), 192
specificity (*SD*), 192
discriminant analysis, 196
canonical analysis, 198
Fisher's criterion of goodness
of classification, 197
Mahalanobis distance, 197
multivariate normal
distribution, 198
probabilistic network model, 191
odds ratio, 191
likelihood ratio, 191
probabilistic expert systems, 187
protected health information (PHI),
64
PSTN network, 24–25. *See also*
BRA; ISDN network; telecare
penetration of, 24–25
PubMed, 130
via KAMATO, 130
pulse oximeters, 294. *See also*
biosignals
Quality of Service (QoS), 5, 207

context-based access control, 76
role-based access control, 75
Common Criteria, 64–70
    access control subsystem, 68
    and functional categories, 67
    evaluation of security functionalities, 66
    identity or credential subsystem, 69
    information flow control subsystem, 69
    security audit subsystem, 67
    security hardware and software, 66
    solution integrity subsystem, 68
HIPAA, 63, 64
mapping design objectives, 70
RAD, 78
    access decision, 80
    GUI interface, 82
    medical portal and, 78, 80, 81
    resource access decision facility, 78
    security policy enforcement, 80
requirements for, 64
service-oriented security architecture, 77
system architecture modeling, 66
techniques, 70
    accountability of changes to protected information, 72
    application and data, 70
    authentication of users, 71
    authorized access to protected information, 71
    basic cryptography, 71
    confidentiality of protected information, 72
    integrity of protected information, 72

    monitoring access and modification of protected information, 73
    networks, 70
    non-repudiation of changes to protected information, 72
    system infrastructure, 70
security audit subsystem, 67
    Common Criteria, 67
semantic nets, 121, 200. *See also* decision support system; expert system
service-oriented architecture, 45–47, 77
    SOSA, 77
Sharable Content Object Reference Model, 307
SIESTA, 299, 300
Simple Object Access Protocol, 52
single sign-on, 53
SME, 311
SMS (short message service), 27, 106
SNMI98, 124
SNOMED, 113, 116, 117–118, 126. *See also* coding systems
SOA. *See* service-oriented architecture
SOAP, 52
    HTTP, 52
    HTTPS, 52
solution integrity subsystem, 68
    Common Criteria, 68
SOSA. *See also* SOA
    interoperable protocols, 78
    policy-based trust, 77
    security policies implementation, 77
    standards, 78
    WS Security, 77
    XML and WS Security merge, 77
speech detection threshold. *See* SDT

universal description, discovery and integration, 52

US images. *See* ultrasound tissue images

User Datagram Protocol, 54, 314
video servers, 314

User Interface Subsystem. *See also* decision support system; expert system

user-based access control, 74

UTRA. *See* UMTS Terrestrial Radio Access

video library, 316

Video Server (Oracle Video Server), 322

virtual private network (VPN), 90. *See also* wireless communication technologies

Virtual Video File System, 320. *See also* distance learning platforms
architecture, 322
MDS, 322
multimedia database, 321
structure, 320
UniTree, 322
user interface, 323

visualisation panel, 107

volume-rendered (VR), 280. *See also* MMVV

VVFS, 320
architecture, 322
MDS, 322
multimedia database, 321
structure, 320
UniTree, 322
user interface, 323

VVFS (Virtual Video File System), 320

WAN. *See also* LAN
data security, 26
distributed geographical region, 26

WAP. *See* wireless application protocol

WCDMA. *See* Wideband CDMA

Web Services Description Language, 52

web services, 51–53, 51–53
architecture, 52
medical environments, 53
SOA, 51–53
WSDL, 52

WEP. *See* Wired Equivalent Privacy

wideband CDMA, 32

Wired Equivalent Privacy, 90

wireless application protocol, 87

wireless communication technologies, 85–89
coding systems, 104, 126
DICOM, 102, 103
GPRS access to database, 103
GSM, 103, 104
in hospital environment, 93
HIS, 94
PACS, 95
RIS, 94, 95
Kerberos, 91
medical environments, 91
radio interference, 91, 92
mobile e-health services, 88
mobile medicine environment, 96
e-soul concept, 97–100
PAN, 85–89
PDA, 101
radiology database access, 101
security aspects, 89
end-to-end encryption, 89
full support for mobility, 89
mutual authentication, 89
per-client keys, 89
secure automated key distribution, 89
VPN, 90
SSID, 90

WEP, 90
wireless devices, 85–89
wireless LAN radios, 92
WLANs, 86–89
WWANs, 86–89
wireless connection, 38–40. *See also*
WLAN
DWL-900AP+, 39
point-to-point link, 39
wireless handheld devices, 101
wireless LAN radios, 92
wireless local area networks, 28–29,
40, 86, 93
authentication
SSID, 90
data transmission, 29
IEEE 802.11, 86
IEEE 802.11a, 29
IEEE 802.11b, 29
network architecture, 39
point-to-point, 39
wired LAN, 86
WLAN. *See* wireless local area
networks
WSDL. *See* Web Services
Description Language
WWAN (wireless wide-area
networks), 86
xDSL networks, 30

Health Informatics Series
(formerly Computers in Health Care)

(continued from page ii)

Advancing Federal Sector Health Care
A Model for Technology Transfer
P. Ramsaroop, M.J. Ball, D. Beaulieu, and J.V. Douglas

Medical Informatics
Computer Applications in Health Care and Biomedicine, Second Edition
E.H. Shortliffe and L.E. Perreault

Filmless Radiology
E.L. Siegel and R.M. Kolodner

Cancer Informatics
Essential Technologies for Clinical Trials
J.S. Silva, M.J. Ball, C.G. Chute, J.V. Douglas, C.P. Langlotz, J.C. Niland, and W.L. Scherlis

Clinical Information Systems
A Component-Based Approach
R. Van de Velde and P. Degoulet

Knowledge Coupling
New Premises and New Tools for Medical Care and Education
L.L. Weed

Healthcare Information Management Systems
Cases, Strategies, and Solutions, Third Edition
M.J. Ball, C.A. Weaver, and J.M. Kiel

Organizational Aspects of Health Informatics, Second Edition
Managing Technological Change
N.M. Lorenzi and R.T. Riley

Information Technology Solutions for Healthcare
K. Zieliński, M. Duplaga, and D. Ingram